Communication and Educational Technology

About the Authors

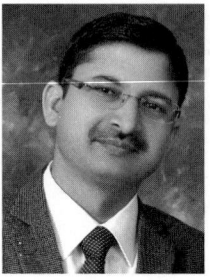

Dr Suresh K. Sharma is Professor-cum-Principal, College of Nursing, All India Institute of Medical Sciences (AIIMS), Rishikesh. He received his bachelor of science degree in nursing from Rajiv Gandhi University of Health Sciences, Bangalore; his master of science degree in medical-surgical nursing from National Institute of Nursing Education, PGIMER, Chandigarh, under Panjab University; and his doctoral degree in administration from Punjab University, Chandigarh. He received his university gold medal for obtaining first position at the university level during his bachelor and master levels of education. He is also registered as an RN with the Board of Registered Nursing, California, USA.

He has been conferred on the prestigious *Florence Nightingale Award-2001* by the Florence Nightingale Nurses' Welfare Association and Anglo-Indian Unity Center, Bangalore. He is member of 15 different national and international nursing societies and associations, including American Association of Critical Care Nursing, Sigma Theta Tau International and International Network for Doctoral Education in Nursing. He is also the fellow of International Network for Doctoral Education in Nursing and Sigma Theta Tau International, USA.

Dr Sharma has taught undergraduate, postgraduate and doctoral program nursing students and worked as a Lecturer, Associate Professor and Professor at College of Nursing, Dayanand Medical College and Hospital, Ludhiana, Punjab. He is also active internationally through his association with Liverpool John Moores University, UK, as external advisor and has acted as invigilator for South African Nursing Council, Pretoria, South Africa, and as adjunct faculty for the prestigious universalities in the USA.

He is a prolific writer and has published seven text books in nursing (Genetics and Genomics in Nursing, Biophysics in Nursing, Pathology for Nurses, Nursing Research and Statistics, Communication and Educational Technology: Contemporary Pedagogy for Health Care Professionals, Biochemistry and Biophysics in Nursing, Pharmacology, and Pathology and Genetics for Nurses). He has reviewed several books, contributed many chapters in books and published more than 50 research papers in national and international nursing journals. His clinical, educational and research interest include generation and dissemination of empirical evidence in nursing to improve the quality of nursing services, education and administration. He has special interest of research in the areas of epidemiology, critical care nursing and basic nursing care, where he has carried out 15 research projects as principle investigator or coinvestigator. He has successfully guided students for six doctoral level theses.

He is currently the editor of the *International Journal of Nursing Research* and *Baba Farid University Journal of Nursing Sciences*. He is also the zonal editor for the *Journal of Nursing Research Society of India* and peer reviewer of *Nursing and Midwifery Research Journal*. In addition, he is also serving as member of editorial board of several national and international health sciences journals, including the *International Journal of Nursing Education, International Journal of Nursing Care* and *International Journal of Nursing Education and Practice*.

Dr Sharma has presented more than 100 research papers/lecturers/talks at international and national level conferences, seminars, symposiums and workshops. He has also chaired the sessions in more than 50 national and international level conferences and participated in more than 100 national and international level conferences. He has also acted as internal and external examiner for undergraduate and post graduate nursing programs in different universities and nursing boards.

He is currently practising as a nurse educator, administrator and researcher with a philosophy of *placing the patient or client before everything, including self*. He is devoted to generating the empirical evidence to provide the quality nursing care at affordable cost and maintaining standards of nursing service, education and nursing administration par excellence.

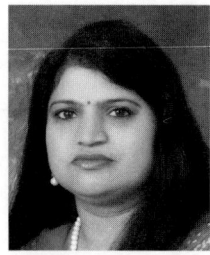

Ms Reena Sharma is an educationist and educational researcher. She received her bachelor degree in arts from Rajasthan University, Jaipur; her master degree in political science from Rajasthan University, Jaipur; and her M.Phil. in Gandhian Thought from Gandhian Study Centre, Rajasthan University, Jaipur. She received her B.Ed. from Rajasthan University, Jaipur, and M.Ed. (Educational Technology) from the Department of Education, Rajasthan University, Jaipur.

Ms Sharma has taught economics and political science in school education at Jaipur for several years. She has also taught *Educational Technology* to undergraduate education students at Baba Kundan College of Education, Ludhiana, Punjab, and Sambal College of Education, Sikar, Rajasthan, for a significant tenure.

She can be considered as a wordsmith or poignant writer, who has published research papers and articles in the field of education, in national and international journals. She is active in participating in and contributing to the academic developments among the educational fraternity.

She is practising as an educationist and educational researcher with a philosophy of *considering education a right of every child and being an educationist with difference, devoting self towards this social cause*. She is devoted to generating the evidence to provide the quality of education to each stratum of society at an affordable cost and maintaining standards of education at par with international standards.

Communication and Educational Technology

Contemporary Pedagogy for Health Care Professionals

SECOND EDITION

Dr Suresh K. Sharma PhD, MScN, RN (USA)
Professor-cum-Principal, College of Nursing,
All India Institute of Medical Sciences (AIIMS),
Rishikesh, Uttarakhand, India

Reena Sharma MPhil, MEd, BEd, MA
Department of Education, Rajasthan University,
Jaipur, Rajasthan, India

ELSEVIER

ELSEVIER

RELX India Pvt. Ltd.

Registered Office: 818, 8th Floor, Indraprakash Building, 21, Barakhamba Road, New Delhi 110001
Corporate Office: 14th Floor, Building No. 10B, DLF Cyber City, Phase II, Gurgaon-122002, Haryana, India

Communication and Educational Technology: Contemporary Pedagogy for Health Care Professionals, 2e
Suresh K. Sharma and Reena Sharma

Copyright © 2016, by RELX India Pvt. Ltd.
First Edition 2012.
All rights reserved.

ISBN: 978-81-312-4374-9
e-Book ISBN: 978-81-312-4654-2

First Printed in India 2016
Reprinted 2018, 2019 (twice), 2020 (twice), 2021, 2022

Content Strategist: Dikshita Khanduja
Sr Project Manager—Education Solutions: Shabina Nasim
Content Development Specialist: Subodh Kumar
Project Manager: Nayagi Athmanathan
Sr Operations Manager: Sunil Kumar
Sr Production Executive: Dhan Singh
Sr Cover Designer: Milind Majgaonkar

Typeset by GW India

Printed in India by Rajkamal Electric Press, Kundli (Haryana)

Dedicated to Parents

Late Smt. Bhagwati Devi Sharma
and
Sh. Badri Narayan Sharma

whose unconditional love and belief in our capabilities
provided us with the power and energy to complete this book

—Authors

International advisors

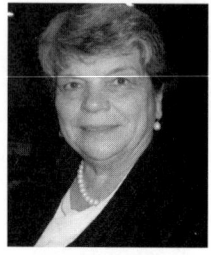

Carol R. Taylor, RN, PhD
Professor in Medicine and Nursing
Georgetown University
Washington DC 20057, USA
Email: taylorcr@georgetown.edu

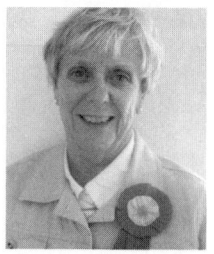

Marylou K. McHugh, RN, EdD, CNE
Professor in Nursing
College of Nursing and Health Professionals
Drexel University, 245 N 15th Street, Bellet Building,
Philadelphia, PA 19102, USA
Email: mm64@drexel.edu

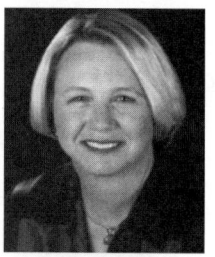

Joan T. Bickes, RN, MSN, PHCNS-BC
Assistant Professor
Wayne State University College of Nursing
262 Cohn Building, 5557 Cass Avenue
Detroit, MI 48202, USA
Email: jbickes@wayne.edu

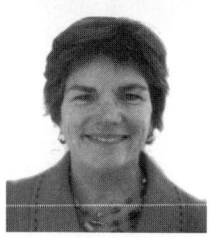

Margaret L. Falahee, APRN, FNP
Assistant Professor
Wayne State University College of Nursing
264 Cohn Building, 5557 Cass Avenue
Detroit, MI 48324, USA
Email: Ab2479@wayne.edu

National advisors

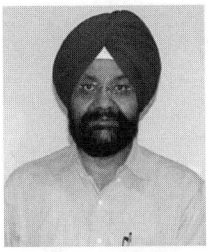

Daljit Singh, MD
Former Principal
Dayanand Medical College and Hospital
Ludhiana, Punjab
Email: dr-daljit-singh@dmch.edu

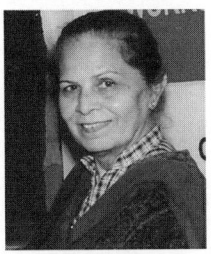

Indarjit Walia, PhD
Former Principal
National Institute of Nursing Education
PGIMER, Chandigarh
Email: indrajitwalia@yahoo.com

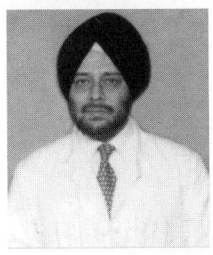

Rajoo Singh Chhina, MD, DM
Dean Academics
Dayanand Medical College and Hospital
Ludhiana, Punjab
Email: drrajoosingh@rediffmail.com

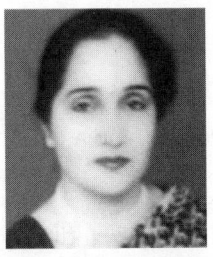

Sandhya Ghai, PhD
Principal
National Institute of Nursing Education
PGIMER, Chandigarh
Email: sandhya.ghai@yahoo.com

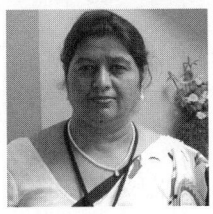

Jasbir Kaur, PhD
Principal
College of Nursing
Dayanand Medical College and Hospital
Ludhiana, Punjab
Email: jksaini1952@yahoo.com

Contributors

Dinesh K. Sharma, MSc (N), RPN (Ireland)
Mental Health Nursing Consultant, St. Brendans Mental Health Hospital, Dublin, Ireland.
Email ID: dineshrajrolia@yahoo.com

Manjulata Evatt, RN, MSc (N), DNP
Assistant Professor, School of Nursing, University of Pittsburg, USA.
Email ID: manjulata-evatt@yahoo.com

Dimple Madan, RN, MSc (N), PhD
Professor and Principal, S.G.R.D. College of Nursing, Hoshiarpur, Punjab, India.
Email ID: principal@sgrdnursingcollege.com

H.C. Rawat, RN, MN
Professor and Principal, University College of Nursing,
Baba Farid University of Health Sciences, Faridkot, Punjab, India.
Email ID: proccrawat@gmail.com

Manpreet Kaur, RN, MSc (N)
Professor, SGRD College of Nursing, SGRDIMSR, Vallah, Amritsar, Punjab, India.
Email ID: manpreet-arora001@rediffmail.com

Nidhi Sagar, RN, MSc (N)
Professor, College of Nursing, Dayanand Medical College and Hospital, Ludhiana, Punjab, India.
Email ID: nidhisagar24@yahoo.com

Vasantha Kalyani, RN, MSc (N)
Assistant Professor, College of Nursing, All India Institute of Medical Sciences, Rishikesh, Dehradun, Uttarakhand, India. Email ID: vasantharaj2003@gmail.com

Prabhjot Kaur, RN, MSc (N)
Clinical Instructor, National Institute of Nursing Education, PGIMER, Chandigarh, India.
Email ID: prab.pgi@gmail.com

Parmees Kaur, RN, MSc (N)
Lecturer, College of Nursing, Govt. Medical College & Hospital, Chandigarh.
Email ID: parmeeskaur@yahoo.com

Harshpunit, RN, MSc (N)
Associate Professor, Guru Nanak College of Nursing, Dahanklera, SBS Nagar, Punjab, India.
Email ID: pariharsh.kauro@gmail.com

Ruchika Rani, RN, MSc (N)
Lecturer, College of Nursing, Dayanand Medical College and Hospital, Ludhiana, Punjab, India.
Email ID: ruchikaheera@gmail.com

Khushveer Kaur, RN, MSc (N)
Child Development Project Officer, Department of Social Security and Women & Child Development, Govt. of Punjab, Kotkapura District- Faridkot, Punjab, India.
Email ID: khushveer767@gmail.com

Bidisha Basu, RN, MSc (N)
Cardiac Nurse Tutor, UN Mehta Institute of Cardiology and Research Center, Ahmadabad, Gujrat, India. Email ID: basubidisha@ymail.com

Foreword

In the last few decades, nursing education in India has undergone tremendous change, from informal bedside hospital-based training to university-based graduate, postgraduate and doctoral nursing education. Furthermore, the rapid growth and development in science and technology has largely influenced the need as well as method of teaching–learning process for nurses in India. Nurses are actively involved in teaching the patients, family and community as well as educating and training the new budding nurses. India has observed a rapid growth and development in nursing education and the Indian nursing faculty has increasing responsibility to educate future nurses using basic and advanced concepts and principles of communication and educational technology. Further, they need to equip the budding nurses, nurse educators and nursing faculty with the basic concepts, principles and methods of communication and educational technology so that they efficiently handle the communication, patient teaching and nursing education and training. However, there was scarcity of literature encompassing the Indian perspective with regard to communication and educational technology in nursing. A sound knowledge of communication and educational technology is essential for the present as well as future nurses that make them capable of offering efficient and effective communication and teaching to their patients.

Therefore, I feel that this textbook, titled *Communication and Educational Technology in Nursing*, will fill the gap in the literature on pedagogy that is tailored to the peculiar needs of teaching–learning process in nursing among developing countries, especially India. This book is a modest attempt to present the content related to communication and educational technology in a lucid manner and includes most of the basic and essential concepts of the communication, interpersonal relationship, educational media and teaching–learning process. I, therefore, commend its author, Dr Suresh K. Sharma, as well as other contributors and advisors for this unique contribution with an Indian background in the area of communication and educational technology. I further commend that this book caters to the needs of the graduate nursing students and their faculty; it may even be used by postgraduate nursing students and other health care professionals.

Dr S.S. Gill
Ex-Vice Chancellor
Baba Farid University of Health Sciences
Faridkot, Punjab, India

Preface to the Second Edition

The focus of the health care education has always been the learning and development of competencies to make a skilful professional. However, the subject content on communication and educational technology remains a neglected area in the health care professionals' teaching–learning pedagogy, which is of paramount importance for them. Effective communication is one of the most important factors in health care services, which facilitates smooth functioning of health care team and ultimately boosts patient satisfaction. The knowledge of educational technology is also essential for health care professionals, as it enables them to produce the better-equipped future generations of health care workers. Therefore, it has been observed in the recent past that the subject content of communication and educational technology has been given its due space in the curricula of health care courses, especially the nursing discipline.

However, there is scarcity of good indigenous literature on communication and educational technology for health care professionals. That precisely is the gap that this book aims to fill in. The development of this book is a modest attempt to provide a comprehensive, lucid and the most-needed indigenous content on subject, which is reviewed and validated by national and international subject experts.

The second edition of this book, *Communication and Educational Technology: Contemporary Pedagogy for Health Care Professionals*, consists of total 10 chapters. It begins with the chapter 'Review of the communication process', followed by the chapters 'Interpersonal relationships', 'Human relations', 'Guidance and counselling', 'Principles and philosophies of education', 'Teaching–Learning process', 'Methods of teaching', 'Educational media', 'Assessment' and 'Information, education and communication for health'. Each chapter begins with Leaning Objectives, followed by the Key Terms and the subject content of the chapter, and ends with Review Questions consisting of long-answer questions, short-answer questions, short notes and multiple-choice questions (MCQs).

This is a simple, comprehensive, lucid and an example-oriented book with indigenous content on communication and educational technology, which will primarily meet the needs of the undergraduate nursing students. However, it can also be used as reference book by the postgraduate nursing, medical, dental, physiotherapy, pharmacy and other paramedical students and faculty members. We are sure that the carefully developed content of this book will find favour with the readers. Furthermore, we invite feedback/suggestions from students or faculty members. It can be sent to us on the email ID: sk.aiims17@gmail.com. Your feedback will help us improve the subsequent editions so that the book can meet your expectations optimally.

—**Authors**

Preface to the First Edition

Most ideas about teaching are not new, but not everyone knows the old ideas.

—Euclid, Circa 300 BC

Nursing education, the science behind teaching and learning in nursing, has been firmly established as a separate discipline. Parallel to the advancement in nursing science, nursing education has seen tremendous progress as a discipline. The beneficial effects of such development are readily evident. Teaching and learning have become more scientific and rigorous curricula are based on good pedagogical principles, and problem-based and other forms of active and self-directed learning are no longer viewed as an anomaly but are now considered to be mainstream. There is a strong emphasis on evidence-based education.

This is a time of great excitement and opportunity for anyone who is interested in teaching and learning in nursing. Parallel to its spectacular growth, nursing education has become more specialized as a discipline. In recent years, there is extensive publication by international and national authors in nursing education. There are several scholarly journals dedicated to nursing education that are published regularly and enjoy a good readership base. Moreover, most clinical professional journals also publish articles on nursing education. There are also many authentic books on the various aspects of nursing education written by renowned scholars and leaders.

But the rapid development and specialization in nursing education has not come without a price. The more developed the discipline became, the more specialized and fragmented became the books and publications on nursing education. Many books are too intimidating and esoteric to meet the needs of general nursing teachers and learners. In contrast to the prolific publication trend in specialized aspects of nursing education, there is a marked paucity of books written for the general reader in nursing education. More importantly, there are few books that are easy to understand, portable as well as affordable for the individual reader. The issue of nonavailability is evident from our interactions with our colleagues. Frequently, we engage our friends and colleagues in a passionate discussion about nursing education and the benefits that they may get from knowing the science of teaching and learning. When we have managed to instill enough interest, our colleagues' response is typical—'It seems nursing education is interesting. Can you name a book where I can read more about it?' Our defeat comes now. It is hard to recommend a book about communication and educational technology that meets all four criteria of syllabus requirement, understandability, portability and affordability.

Therefore, in this simple nonintimidating book, we promise to tell the undergraduate-level nursing students and teachers what they need to know about communication and educational technology. We strive towards making the book a readable, jargon-free, precise yet complete guide to communication and educational technology in nursing, which is written exactly as per the syllabus prescribed by the Indian Nursing Council.

—Authors

Contents

Review of the communication process

Words are singularly the most powerful force available to humanity. We can choose to use this force constructively with words of encouragement, or destructively using words of despair. Words have energy and power with the ability to help, to heal, to hinder, to hurt, to harm, to humiliate and to humble.
—**Yehuda Berg**

LEARNING OBJECTIVES

This chapter is designed to enable the reader to
- Understand the meaning and concept of communication
- Describe the process of communication
- Classify the types of communication and recite relevant examples
- Recognize the facilitators of communication
- Appraise the barriers of communication and methods to overcome these barriers
- Identify techniques of effective communication
- Discuss the techniques of therapeutic communication

KEY TERMS

INTRODUCTION

The term *communication* is derived from the Latin word *communis*, meaning common. In general, communication refers to the reciprocal exchange of information, ideas, facts, opinions, beliefs, feelings and attitudes through verbal or nonverbal means between two people or within a group of people. It can be

---

BOX 1.1 WATZLAWICK'S FOUR BASIC PRINCIPLES OF COMMUNICATION

1. One alone cannot communicate.
2. Every communication has a content and relationship aspect and the latter classifies the former and, therefore, it is a meta communication.
3. A series of communication can be viewed as an uninterrupted series of interchanges.
4. All communication relationships are either symmetrical or complementary depending on whether they are based on equality or inequality.

---

defined as a two-way process of exchanging or sharing ideas, feelings and information. Broadly speaking, communication refers to the way people interact and keep in touch. It is more than merely the sharing of information and is necessary for paving the way for desired changes in human behaviour and providing others with information for achieving predetermined goals. Communication is essential for an individual's progress and is considered the foundation for good interpersonal human relationship. Recently, communication has been recognized as an integral part in each field of practice and has therefore matured into an interdisciplinary science, with the development of newer methods of communication and information. The basic principles of communication, however, remain the same and are depicted in Box 1.1 (Watzlawick, Beavin, & Jackson, 1967).

Nursing is a discipline that compels its professionals to continuously use communication in their day-to-day duties as bedside nurse, nurse administrator or nurse educator. Nursing practices involve three kinds of communication: social, structured and therapeutic communication. An eminent nurse thinker, Dr Indarjit Walia, has pointed out that the success of the nursing profession largely depends on the way nurses communicate with their patients as well as within and between health care teams. Research findings also suggest that patient satisfaction largely depends on nurses' communication skills. Therefore, nurses must have sound knowledge of communication so that they can focus on a patient's outcome-oriented care. Unfortunately, most Indian studies report that nurses possess poor communication skills and recommend an emphasis on providing communication skills training for nurses (Sharma, 2009). Today, nurses need to have a good understanding of verbal, nonverbal, written and electronic communication to carry out their professional responsibilities in an efficient manner.

DEFINITIONS OF COMMUNICATION

Communication is a process by which information is exchanged between individuals through a common system of symbols and signs of behaviour.
—**Webster's Dictionary**

Communication is interchange of thoughts, opinions or information by speech, writing or signs.
—**Robert Anderson**

Communication is the transmission and interchange of facts, ideas, feelings or course of action.
—**Leland Brown**

Communication is sharing of ideas and feelings in a mood of mutuality.
—**Edgar Dale**

Communication is the process of passing information and understanding from one person to another. It is the process of imparting ideas and making oneself understood by others.

—**Theo Haimann**

MEANING OF COMMUNICATION

From the discussion and definitions in the previous section, we can describe communication as:

- A process through which individuals mutually exchange their ideas, values, thoughts, feelings and actions with one or more people.
- The transfer of information from the sender to the receiver so that it is understood in the right context.
- The process of initiating, transmitting and receiving information.
- The means of making the transfer of information productive and goal oriented.
- The process of sharing information, ideas and attitudes between individuals.

PROCESS OF COMMUNICATION

The process of communication is a complex, ongoing, dynamic and multidimensional human interaction as depicted in Fig. 1.1. It is a two-way process between the sender and the recipient of the message or information, and has several components such as the referent, sender, message channels, receiver and feedback. The communication process begins with a *referent* who gives stimulus to the *sender* to send a *message*, followed by the sender encoding the message and sending it through appropriate *channel(s)* to the *recipient*. Finally, the recipient encodes the message, interprets it and sends *feedback* to the sender using an appropriate channel. This cyclic process continues till the desired purpose of communication is achieved by the sender and/or the recipient.

I. ELEMENTS OF COMMUNICATION PROCESS

Some important elements of the communication process are explained below:

1. *Referent:* A referent motivates the sender (or receiver) to share information (message, objects, sounds, sights, time schedules, ideas, perceptions, sensations, emotions, odour, etc.) that may initiate

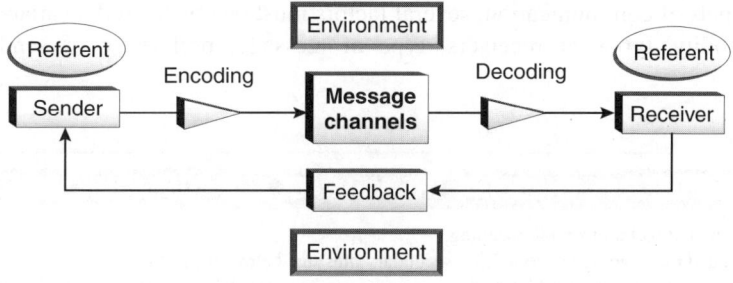

FIGURE 1.1

Process of communication.

communication. Referents are the triggering factors of the communication process. Knowledge of the referent helps the sender (or the receiver) perceive, develop and organize the communication process more effectively. Referents play a significant role in the nurse's professional communication process. For example, a nurse sighting a patient with difficulty in breathing may serve as a referent to the nurse prompting her to initiate communication with the patient.

2. *Sender:* A sender is a person who encodes and sends the message to the expected receiver through an appropriate channel. In other words, a sender is a source or an encoder who wishes to convey a message or information to another individual or a group of individuals. A sender is the source of the message that is generated to be delivered to the receiver after an appropriate stimulus from the referent. The message delivered by the sender serves as a referent to the receiver. The sender encodes the information to be shared in a transmissible form and delivers it to the receiver. Primarily, the sender remains responsible for the content and emotions involved in a message. It is generally believed that the sender and receiver need to have similar communication skills, attitude, knowledge, social system, culture and the same understanding level for smooth communication to occur. Encoding is a subelement of the communication process and involves the selection of specific words or symbols articulated to form a message that can be transmitted to the receiver.

3. *Message:* The message is the content of communication and may contain verbal, nonverbal or symbolic language. It is an essential element of the communication process. Perception and personal factors of the sender and receiver may sometimes distort this element and the intended outcome of communication may not be achieved. For example, the same message may be communicated or perceived differently by two individuals. Therefore, a message must be well-planned and delivered so that the actual purpose of communication is achieved. A message comprises of a message code (symbols) and message content that must be precise, clear, comprehensive, correct, complete, relevant, interesting and useful to both the sender and the receiver. A message may be delivered using the four modes of encoding for communication as illustrated in Box 1.2.

4. *Channel:* A channel is a medium through which a message is sent or received between two or more people. Several channels can be used to send or receive the message, i.e. seeing, hearing, touching, smelling and tasting. It is believed that when a sender uses more than one channel, the message is delivered more effectively and communication is smoother. For example, when teaching a patient about the use of incentive spirometry, the patient will understand more easily if a nurse uses conversation along with the demonstration of techniques. Therefore, experts recommend the use of more than one channel of communication for more fruitful results in the communication process. While selecting channels of communication, several factors must be considered: availability of channel(s), purpose, suitability, types of receivers, type of message, preference of sender and receivers,

---

BOX 1.2 FOUR MODES OF ENCODING THE MESSAGE FOR COMMUNICATION

1. Surface message with direct and simple meaning.
2. Consciously encoded message which contains a secondary message below the surface.
3. Unconsciously encoded message in which feelings are unconsciously disguised to protect experiences or emotions.
4. Dumping; where an individual gets rid of disturbing experiences or emotions by dumping them on someone else.

communication skills of the sender, cost, etc. A brief classification and description of the channels of communication is given below (Box 1.3).

- *Visual channels:* Visual channels of communication are considered to be the most primitive because they have been used since before languages were developed. They are primarily used to send messages through nonverbal communication. Some of the nonverbal channels are facial expressions, body language, posture, gestures, pictures, written symbols, words, etc. Nurses are commonly found using visual channels to send or receive messages to their patients or health care team. For example, when a nurse in a medical unit observes a patient sleeping in an awkward position and repeatedly touching his or her abdomen, the nurse receives a message (through visual channels) that the patient is not comfortable and may be experiencing pain or discomfort in the abdomen. In another instance, when a scrubbed nurse involved in assisting with a surgical procedure needs gauze pieces, she asks the circulatory nurse to supply them by showing her four fingers indicating the number of gauzes to be supplied. In large organizations, most communication is carried out by written circulars, memos, e-mails, personal letters and notices. However, visual channels of communication are used most frequently and promptly in the general as well as health care scenario.
- *Auditory channels:* Auditory channels are used to send or receive verbal communication messages. Auditory channels are the most frequently used channels of communication and involve using spoken words and sounds to transmit messages between two or more individuals. Auditory channels are the cheapest, easiest, quickest and universally available channels of communication. For example, when nurses want to collect the health-illness history from patients and their families, they prefer to use auditory channels of communication so they can promptly, easily and cost-effectively communicate with the patients and their family.
- *Tactile channels:* Tactile channels involve conveying messages through touch. For example, nurses wanting to show sympathy towards a patient in grief and loss will use touch to show their concern. This channel of communication is less frequently used, but is considered one of the most powerful of channels for conveying emotions.
- *Combined channels:* As the name suggests, these are the use of more than one channels of communication at any given instance to send or receive messages. It is widely believed and proven by research that the use of combined channels of communication is a stronger means for effective communication. Marry et al. (2003) stated that the meaning of words may be enhanced or changed with the use of gestures or postures.

5. *Receiver:* A receiver is an individual or a group of individuals intended to receive, decode and interpret the message sent by the sender/source of message. A receiver is also known as a *decoder*

BOX 1.3 CHANNELS OF COMMUNICATION	
Channels	**Types of Message**
1. Visual	Facial expressions, body language, posture, gestures, pictures and written words, electronic mails, mass media, etc.
2. Auditory	Spoken words, sounds, telephone or mobile communications, delivering audio content (radio, voicemail), etc.
3. Tactile	Touch sensations, therapeutic touch, etc.
4. Combined	Audiovisual media, consoling a person with touch and spoken words.

and is considered as another end of the communication process. He is expected to have the ability and skills to receive, decode and interpret the message. Some experts believe that the sender and the receiver are two faces of a coin, and both are essential and inseparable elements of the communication process. The sender and the receiver interact back and forth so spontaneously and simultaneously that mutual and reciprocal relation consistently exists for efficient communication. Depending on the purpose of communication, a receiver could be an individual, a homogenous group or a free group.

6. *Feedback:* Feedback is a return message sent by the receiver to the sender. It is the most essential element of the communication process as it shows that the receiver has understood the primary message sent by the sender and the communication process is now considered complete. A successful communication must be a two-way process where the sender sends the message and receives feedback from the receiver. This feedback could be verbal or nonverbal. For example, a nurse receiving a phone message from the nursing superintendent to report for a morning meeting gives feedback that she will get there at the earliest possible time. The loop as well as the purpose of communication is considered complete after the sender receives feedback from the receiver.

7. *Confounding elements:* These elements are not a direct part of the flow of the communication process but influence the communication process significantly indirectly. These elements are *interpersonal variables* of the sender and the receiver and the *environment* where the communication process takes place. Interpersonal variables, such as perception, beliefs, values, sociocultural backgrounds, educational and developmental levels, emotions, gender, physical and mental health, etc., may significantly affect the communication process. For example, an Indian woman will be unable to communicate freely about her reproductive problems with a male nurse or a male gynaecologist. In this case, the sociocultural values of Indian women affect communication. Similarly, the environment also plays a pivotal role in the communication process. The environment comprises of noise, temperature, destruction, lack of privacy or space, discomfort, etc. For example, it is difficult for a nurse to communicate with health care team members or a patient in a noisy ward. Nurses must, therefore, ensure a favourable environment for effective nurse–patient communication.

TYPES OF COMMUNICATION

There is a lack of consistency about the types of communication in literature. To avoid such confusion and provide clarity, this book offers a clear, comprehensive and simple classification of the types of communication (Table 1.1).

I. BASED ON THE MEANS OF DELIVERING THE MESSAGE

Communication may be broadly categorized into verbal, nonverbal, symbolic and meta communication based on the means of delivering the message from the sender to the recipient.

A. Verbal communication

Verbal communication occurs through the medium of spoken or written words. A combination of several words is used and each word conveys a specific meaning. It is a traditional way of communication to convey factual information accurately and effectively. Some of the important elements of verbal communication are language, vocabulary, denotative and connotative meaning, pacing, intonation, clarity,

Table 1.1 Types of Communication with a Brief Description

I. *Based on the Means of Delivering the Message*	

• Verbal communication
  – Spoken communication
  – Written communication
  – Telecommunication
  – Electronic communication
	It occurs through the medium of spoken or written words. Verbal communication occurs directly and face to face using spoken words or a telephonic device. It may also occur through written words using a paper and a pencil. Today, written words may be communicated using electronic means such as a computer and e-mail facility.

• Nonverbal communication	This communication occurs without words, where the five senses and a whole range of body movements, posture, gesture, facial expressions and silence are used for sending and receiving the message.
• Symbolic communication	It involves verbal as well as nonverbal symbols to convey a message (such as music).
• Meta communication	The communication within the message is uncovered and understood in meta communication. For example, when someone says. 'I am ok', meta communication helps in understanding if he or she is actually alright or not.
II. *Based on the Purpose of Communication*	
• Formal communication	Formal communication follows lines of authority such as organizational meetings.
• Informal communication	Informal communication does not follow lines of authority such as gossip.
• Therapeutic communication	It is a formal process where the patient and health care provider get an opportunity to learn about each other to modify the patient's behaviour.
III. *Based on the Levels of Communication*	
• Intrapersonal communication	The communication that takes place within an individual (or self-talk); crucial to understand oneself.
• Interpersonal communication	Where two or more people share ideas or messages with each other.
• Transpersonal communication	The communication that takes place within a person's spiritual domain, e.g. communicating with one's inner self-conscious.
• Small-group communication	Communication in a small-group, consisting of 3–4 people interacting face to face or using electronic means.
• Public communication	Interaction of one or more people with a large audience, such as health education by a nurse (or nurses) to a group of people.
• Organizational communication	It takes place when individuals and groups within an organization communicate to achieve established organizational goals.
IV. *Based on the Patterns of Communication*	
• One-way communication	It is a unidirectional process where the message flows from the sender to the recipient without feedback, such as in public speeches.
• Two-way communication	It is a bidirectional process where the message flows from the sender to the recipient with due feedback from the recipient to the sender.
• One-to-one communication	Communication between one sender and one recipient at the same time, e.g. a nurse providing discharge information to a patient.
• One-to-many communication	One person communicating with many people at the same time, such as a nurse providing health education to a group of people in a community.
• Many-to-one communication	Many people communicating with one person at the same time, e.g. a group of experts taking an interview.

conciseness, preciseness, comprehension, brevity, timing and relevance. Verbal communication may be further classified into the following subtypes:

- *Spoken communication:* This is the most primitive method of verbal communication; other methods of verbal communication were developed with the advancement of human existence. In spoken communication, the message is exchanged through spoken words face to face.
- *Written communication:* This form of communication ensures the exchange of facts, ideas and opinions through written means. The sender and the recipient come in contact with each other through written means and share meaning and understanding. It is the best method of verbal communication when it is not possible for the sender and the recipient to exchange spoken words because of the distance between them.
- *Telecommunication:* Telecommunication is carried out through the use of specific electronic devices such as telephones, mobile phones, televisions, videoconferencing facilities, etc. In this method, verbal messages are exchanged between the sender and the recipient with the help of specific electronic devices based on availability and the purpose of communication. Telecommunication is generally used when immediate communication is desired and face-to-face verbal communication is not possible. Recent developments in science and technology have revolutionized telecommunication with the availability of more and more advanced and sophisticated electronic devices for faster and better communication.
- *Electronic communication:* Electronic communication has become more popular recently because it is speedy, accurate and confidential and a large number of messages can be exchanged at a faster speed. This is why electronic mail (e-mail) communication has become a more popular means of communication. Electronic communication is usually accomplished through a computer and internet facility.

B. Nonverbal communication

Nonverbal communication takes place without the use of spoken or written words. It includes all five senses and the whole range of body movements, posture, gestures and facial expressions (e.g. smile, raised eye-brow, frown, staring and gazing) including silence. Nonverbal communication is a more accurate way of communication because it conveys the true and intended meaning of the message. For example, a gloomy facial expression of a patient who says he is alright will urge the nurse to focus and rely more on the patient's facial expressions to judge his actual mood. Research supports this opinion as well; Stuart and Laraia (2005) documented that 7% of a message is transmitted by words, 38% through vocal cues and 55% by body cues. Nonverbal communication may be accomplished by the following means:

- *Touch:* Touch is a personal behaviour and means different things to different people. Studies have shown that tactile experiences are largely shaped by families and regional, class and cultural influences. Factors such as age and sex also play an important role in individual meanings associated with touch. Despite its individuality, touch is viewed as one of the most effective nonverbal ways of expressing feelings such as comfort, love, affection, security, anger, frustration, aggression and excitement.
- *Eye contact:* Communication often begins with eye contact. Eye contact also suggests respect, willingness to listen and keeps the communication open. Absence of eye contact often indicates anxiety, defensiveness or an avoidance of communication. In some cultures, however, young children and adolescents are taught it is disrespectful to look an adult in the eyes. In others, people are taught to

avoid eye contact or not to make eye contact with elders. The eyes carry a large number of nonverbal messages that can easily be assessed on eye contact.

- *Facial expression:* The face is the most expressive part of the body. Facial expressions convey feelings such as anger, joy, suspicion, sadness and fear. Some people have an extremely expressive face whereas others are able to mask their feelings, making it difficult for others to determine what the person is really thinking.
- *Posture:* The way a person holds his or her body carries a nonverbal message. People in good health and with a positive attitude usually hold their bodies in good alignment. Depressed or tired people are more likely to slouch. Posture also often provides nonverbal clues concerning pain and physical limitations. For example, a rigid and stiff appearance may be a good indicator of tension and pain.
- *Gait:* A bouncy, purposeful walk usually carries a message of well-being. A less purposeful, shuffling gait is associated with illness.
- *Gesture:* A gesture using various parts of the body can carry numerous messages. For example, thumbs up means victory and a thumb down carries a negative implication. Kicking objects often expresses anger. Wringing hands or tapping a foot usually indicates anxiety or anger, and a waving hand signifies beckoning someone to come or leave. Gestures are used extensively when two people speaking different languages communicate with each other.
- *Physical appearance:* Illnesses result in an alteration in the general physical appearance. On the other hand, a person in good health tends to put it across through general physical appearance.
- *Sound:* Crying, moaning, gasping and sighing are oral but nonverbal forms of communication. Such sounds can be interpreted in numerous ways. For example, a person may cry because of sadness or joy.
- *Silence:* A period of silence during a conversation often carries important nonverbal messages. For example, someone sitting silently in a group discussion suggests disinterest in the discussion or preoccupation with other thoughts.

The nonverbal signal of friendly attitude may be understood from the findings reported by Argule (1992) in his qualitative study on the ways of nonverbal expression in a friendly attitude (Box 1.4).

II. BASED ON THE PURPOSE OF COMMUNICATION

Communication may be categorized into formal, informal and therapeutic communication based on the purpose of communication.

BOX 1.4 NONVERBAL SIGNALS OF A FRIENDLY ATTITUDE (ARGULE, 1992)	
Proximity	Closer, leaning forward if seated directly but side to side in some situations
Gaze	More and mutual gaze
Facial expression	More smiles
Gestures	Nodding heads, lively movements, opening arms straight towards each other rather than folded arms or on hips
Touch	More touching in an appropriate manner
Tone of voice	Higher pitch, upwards contour, pure tone

A. Formal communication

Formal communication follows lines of authority and is generally used in organizations to achieve organizational objectives. For example, the nursing superintendent of a hospital will communicate with staff nurses through assistant nursing superintendents, supervisors and ward-in-charge nurses. The channels of communication may be more formal and active through the use of circulars, memos and formal meetings in this method of communication. In formal communication, the purpose of communication is to share official or organizational information with members in an organization to achieve specific organizational goals.

B. Informal communication

Informal communication does not follow lines of authority. Some examples of informal communication are gossip, chitchat and kitty parties. Informal communication is very fast and usually takes place in social groups such as friends, family and peer groups. The main purpose of informal communication is to share individual information with familiar people in a social group.

C. Therapeutic communication

Therapeutic communication takes place between a health care personnel and a patient, with the purpose of modifying the patient's behaviour. This is accomplished with repeated interactions using certain essential attributes such as trust, empathy, tenderness, concern and a nonjudgemental attitude.

III. BASED ON THE LEVELS OF COMMUNICATION

Communication may be categorized into intrapersonal, interpersonal, transpersonal, small-group, public and organizational communication based on the levels of communication.

A. Intrapersonal communication

Intrapersonal communication takes place within an individual; we may also say it is self-talk. It is crucial because it provides a person with an opportunity to assess self and/or a situation, before acting on it, ultimately affecting the person's behaviour.

B. Interpersonal communication

Interpersonal communication takes place whenever two or more people interact and exchange messages or ideas. This is also one of the most common forms of communication in our daily lives. Good interpersonal skills equip nurses with sharing, problem solving, team building, health teaching, caring, counselling and advocating for patients more efficiently. Interpersonal communication may be further categorized into assertive, nonassertive and aggressive communication.

C. Transpersonal communication

Transpersonal communication takes place within a person's spiritual domain. The purpose of transpersonal communication is to realize selfhood, enhance spirituality and answer questions that are spiritual in nature.

D. Small-group communication

An example of a small-group communication is when nurses interact with two or more individuals face to face or use a medium (like a conference call). To be functional, the members must communicate with each other to achieve their goals. Patient-care conferences, staff meetings and reports are good examples of small-group communication.

E. Public communication

Public is generally defined as a large group of people. Communication with such a large group of people is known as *public communication*. In health care, public communication becomes essential when a message needs to be disseminated to a large group at once. Public communication requires essential skills to influence people at large and media material to reach out to each member of the public clearly and loudly.

F. Organizational communication

Organizational communication takes place when individuals and groups within an organization communicate with each other to achieve established organizational goals. The success of an organization depends largely on the effectiveness of organizational communication.

IV. BASED ON THE PATTERN OF COMMUNICATION

Communication may be categorized into one-way, two-way, one-to-one, one-to-many and many-to-one communication based on the levels of communication.

A. One-way communication

One-way communication takes place when messages are delivered to the audience from the communicator only without constant feedback. A common example of one-way communication is a lecture delivered in a classroom. There are plenty of drawbacks in one-way communication including the absence of constant feedback, the message being imposed on the receiver, the delivery of message being authoritative and little participation of audience.

B. Two-way communication

Two-way communication takes place when both the communicator and audience take part in the process. The audience may raise questions and add information, ideas and opinions on the subject. In two-way communication, the process of learning is active and democratic.

C. One-to-one communication

Communication between one sender and one recipient at one time is termed as *one-to-one communication*. A nurse providing discharge information to a patient is an example of one-to-one communication. This method of communication is used when a more focused and individualized method of communication is required.

D. One-to-many communication

Where one person communicates with many people at the same time, it is termed as *one-to-many communication*. A nurse providing health education to a community is an example of one-to-many communication. In one-to-many communication, the communicator gets an opportunity to communicate with a large number of people at the same time, saving money and effort.

E. Many-to-one communication

Many-to-one communication takes place when several people communicate with one person at the same time. A panel of experts taking an interview is an example of many-to-one communication. This method is used when several people want to explore a single individual extensively at the same time.

FACILITATORS OF COMMUNICATION

Facilitators help achieve smooth and hurdle-free communication between two or more people. The facilitators of communication are discussed in this section.

SEVEN Cs OF EFFECTIVE COMMUNICATION

The seven Cs of communication are considered essential for effective written and oral communication (Fig. 1.2). These seven attributes are as follows:

1. *Clarity:* A clear message helps the receiver understand the message easily and appropriately avoiding any possible misunderstandings.
2. *Completeness:* Incomplete communication has no use; therefore, a message sent by the sender (or receiver) must be complete to achieve the desired purpose of communication.
3. *Conciseness:* Communication can be more effective if the message is as concise as possible so the meaning is not lost in a large amount of content and can be easily understood by the receiver. This also makes communication less time-consuming and crystallized.
4. *Concreteness:* Concrete communication is specific, clear and free from fuzziness. Concreteness makes communication more specific and meaningful.
5. *Correctness:* Correct communication helps in having an error-free message or content in communication. Correctness could be in reference to grammar or in the use of right words at the right place.
6. *Courtesy:* Courtesy helps the senders/receivers express their politeness, empathy, enthusiasm, sincerity, etc., in communication.
7. *Consideration:* Consideration helps in the understanding of others' problems by stepping into others' shoes. A message delivered following the principles of consideration is accepted by the recipient more openly and easily.

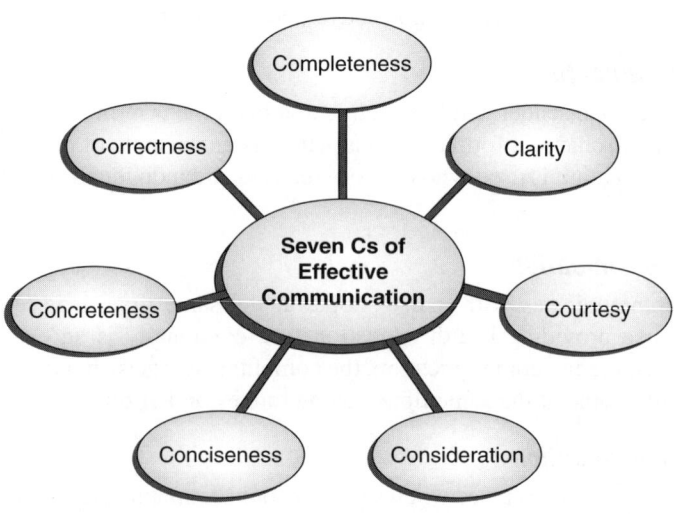

FIGURE 1.2

Seven Cs of effective communication.

In addition to the above attributes, communication can be facilitated by using the following strategies or general guidelines:

- *Positive attitude:* A positive attitude facilitates communication. Defensiveness interferes with communication.
- *Improving communication skills:* Improving communication skills takes knowledge and work. Increased awareness of the potential for improving communication is the first step for better communication.
- *Getting feedback of communication skills:* Including communication as a skill to be evaluated along with other skills facilitates communication. It helps other people improve their communication skills by helping them understand their communication problems.
- *Goal-oriented communication:* Making communication goal-oriented boosts communication. Relational goals come first and pave the way for other goals. When the sender and the receiver have a good relationship, they are much more likely to accomplish their communication goals.
- *Using creative alternative approaches:* Approaching communication as a creative process rather than simply as a part of the chore of working with people facilitates communication. Experimenting with communication alternatives (various channels, listening techniques and feedback techniques) is a good idea as what works with one person may not work well with another.
- *Minimizing negative impact:* Accepting the reality of miscommunication helps in minimizing the impact of communication failure. The best communication may sometimes fail, so we should accept miscommunication and work towards minimizing its negative impact.
- *Warmth and friendliness:* Good communication maintains qualities of warmth and friendliness throughout the communication process.
- *Openness and respect:* An attitude of acceptance, frankness, respect and lack of prejudice helps in improving communication.
- *Empathy:* Empathy is identifying with the way another person feels. An empathetic nurse is sensitive to the patient's feelings and problems but remains objective enough to help the patient achieve positive outcomes.
- *Comfortable environment:* A comfortable environment is one that is trustworthy and safe for communication to take place.

BARRIERS OF COMMUNICATION

Communication is not an easy process and can be hindered by several factors including personal, physiological, physical, environmental, psychological, social, cultural, semantic, and organizational and communication process-related barriers (Fig. 1.3). The barriers of communication are discussed in detail below (Table 1.2).

I. PHYSIOLOGICAL BARRIERS

- Poor retention due to memory problems
- Lack of attention
- Discomfort due to illness
- Poor sensory perception

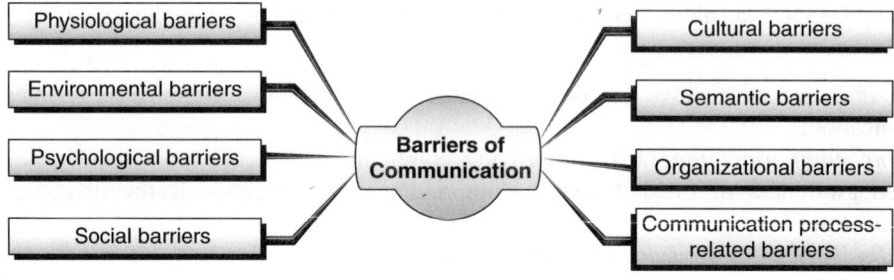

FIGURE 1.3

Barriers of communication.

Table 1.2 Barriers of Communication and Methods of Overcoming the Barriers

Categories of Barriers	Description of Barriers of Communication	Methods to Overcome the Barriers of Communication
1. Physiological barriers	Poor retention due to memory problems Lack of attention Discomfort due to illness Poor sensory perception Hearing problems Poor listening skills Information overload Gender physiological differences	Sender and recipient must keep in mind each other's retention and memory abilities. Sender and recipient must have each other's complete attention. Before initiating communication, the sender and the recipient must ensure each other's comfort. Intactness of sensory perception between the sender and the recipient must be considered. Limitations of hearing ability must be kept in mind. In addition to hearing, the sender and the recipient must ensure active listening between each other. Information overload must be avoided. Gender differences must be kept in mind.
2. Environmental barriers	Loud background noise Poor lighting Uncomfortable setting Unhygienic surroundings and bad odour Very hot or cold room Distance	Background noise must be kept at lowest possible level. Good lighting must be ensured to facilitate nonverbal communication. Comfortable seating arrangement must be provided for effective communication. Hygienic and odour-free environment must be ensured. Optimal environmental temperature must be maintained.
3. Psychological barriers	Misperception and misunderstanding Distrust and unhappy emotions Emotional disturbance such as anger, jealousy and suspicion Prejudiced, resentment and antagonism Psychotic or neurotic illness Worry and emotional disturbance Fear, anxiety and confused thinking	Communication must be carried out in a happy and trustworthy manner. The sender and the recipient must refrain from negative emotions such as anger, jealousy and suspicion. Sender and recipient must avoid feelings of prejudice, resentment and antagonism. The sender and the recipient must be free from fear, anxiety and confused thinking.

Table 1.2 Barriers of Communication and Methods of Overcoming the Barriers—cont'd

Categories of Barriers	Description of Barriers of Communication	Methods to Overcome the Barriers of Communication
4. Social barriers	Diffidence in social norms, values and behaviour Social taboos Different social strata	Diffidence in social norms, values and behaviour must be given due consideration. Social beliefs of the sender and recipient must be kept in mind while communicating.
5. Cultural barriers	Ethnic, religious and cultural differences Cultural traditions, values and behaviour	Cultural difference must be given due consideration. Cultural traditions, values and behaviour must be kept in mind.

- Hearing problems
- Poor listening skills
- Information overload
- Gender physiological differences

II. ENVIRONMENTAL BARRIERS

- Loud background noise
- Poor lighting
- Uncomfortable setting
- Unhygienic surroundings and bad odour
- Very hot or cold room
- Distance

III. PSYCHOLOGICAL BARRIERS

- Misperception and misunderstanding
- Distrust and unhappy emotions
- Emotional disturbances such as anger, jealousy and suspicion
- Prejudice, resentment and antagonism
- Psychotic or neurotic illness
- Worry and emotional disturbance
- Fear, anxiety and confused thinking

IV. SOCIAL BARRIERS

- Diffidence in social norms, values and behaviour
- Social taboos
- Different social strata

V. CULTURAL BARRIERS

- Ethnic, religious and cultural differences
- Cultural traditions, values and behaviour

VI. SEMANTIC BARRIERS

- Language barriers
- Language jargons
- Faulty language translations
- Individual differences in expression and perception
- Past experiences of an individual
- Failure to listen

VII. ORGANIZATIONAL BARRIERS

- Organizational policy, rules and regulations
- Technical failure
- Time pressure
- Complexity of organizational structure due to hierarchy
- Size of the organization

VIII. COMMUNICATION PROCESS-RELATED BARRIERS

- Unclear and conflicting messages
- Stereotypical approach
- Inappropriate channels
- Lack of or poor feedback

METHODS TO OVERCOME BARRIERS OF COMMUNICATION

Several strategies or guidelines may be used to overcome the barriers of the communication. Some essential guidelines to overcome these barriers are discussed below.

I. METHODS TO OVERCOME PHYSIOLOGICAL BARRIERS

- The sender and the recipient must keep in mind each other's retention and recollection abilities.
- The sender and the recipient must pay complete attention during the sharing of information.
- Before initiating communication, the sender and the recipient must ensure each other's comfort.
- The intactness of sensory perception between the sender and the recipient must be ensured.
- The limitations of hearing ability must be kept in mind while communicating.
- In addition to hearing, the sender and the recipient must ensure active listening between each other.
- Information overload must be avoided.
- Difference in communication on account of gender must be kept in mind while communicating.

II. METHODS TO OVERCOME ENVIRONMENTAL BARRIERS

- Good lighting must be ensured to facilitate nonverbal communication.
- A comfortable seating arrangement must be ensured.
- A hygienic and odour-free environment must be encouraged.
- Optimal environmental temperature must be ensured.

III. METHODS TO OVERCOME PSYCHOLOGICAL BARRIERS

- Communication must be carried out in a happy and trustworthy manner.
- The sender and the recipient should not harbour negative emotions such as anger, jealousy and suspicion.
- The sender and the recipient must avoid feelings of prejudice, resentment and antagonism.
- The sender and the recipient must be free from fear, anxiety and confusion during communication.

IV. METHODS TO OVERCOME SOCIAL BARRIERS

- The difference in social norms, values and behaviour must be given due consideration during communication.
- Social beliefs must be kept in mind while communicating.

V. METHODS TO OVERCOME CULTURAL BARRIERS

- Cultural difference must be given due consideration while communicating.
- Cultural traditions, values and behaviour must be kept in mind during communication.

VI. METHODS TO OVERCOME SEMANTIC BARRIERS

- The sender and the recipient must use the same language during communication.
- Individual differences in the expression and perception of messages must be considered.

VII. METHODS TO OVERCOME ORGANIZATIONAL BARRIERS

- Organizational policy, rules and regulations must be procommunication.
- The organizational structure must be simple and noncomplex for smooth communication.
- The organization must be technically strong with respect to communication.
- Large organizations must be divided into smaller subsets to promote effective communication.

VIII. METHODS TO OVERCOME COMMUNICATION PROCESS-RELATED BARRIERS

- An appropriate channel must be used.
- A stereotypical approach must be avoided in communication.
- The message must be clear and nonconflicting.
- Proper feedback must be ensured by the recipients.

TECHNIQUES OF EFFECTIVE COMMUNICATION

Although we are involved in communication at all times, the therapeutic use of communication requires training and practice to develop necessary skills. The following techniques/skills are considered essential in ensuring effective communication (Fig. 1.4).

I. CONVERSATIONAL SKILLS

Conversation or an exchange of verbal communication is a social interaction. As social beings, we learn how to converse with others as children. The techniques discussed below may be used for effective verbal communication.

- *Focusing:* Focusing is a central or key element of communication. It helps individuals come down to reality and builds trust between the two communicating individuals.
- *Paraphrasing:* Paraphrasing is restating another person's message more briefly using one's own words. It helps individuals in sending reciprocal feedback showing they are keen to listen to and understand each other's message.

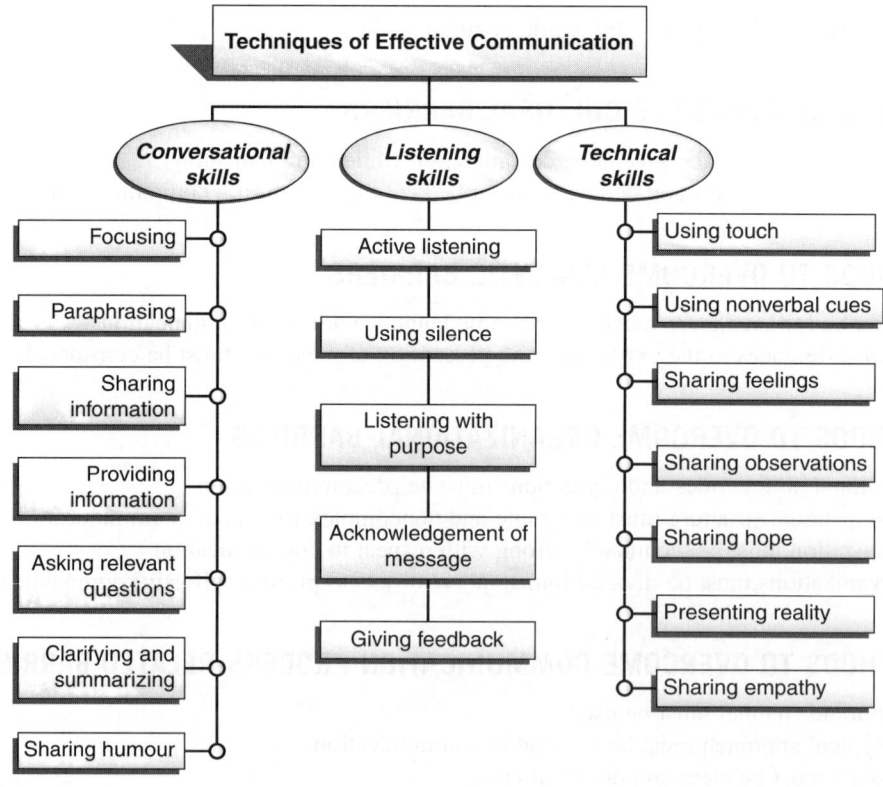

FIGURE 1.4

Techniques of effective communication.

- *Sharing information:* Sharing information is a fundamental technique of effective communication. It helps individuals to reciprocally understand each other.
- *Providing information:* The skills of providing information equip the individuals to deliver the information to other individual(s) without naming or causing undue anxiety and disturbance with an ease of relaxation, safe and secure with fellow members in loop of communication.
- *Asking relevant questions:* Asking relevant questions helps individuals in getting more appropriate and relevant information. This helps them collect and complete basic and specific information to take an appropriate decision on a particular matter.
- *Clarifying and summarizing:* Clarifying is restating and seeking further information about subject matter that is unclear and ambiguous, whereas summarizing is a concise review of the key aspects of interaction. Clarification helps individuals avoid invalid assumptions and misunderstandings. Summarizing helps provide a sense of satisfaction to individuals and aids in the termination of communication.
- *Sharing humour:* Humour is considered an important skill in communication. It is generally believed that using humour while conveying a message may help in establishing a cardinal relationship between the interacting individuals. Furthermore, humour also helps in increasing the ease of sending and receiving messages, by minimizing the likelihood of anxiety between the sender and the recipient.

II. LISTENING SKILLS

Listening involves both hearing and interpreting what others say. It requires attention and concentration to sort out, evaluate and validate clues to better understand the true meaning of what is being said. The following recommended techniques may help improve listening skills:

- *Active listening:* Attentive and active listening is the key to effective communication. It enhances trust and understanding between the communicating individuals.
- *Using silence:* Silence during communication can carry a variety of meanings. It provides an opportunity for the communicator to explore his or her inner thoughts or feelings comfortably. It can also promote patient exploration when he or she gets more opportunity to talk.
- *Listening with purpose:* It is said that one must not only hear but listen with a purpose during communication so that information may be appropriately received and understood.
- *Acknowledgement of message:* Verbal or nonverbal acknowledgement helps individuals in the loop of communication show they are interested and keen to participate in the communication process.
- *Giving feedback:* Providing feedback to the sender helps in completing one cycle of communication and it may further extend without any hindrance. Without feedback, the cycle of communication cannot be completed.

III. TECHNICAL SKILLS

There are several technical skills an individual may use to improve communication which includes using touch, nonverbal cues and sharing feelings, observation, hope, reality, etc. None of the single techniques, however, is enough to promote communication.

- *Using touch:* Touch is the most potent technical skill in communication. It can help individuals translate multiple messages such as ensuring comfort, affection, personal attention and encouragement.

- *Using nonverbal cues:* Nonverbal cues are important aspects of effective communication as they may help individuals develop a sense of reciprocal containment.
- *Sharing feelings:* Thoughts of someone give rise to emotions and feelings that must be shared and can help individuals understand the inner context of their thoughts.
- *Sharing observations:* Individuals in the loop of communication observe how other people look, sound and act. The sharing of such observations helps individuals communicate without the need of questioning, focusing or clarification.
- *Sharing hope:* Hope is essential to continuously move on in life. In health care, it is essential to keep the patient's hopes alive. It helps individuals utilize their positive aspects in terms of behaviour, performance or response.
- *Presenting reality:* It is a technique used to convey to the individuals real facts without confrontation. It helps individuals come down to reality and build further trust.
- *Sharing empathy:* Empathy is the ability to understand and accept another person's reality. It is the accurate perception of others' feelings and communicating this understanding to others helps establish trust in difficult situations.

IV. GENERAL SKILLS

Individuals must keep the following essential points in mind for effective communication:

- Control the tone of your voice, so that you are conveying exactly what you mean and not a hidden message.
- Be knowledgeable about the subject of conversation and have accurate information.
- Be flexible in adapting to the needs of the situation.
- Be clear and concise while conveying the message.
- Avoid words that may be interpreted differently.
- Keep an open mind while receiving information; bias may lead to misunderstanding.
- Take advantage of an available opportunity.
- Whenever possible, sit with the person. While communicating, do not cross your arms or legs because it conveys a message of approaching the conversation with a closed mind.
- Be alert and relaxed and take sufficient time to make the patient feel at ease during the conversation.
- Keep the conversation as natural as possible and avoid being overly eager.
- If culturally appropriate, maintain eye contact with the person.
- Indicate you are paying attention to what the patient is saying by using appropriate facial expressions and body gestures.
- Think before giving feedback and ensure constant feedback.
- No single technique is complete; one should use a combination of all of these techniques to ensure effective communication.

TECHNIQUES OF THERAPEUTIC COMMUNICATION

Nurses are key members of the health care team. They must be knowledgeable and competent in therapeutic communication so that the quality of nursing care can be ensured. Some of the key techniques of therapeutic communication are discussed in Table 1.3. Table 1.4 presents the techniques which may block therapeutic communication so they must be avoided.

Table 1.3 Techniques of Therapeutic Communication

Listening	The process of consciously receiving another person's message. It includes listening eagerly, actively, responsively and seriously
Acknowledgement	Recognizing the other person without inserting your own values or judgements. Acknowledgement may be simple and with or without understanding. For example, in the response 'I hear what you are saying', the person acknowledges a statement without agreeing with it. Acknowledgement may be verbal or nonverbal.
Feedback	The process where the receiver relays the effect of the message to the sender, which either helps keep the sender on course or alters his course. It involves acknowledging, validating, clarifying, extending and altering. Nurse's feedback to patient: 'You did that well' involves giving constructive information to patients about how the nurse perceives and hears them.
Mutual or congruence	Harmony of verbal and nonverbal messages. For example, a patient is crying and says, 'I feel okay'. The nurse says, 'you say you feel okay, but you are crying. Let's talk about what's going on'.
Clarification	The process of checking out or making the intent or the hidden meaning of the message clear or of determining if the message sent was the message received. Nurse: 'You said you feel funny. Can you describe what funny means?'
Focusing or refocusing	Picking up on central topics or 'cues' given by the individual; concentrating attention on a single point. Nurse: 'You were telling me how hard it was to talk to your mother'.
Validation	The process of varying the accuracy of the sender's message. Nurse: 'Yes, it is confusing with so many people around'.
Reflection	Identifying and sending a message back acknowledging the feeling expressed or reflecting back the last few words of the message; directing question, feelings and ideas back to the patient (conveys acceptance and great understanding) Nurse: 'You feel depressed?' or 'Depressed?'
Open-ended questions	Asking questions that cannot be answered in a 'yes' or 'no' or 'maybe'; generally requiring an answer of several words in order to broaden conversational opportunities and to help the patient communicate. Do not ask 'Did you have a good time on your pass?' rather ask, 'How did your pass go?'
Nonverbal encouragement	Using body language to show interest, attention, understanding, support, caring and/or listening in order to promote data gathering. Nurse: 'Nod appropriately as someone talks'.
Restatement	Restating what the patient says; repeating the main idea expressed. Nurse: 'You said that you hear voices'.
Paraphrase	Summarizing or rewording what has been said. Nurse: 'What I hear you saying is that you can't live comfortably at home'
Neutral response	Showing interest and involvement without saying anything else. Nurse: 'Yes . . .' 'Uh hmm . . .'.
Incomplete sentences	Encouraging the patient to continue. Nurse: 'Then your life is . . .'.
Minimum verbal activity	Keeping your own verbalization minimal and letting the patient lead the conversation. Nurse: 'You feel . . .?'
Broad coining statements	Opening the communication by allowing the patient freedom to talk and focus on himself. Nurse: 'How have you been feeing?' 'What would you like to talk about today?'

Table 1.4 Techniques that Block Communication

Internal validation	Making an assumption about the meaning of someone else's behaviour that is not validated by the other person (jumping to conclusions). The nurse finds the suicidal patient smiling and tells the staff he is in a cheerful mood.
Giving advice	Telling the patient what to do. Giving your opinion, or making decisions for the patient. Implies the patient cannot handle his or her own life decisions and that you are accepting responsibility for the patient. Nurse: 'If I were you . . .'.
Changing the subject	Introducing new topics inappropriately, a pattern indicating anxiety. The patient is crying and discussing her fear of surgery, when the nurse asks, 'How many children do you have?'
Social response	Responding in a way that focuses attention on the nurse instead of the patient. Nurse: 'This sunshine is good for my roses, I have a beautiful rose garden'.
Invalidation	Ignoring or denying another's presence, thoughts or feelings. Patient: 'Hi, how are you?' Nurse: 'I can't talk now. I'm on my way to lunch'.
False reassurance/agreement	Using clichés, pat answers, cheery words, advice and comforting statements as an attempt to reassure the patient. Most of what is called *reassurance* is really false reassurance. Nurse: 'It's going to be all right'.
Overloading	Talking rapidly, changing subjects or asking for more information than can be absorbed at one time. Nurse: 'What's your name? I see you're 48 years old and that you like sports, where do you come from?'
Underloading	Remaining silent and unresponsive, not picking up cues and failing to give feedback. Patient: 'What's your name?' Nurse smiles and walks away.
Incongruence	Sending verbal and nonverbal messages that contradict one another, two or more messages sent via different levels seriously contradicting one another. The contradiction may be between the content, verbal or nonverbal message. This contradiction is labelled a double message. Nurse: 'I'd like to spend time with you', then turns and walks away.
Value judgements	Giving one's own opinion evaluating, moralizing or implying one's own values by using words such as 'nice', 'good', 'bad', 'right', 'wrong', 'should' and 'ought'. Nurse: 'You should not do that, it's not "right," that's good'.

REVIEW QUESTIONS

Long-Answer Questions

1. Describe therapeutic communication techniques and phases of IPR.
2. Identify the elements required for communication.
3. Explain any four techniques of communication.
4. Explain the communication process.
5. Explain the facilitators and barriers of communication.
6. List the four techniques of communication with examples.
7. Describe the barriers of communication.
8. Explain the channels of communication.
9. Describe therapeutic communication techniques.
10. Describe the nonverbal communication methods.
11. Explain communication process. What are the barriers of communication?

Short-Answer Questions

1. Write four factors essential for sound communication.
2. List down the types of communication.
3. Discuss briefly the techniques of effective communication.

Short Notes

Write short notes on the following:

1. Communication.
2. Barriers of communication.

Multiple-Choice Questions (MCQs)

1. The 2-way process of exchange of information between individuals through a common system can be termed as
   (a) Interaction
   (b) Interpersonal relationship
   (c) Communication
   (d) Sharing
2. All are important elements of communication process, except
   (a) Sender and receiver
   (b) Referent and message
   (c) Channels and feedback
   (d) Time and environment
3. Which type of channels is considered as the best ones for effective communication?
   (a) Combined
   (b) Visual
   (c) Auditory
   (d) Tactile
4. Line of authority is followed under
   (a) Symbolic communication
   (b) Informal communication
   (c) Formal communication
   (d) Therapeutic communication
5. Health education by a nurse to a group of people can be termed as
   (a) Small-group communication
   (b) Interpersonal communication
   (c) Intrapersonal communication
   (d) Public communication
6. All are considered as types of communication on the basis of purpose, except
   (a) Formal communication
   (b) Meta communication
   (c) Informal communication
   (d) Therapeutic communication

7. Semantic barriers of communication involve
   (a) Language jargons
   (b) Poor sensory perception
   (c) Psychotic and neurotic illness
   (d) Different social strata

8. Methods to overcome process-related barriers include
   (a) Use of appropriate channels
   (b) Ensuring proper feedback by recipients
   (c) Procommunication of organizational policy, rules and regulations
   (d) Both (a) and (b)

9. Technical skill to improve communication
   (a) Using silence
   (b) Using touch
   (c) Active listening
   (d) Focusing on key elements

10. The process of verifying the accuracy of sender's message is termed as
    (a) Reflection
    (b) Clarification
    (c) Validation
    (d) Restatement

11. Communication that involves distance along with nonpossibility of face-to-face verbal communication and requires immediate response is
    (a) Electronic communication
    (b) Informal communication
    (c) Written communication
    (d) Telecommunication

12. Restating another's message more briefly in one's own words, which helps in clear understanding is termed as
    (a) Focusing
    (b) Paraphrasing
    (c) Clarifying
    (d) Acknowledgement

13. Techniques of effective communication include
    (a) Conversational skills
    (b) Listening skills
    (c) Technical skills
    (d) All of these

14. During a communication with patient, the nurse says, 'You said you feel shaking, can you describe what shaking means?' Which type of communication technique is being used here?
    (a) Clarification
    (b) Focusing
    (c) Paraphrasing
    (d) Restating

15. During communication with patient, the nurse says, 'Yes, hmm . . .' while nodding her head. Which technique is this?
(a) Nonverbal encouragement
(b) Incomplete sentences
(c) Neutral response
(d) Minimum verbal activity

Answers of the Multiple-Choice Questions

1. (c), 2. (d), 3. (a), 4. (c), 5. (d), 6. (b), 7. (a), 8. (d), 9. (b), 10. (c), 11. (d), 12. (b), 13. (d), 14. (a), 15. (c)

FURTHER READING

Argule, M. (1992). *The social psychology of everyday life*. London, UK: Routledge.

Baluška, F., Stefano, M., & Volkmann, D. (2006). *Communication in plants: neuronal aspects of plant life*. Berlin: Springer.

Barnlund, D. C. (2008). A transactional model of communication. In C. D. Mortensen (Ed.), *Communication theory* (2nd ed.). New Brunswick, NJ: Transaction.

Bateson, G., Jackson, D. D., Haley, J., & Weakland, J. (1956). Toward a theory of schizophrenia. *Behavioral Science*, 1, 251.

Becker, F. E., & Wortmann, J. (2009). *Mastering communication at work: How to lead, manage and influence*. New York McGraw Hill.

Berko, R. M., Wolvin, A. D., & Wolvin, D. R. (2010). *Communicating* (11th ed.). Boston, MA: Pearson Education.

Berlo, D. K. (1960). *The process of communication*. New York Holt, Rinehart, and Winston.

Bradely, J. C., & Edinberg, M. A. (1990). *Communication in the nursing context* (3rd ed.). Norwalk, CT: Appleton & Lange.

Chandler, D. (1994). *The Transmission Model of Communication*. Available online at: www.aber.ac.uk.

Davis, M., Paleg, K., & Fanning, P. (2004). *The message workbook: Powerful strategies for effective communication at work and home*. Oakland, CA: New Harbinger Publications.

Dimbleby, R., & Burton, G. (1992). *More than words: An introduction to communication* (2nd ed.). London, UK: Routledge.

Donaghue, P. J., & Siegel, M. E. (2005). *Are you really listening? Keys to successful communication*. Notre Dame, IA: Sorin Books.

Ellis, R., & McClintock, A. (1990). *If you take my meaning: Theory and practice in human communication*. London, UK: Edward Arnold.

Garner, A. (1997). *Conversationally speaking: Tested new ways to increase your personal and social effectiveness* (3rd ed.). Los Angeles, CA: Lowell House.

Hein, E. C. (1980). *Communication in nursing practice* (2nd ed.). Boston, MA: Little, Brown and Company.

Heyman, R. (1994). *Why didn't you say that in the first place? How to be understood at work*. San Francisco, CA: Jossey-Bass Publishers.

Kruijver, I., Kerkstra, A., Francke, A., & Bensing, J. (2000). Evaluation of communication training programs in nursing care: A review of the literature. *Patient Education and Counseling*, 39(1), 129–145.

Kübler-Ross, E. (1970). *On death and dying*. London, UK: Tavistock/Routledge.

Maxwell, J. C. (2000). *Everyone communicates few connect: What the most effective people do differently*. Nashville, TN: Thomas Nelson.

Merry GD, Fleischer, S.; Berg, A.; Zimmermann, M.; Wüste, K.; Behrens, J. (2003). "Nurse-patient interaction and communication: A systematic literature review". *Journal of Public Health* 17(5): 339–353.

Montana, P. J., & Charon, B. H. (2008). *Management* (4th ed.). New York Barron's Educational Series.

Morrison, P., & Burnard, P. (1991). *Caring and communicating*. London, UK: Macmillan.

Schramm, W. (1954). How communication works. In W. Schramm (Ed.). *The process and effects of communication*. Urbana, IL: University of Illinois Press.

Shannon, C. E., & Weaver W. (1949). *The mathematical theory of communication*. Urbana, IL: University of Illinois Press.

Sharma, S. K. (2009). Nursing Care Administration: Patients' satisfaction in public and private hospitals at Ludhiana, Punjab. Unpublished PhD dissertation of Panjab University, Chandigarh.

Shedon, L. K. (2009). *Communication for nurses* (2nd ed.). Sudbury, MA: Jones and Bartlett.

Stanley, A., & Jones, L. (2006). *Communicating for a change: Seven keys to irresistible communication*. Liverpool: Multnomah Publishers.

Stuart, G. W., & Laraia, M. (2009). *Principles and Practice of Psychiatric Nursing* (8th ed., pp. 22-27). St. Louis: Mosby Elsevier Publications.

Wainwright, G. R. (1985). *Body language*. Kent, UK: Hodder and Stoughton.

Watzlawick, P., Beavin, J., & Jackson, D. (1967). *Pragmatics of human communication*. New York WW Norton.

Interpersonal relationships

A cardinal principle of Total Quality escapes too many managers: you cannot continuously improve interdependent systems and processes until you progressively perfect interdependent, interpersonal relationships.
—**Stephen R. Covey**

LEARNING OBJECTIVES

This chapter is designed to enable the reader to

- Define the interpersonal relationship
- Explain dynamics of interpersonal relationship
- Discuss purposes of interpersonal relationship
- Classify the types of interpersonal relationship
- Describe the phases of interpersonal relationship
- Identify the barriers of interpersonal relationships and methods to overcome these barriers
- Discuss the concept, functions, description of Johari window and its applications in nursing

KEY TERMS

INTRODUCTION

One of the most distinctive aspects of human beings is that we are social beings. We meet a number of people in a variety of settings and share a variety of experiences every day. Each individual is affected by the presence of other individuals. We start developing an association with each other and join groups with other people to adapt well and meet our several needs.

Interpersonal relationships (IPRs) are and have been the core of our social system since the dawn of civilization. Our ancestors formed associations and alliances to ensure survival in a hostile environment and passed on this need for human companionship as an integral part of our physical and emotional composition. Today friends, lovers, companions and confidants make valuable contributions to our daily lives.

Nursing is a therapeutic process and demands an association between the nurse and the patient. A therapeutic nurse–patient relationship can be established only when each of them views the other as a unique human being. Both participants have needs that are met by this relationship. 'The essence of professional nursing is the therapeutic relationship with the patient' (McCormack, 1997).

Nurses must understand the dynamics of therapeutic relationships as their professional responsibility to establish and maintain a relationship within therapeutic boundaries by considering the patient's cultural, spiritual, emotional and biophysical needs. If a nurse is not able to understand the difference between a therapeutic and a social or personal relationship, then it will be difficult for a nurse and the patient to initiate or terminate the relationship therapeutically.

DEFINITIONS OF INTERPERSONAL RELATIONSHIP

Interpersonal relationships refer to reciprocal social and emotional interactions between two more individuals in an environment.

Interpersonal relationship is defined as a close association between individuals who share common interests and goals.

Interpersonal relationship means interaction or relations between two or more individuals.

Interpersonal relationship is an interpersonal process that involves two or more people, which is the end result of a series of planned and purposeful interaction between them.

DYNAMICS OF INTERPERSONAL RELATIONSHIP

Interpersonal relationships are *dynamic systems* that keep changing continuously during their existence. Like living organisms, relationships have a beginning, a lifespan and an end. The three major dynamics of interpersonal relationships are discussed next (Fig. 2.1).

I. DYAD

- A dyad consists of two interacting people.
- It is the simplest of the three interpersonal dynamics.
- One person relays a message and the other listens.
- It is one of the most unstable interpersonal dynamic. The interaction ends when one constituent of the dyad refuses to listen or share his or her message.
- It is also one of the most intimate interpersonal dynamic as the focus of listening and communicating is centred on only one person.

II. TRIAD

- A triad consists of three interacting people.
- The members engage in relay and reception of thoughts and ideas.
- It is more stable than the dyad as the third member may act as a mediator when there is conflict between the other two.

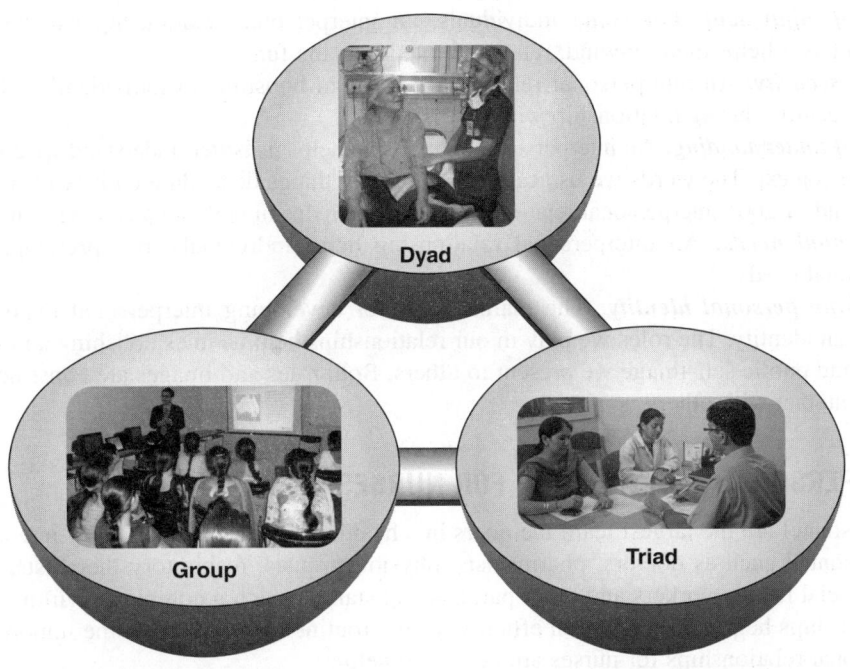

FIGURE 2.1

Dynamics of the interpersonal relationship.

III. GROUP

- A group consists of more than three members and is a collection of triads and/or dyads.
- It is the most stable form of interpersonal relationship.
- It is one of the least intimate relationships, as there is a diffusion of attention and focus.
- The members engage in the relay and reception of thoughts and ideas.
- It is more stable than the dyad and triad as many members may act as a mediator when there is conflict between the other members.
- Triads and/or dyads in a group share a certain association with one another.

PURPOSES OF INTERPERSONAL RELATIONSHIP

The major purposes of interpersonal relationship are discussed in the following section.

I. INTERPERSONAL RELATIONSHIP FOR AN INDIVIDUAL

An interpersonal relationship aids in personal growth and development, is a source of enjoyment, provides a sense of security, boosts self-esteem, builds a context of understanding, meets interpersonal needs and helps establish an identity for an individual. These are discussed in detail below.

- *Personal growth and development:* A good interpersonal relationship actively and continually facilitates personal growth and development of people by sharing vivid experiences of life.

- **Source of enjoyment:** For some individuals, an interpersonal relationship can be a source of enjoyment as it helps them unwind, relax and maximize the fun.
- **Sense of security:** An interpersonal relationship helps in boosting an individual's self-esteem and sense of security during relationship with others.
- **Context of understanding:** An interpersonal relationship helps us better understand what someone says in a given context. The words we use can mean different things depending on how or in what context they are said. A good interpersonal relationship, however, helps in building a context of understanding.
- **Interpersonal needs:** An interpersonal relationship helps individuals in expressing and meeting interpersonal needs.
- **Establishing personal identity:** The main reason for developing interpersonal relationships is to establish an identity. The roles we play in our relationships help us in establishing an identity. So do the face and public self-image we present to others. Both roles and images are constructed based on how we interact with others.

II. INTERPERSONAL RELATIONSHIP FOR NURSES

Nursing personnel are the largest team members in a health care organization. They interact with a variety of personnel such as doctors, pharmacists, physiotherapists, respiratory therapists, occupational therapists, social health workers and other paramedical staff. In such a complex environment, interpersonal relationships help nurses function efficiently on a routine basis. Some of the important functions of interpersonal relationships for nurses are described below.

- **Building a positive functional multidisciplinary team:** A hospital is a complex system where many people work together for a common purpose, i.e. offer quality care. Interpersonal relationships help nurses in building a positive functional multidisciplinary team both personally and professionally.
- **Improving intra- and/or inter-team communication, coordination and cooperation:** Interpersonal relationships help nurses establish intra- and/or inter-team communication, coordination and cooperation, which is very important for functioning efficiently.
- **Building mutual understanding and cooperation:** Interpersonal relationships help nurses build mutual understanding and cooperation that helps them accomplish their personal and professional tasks more efficiently.
- **Understanding self:** Interpersonal relations not only help understand others but also help in understanding oneself more effectively and efficiently. Interpersonal relations help individuals introspect as well as receive positive criticism from others. The use of effective interpersonal relationship is a continuous process that improves self-awareness and insight. Interpersonal relationships enable us become interpersonally effective.
- **Improved decision making and problem solving:** Interpersonal relationships help nurses in taking right decisions and solve problems effectively. It also acts as a tool in achieving common goals in administration and management processes.

III. INTERPERSONAL RELATIONSHIP FOR PATIENTS

Patients are a core aspect in health care practices and each activity evolves and revolves around them. Interpersonal relationship, therefore, certainly benefits patients as well as their families and is discussed below in detail.

- **Developing a sense of security and comfort:** Good interpersonal relations help patients and their families develop a sense of nonthreatening feelings in hospitals and also develop a sense of security and comfort during their stay in hospital.

- *Fostering trust and cooperation:* Trust is a key factor in personal, social and professional functionings. Interpersonal relationship is an essential strategy to foster feelings of trust between patients and the health care team. This plays an important role in seeking the cooperation of patients and their families in health care practices.
- *Facilitating communication:* Interpersonal relationships are essential to foster communication between patients, family and the health care team. Good interpersonal relations also help patients express their distress and disappointment, which ultimately helps in their recovery from the present state of morbidity.
- *Improving socialization:* Man is a social animal and each one of us requires good socialization for effective personal and social functioning. Interpersonal relationships act as a tool for improving socialization between the patients admitted in hospitals or health care facilities.
- *Developing and maintaining positive feelings:* Interpersonal relations are necessary to develop and maintain positive feelings. Furthermore, positive feelings between patients have multidimensional benefits.

TYPES OF INTERPERSONAL RELATIONSHIPS

Interpersonal relationships are classified based on relational contexts of interaction and the types of mutual expectations between communicators. Some common types of interpersonal relations are friendship, family, marriage, acquaintances, work, clubs, neighbourhoods, churches, etc. They are discussed in detail as follows.

I. FRIENDSHIP

Theories of friendship emphasize the concept as a freely chosen association where individuals develop a common ground of thinking and behaving when they enter into the relationship by including mutual love, trust, respect and unconditional acceptance for each other. This usually leads to the establishment of true friendship. In other words, it is an unconditional interpersonal relationship individuals enter into by their own will and choice. Friendship is a relationship with no formalities and the individuals enjoy each other's presence. Friendship can be between man and woman, man and man or woman and woman. The significance of friendship in nursing is depicted in Box 2.1.

II. FAMILY AND KINSHIP

Individuals related by blood or by marriage are said to form a family. Family communication patterns establish roles and identify and enable personal and social growth of individuals. The significance of family and kinship in nursing is depicted in Box 2.2.

BOX 2.1 SIGNIFICANCE OF FRIENDSHIP IN NURSING

A nurse must enquire about a patient's friendly relations as this type of interpersonal relationship provides a great sense of security to an individual and boosts his or her self-esteem. In an absence of these relations, an individual may develop feelings of loneliness, low self-esteem, lack of relaxation in life, etc.

BOX 2.2 SIGNIFICANCE OF FAMILY AND KINSHIP IN NURSING

- Family discord can decrease the security level and self-esteem of a person leading to the development of psychological problems.
- Family relationships can get distorted if there is an unresolved conflict between members. Most of the time, a significant family member senses other family members (especially children) have significant emotional difficulties but fails to bring them out unless the physician or nurse enquires. So, a nurse must use open-ended questions to enquire about a patient's family relationships (i.e. interaction of the patient with other significant family members) in order to rule out a connection between his or her symptomatology and distorted family relationships, particularly when the presenting problem is a psychophysiologic one (such as asthma or peptic ulcer).

III. PROFESSIONAL RELATIONSHIP

Individuals working for the same organization are said to share a professional relationship and are called *colleagues*. Colleagues may or may not like each other. The significance of professional relationships in nursing is illustrated in Box 2.3.

IV. LOVE

An informalized intimate relationship characterized by passion, intimacy, trust and respect is called *love*. Individuals in a romantic relationship are deeply attached to each other and share a special bond. The significance of love in nursing is presented in Box 2.4.

BOX 2.3 SIGNIFICANCE OF PROFESSIONAL RELATIONSHIPS IN NURSING

Work is a universal human experience so it is not surprising that it can be a major source of stress. Work may be deceived as a problem-free area for a patient, but indirect effects of the occupation on other aspects of life-experience may not have been recognized by the person. For a nurse, this information can be gathered by asking the patient direct open-ended questions that can help the nurse understand the psychopathology behind the individual's low self-esteem. The nurse can improve a patient's professional relationships, if distorted in anyway. Asking about the childhood ambitions may lead to a comparison of current status with what the patient would have preferred to become. If the patient describes difficulties, either dissatisfaction with advancement, personality clashes or a failure to see meaning in his or her work, this area should be explored in as much depth as the patient is willing to pursue. Good cordial professional relationships with colleagues can help a person give the best outcome for the organization. In turn, it can provide a person with monetary rewards as well as a sense of satisfaction and high self-esteem.

BOX 2.4 SIGNIFICANCE OF LOVE IN NURSING

Distorted love relationships contribute a lot to the development of psychological problems in an individual as people in this type of relationship have great intimacy with each other. A nurse must understand this special bond of intimacy and try to resolve the associated conflict.

BOX 2.5 SIGNIFICANCE OF MARRIAGE IN NURSING

While providing care to a married person, a nurse must enquire about his or her marital relationship as distortion in this relationship can lead to the development of various somatoforms as well as psychosomatic disorders, especially due to lack of love, attention, trust and sexual satisfaction.

V. MARRIAGE

Marriage is a formalized intimate relationship or a long-term relationship where two individuals decide to enter into wedlock and stay together life-long after knowing each other well. The significance of marriage in nursing is depicted in Box 2.5.

VI. PLATONIC RELATIONSHIP

A relationship between two individuals without feelings of sexual desire for each other is called a *platonic relationship*. In such a relationship, a man and a woman are just friends and do not mix love with friendship. Platonic relationships might end in a romantic relationship with both partners developing feelings of love for each other.

VII. CASUAL RELATIONSHIPS

In these relationships, the individuals usually develop a relationship that exclusively lacks mutual love and consists only of sexual behaviour that does not extend beyond one night. These individuals may be known as *sexual partners* in a wider sense or friends with benefits who consider only sexual intercourse in their relationship.

VIII. BROTHERHOOD AND SISTERHOOD

Individuals united for a common cause or a common interest (may involve formal memberships in clubs, organizations, associations, societies, etc.) may be termed as a brotherhood or a sisterhood. In this relationship, individuals are committed to doing good deeds for fellow members and people. For example, India is expecting a brotherhood relationship with neighbouring countries including Pakistan.

IX. ACQUAINTANCES

An acquaintance is a relationship where someone is simply known to someone by introduction or by a few interactions. There is an absence of close relationship and the individuals lack in-depth personal information about each other. This could also be a beginning of a future close relationship.

PHASES OF INTERPERSONAL RELATIONSHIP

Hildegard Peplau (1952) gave the interpersonal relationship model described in Fig. 2.2. Her model describes the phases in a nurse–patient relationship in terms of the interpersonal process used in

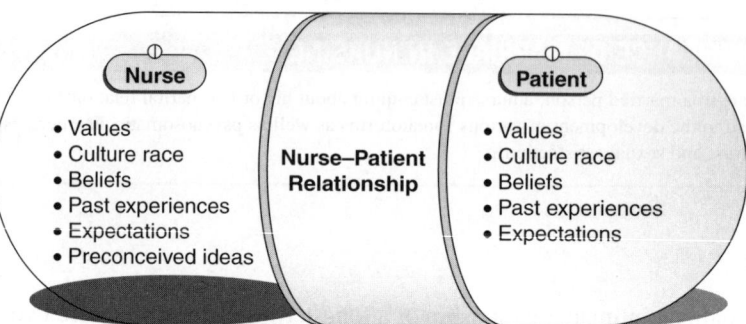

FIGURE 2.2

Factors influencing the orientation phase.

psychodynamic nursing. Peplau's model comprehensively described the four major phases of a nurse–patient relationship which is discussed in detail next (Fig 2.3A and 2.3B).

Fig. 2.4 illustrates the major concepts in Peplau's framework and their relationships in a nurse–patient relationship.

I. ORIENTATION PHASE

- The phase starts with an initial encounter between a nurse as a stranger and the patient having problems.
- The pact formulation begins between the nurse and the patient. The pact states the duration of the therapeutic relationship, frequency of sessions to be conducted by the nurse with the patient and details of termination of the relationship.

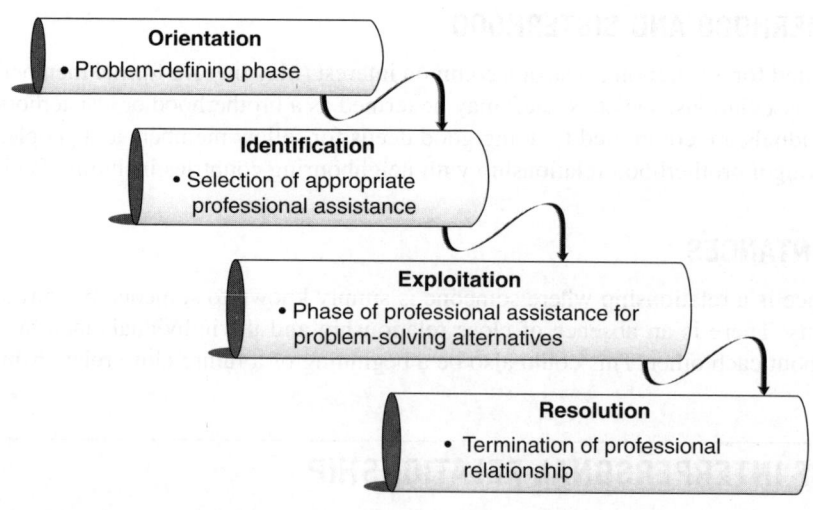

FIGURE 2.3 (A)

Phases of interpersonal relationships.

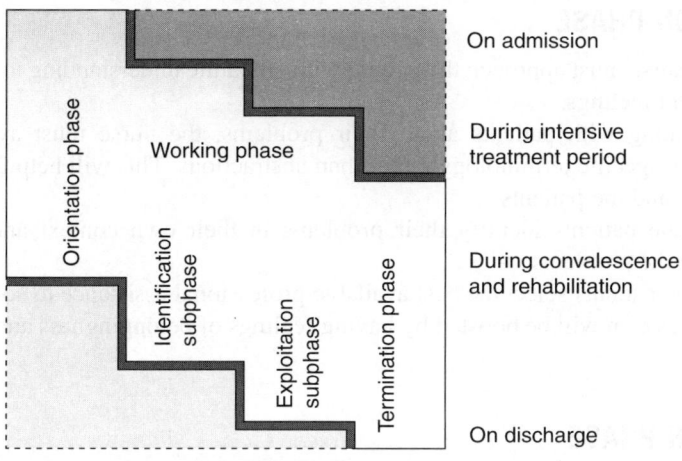

FIGURE 2.3 (B)

Phases of an interpersonal relationship with stages of hospitalization.

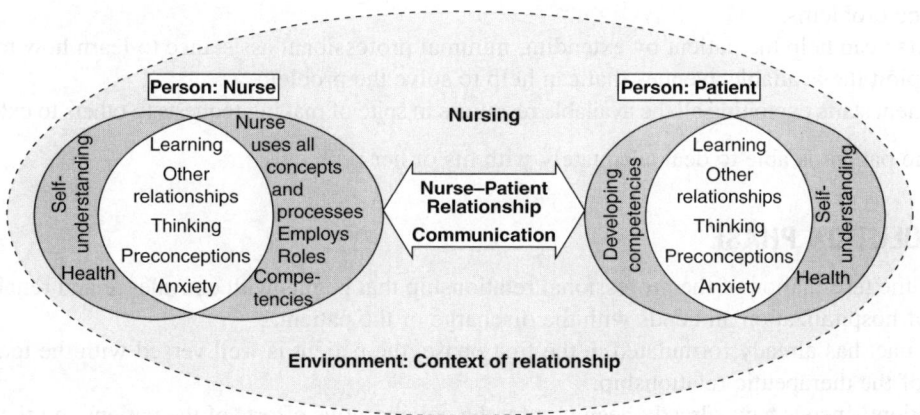

FIGURE 2.4

Peplau's framework: Major concepts and their relationships.

- The nurse clarifies his or her roles and responsibilities within the therapeutic boundary to the patient with a view to avoid the development of psychological bonding or dependence on each other.
- The nurse identifies the patient's problems, defines the problems after understanding them and settles on the type of nursing services needed.
- After developing a trustworthy relationship, the patients start clarifying doubts, share preconceptions and convey their needs and expectations to the nurse.
- There are several factors, such as values, cultural background, beliefs, past experiences, expectations and preconceived ideas of both the nurse and the patient, that may affect the orientation phase in a nurse–patient relationship. These are presented in Figure 2.2.

II. IDENTIFICATION PHASE

- In this phase, the nurse must approach the patient with empathic understanding to accurately perceive the patient's current feelings.
- While communicating with patients about their problems, the nurse must avoid vagueness and ambiguity by using specific terminology rather than abstractions. This will help foster understanding between the nurse and the patients.
- The nurse helps the patients identify their problems in their own context and use the available resources to solve the problems.
- The nurse helps the patients select the best available professional assistance to solve their problems.
- The patient's self-esteem will be boosted by having feelings of belongingness and the ability to solve problems.

III. EXPLOITATION PHASE

- The dictionary meaning of *exploitation* is the process of making use of something to gain as much as possible from it. But during the problematic phase, one feels that there are no resources available which can help the person solve the problem.
- In this phase, the patients are made to understand the problems by exploring all available avenues to solve the problems.
- The nurse can help the patient by extending minimal professional assistance to learn how to explore and exploit the available avenues that can help to solve the problem.
- The patient starts exploiting all the available resources in spite of making requests to others to extend help.

Finally, the patient is able to deal adequately with his or her problems.

IV. RESOLUTION PHASE

- This is the termination of the professional relationship that begins with convalesce and rehabilitation stage of hospitalization and ends with the discharge of the patient.
- As the pact has already formulated in the first phase, the patient is well versed with the termination phase of the therapeutic relationship.
- The patient's needs have already been met by the collaborative efforts of the patient and the nurse in previous phases, so this is the phase to depart from each other therapeutically.
- If psychological dependence persists between both of them, it becomes difficult to resolve the transference or counter transference. A nurse must be aware of the techniques to resolve it.
- The relationship must be terminated by maintaining a healthier emotional balance by both the parties involved and no one should remain dependent on each other.

BARRIERS OF INTERPERSONAL RELATIONSHIPS

A barrier can be anything that restrains or obstructs progress, access, etc. The barriers of interpersonal relationships interrupt the development of a relationship between individuals. Personal factors, situational factors and sociocultural factors may hinder the development and maintenance of interpersonal relationships (Fig. 2.5 and Table 2.1).

I. PERSONAL BARRIERS

The major personal factors that can influence the development or maintenance of an interpersonal relationship between two or more people are discussed below.

- *Gender:* Gender may influence an interpersonal relationship. A strange man may establish a prompt and intimate interpersonal relation with another man. However, the same may not ensue between a man and a woman and vice versa.
- *Lack of honesty and trust:* Absence of honesty and trust between two or more individuals may affect their interpersonal relationships. Therefore, the presence of honesty and trust are essential factors in the development of interpersonal relationships. In the absence of honesty, an inner positive feeling of closeness may not be established and trust cannot be built, which is one of the fundamental prerequisites for building strong interpersonal relationships.

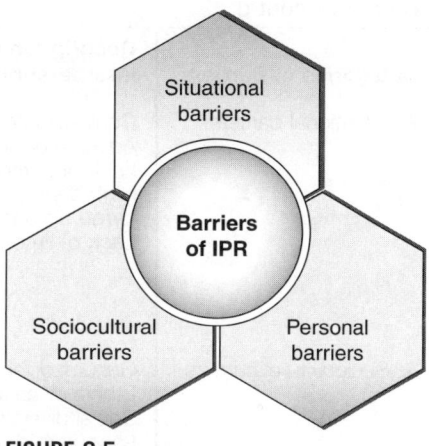

FIGURE 2.5

Barriers of interpersonal relationships.

Table 2.1 Barriers of Interpersonal Relationship and Methods of Overcoming These Barriers

Categories of Barriers	Description of Barriers of Interpersonal Relationship	Methods to Overcome Barriers of Interpersonal Relationship
1. Personal barriers	Gender variation Lack of honesty and trust Lack of compatibility Feelings of insecurity Ineffective communication Distorted self-concept Lack of flexibility Lack of respect for others rights Fear of rejection Pre-existing psychiatric problems	In interpersonal relationships, gender must be given due considerations. Honesty and trust must be maintained while establishing and building interpersonal relationships. Compatibility between the individuals involved in interpersonal relationship must be ensured. A sense of security must be ensured between the people involved in an interpersonal relationship. Effective communication is a key aspect of efficient interpersonal relationships. Therefore, effective communication must be ensured. Individuals involved in interpersonal relationships must have a sound self-concept and positive self-esteem. There must be flexibility in ideology and philosophy of the individuals in a relationship for an effective adaptation and success of the interpersonal relationship. A mutual sense of respect must be ensured by the people involved in personal and professional relationships. Fear of rejection must be eliminated between the individuals involved in a relationship. Skilled therapeutic communication is required to interact with individuals suffering from psychiatric or personality problems.

Continued

Table 2.1 Barriers of Interpersonal Relationship and Methods of Overcoming These Barriers—cont'd

Categories of Barriers	Description of Barriers of Interpersonal Relationship	Methods to Overcome Barriers of Interpersonal Relationship
2. Situational barriers	Complex interaction settings Adverse environmental situations Lack of territoriality High density of individuals Large distance Lack of time	The individuals must try to make the interaction setting simple and familiar and must make the other person feel important. Special care must be taken while developing a relationship between individuals of diversified territories and high density or interaction in adverse environmental situations. Even in an organization, individuals must spend quality time with their co-workers to strengthen the bond between them.
3. Sociocultural barriers	Cultural diversity Ethnic diversity Social diversity Language diversity	Individuals can try to overcome cultural diversity by trying to enhance the four primary factors that decide interaction patterns (such as openness, trust, owing and risk to experiment). Individuals must try to enhance interpersonal communication skills (such as maintaining good eye contact, appropriate body language and listening with patience)

- *Lack of compatibility:* Reciprocal compatibility is essential for a strong interpersonal relationship. Two individuals with a contrasting personality, who are not at all compatible, may face difficulties in getting along with each other and may not be able to establish a good interpersonal relationship.
- *Feelings of insecurity:* When individuals lack security in a relationship, they may fail to establish a good interpersonal relationship because of feelings of threat and anxiety that may hinder a strong interpersonal relationship.
- *Ineffective communication:* Effective communication is a primary tool for establishing good interpersonal relationships. Where active listening, effective and helpful responding and open problem-solving is absent, a positive interpersonal relationship cannot be established. Therefore, effective communication is most essential for the establishment of good interpersonal relationships.
- *Distorted self-concept:* Self-concept is a reflection of the past experiences of an individual with others and includes characteristics which differentiate him from others. Self-concept, if developed in a distorted way (by adopting specific patterns of behaviour due to past experiences), tends to resist change in a person and acts as a barrier in an interpersonal relationship. To maintain interpersonal environment and to maximize the congruence of harmony, a positive self-concept or strong self-esteem is needed.
- *Lack of flexibility:* Rigidity in personality may become a cause of concern in interpersonal relationships because rigidity blocks the adaptability of an individual to desired situations. Individuals, therefore, may not able to establish a congruent interpersonal relationship.
- *Lack of respect for the rights of others:* An individual's conscious and unconscious feelings of insecurity about his rights and freedom may become a barrier in an interpersonal relationship. Individual rights must, therefore, be safeguarded by the people involved in an interpersonal relationship.
- *Fear of rejection:* An individual's preoccupation with the fear of rejection may block the development of strong interpersonal relationship. People proceeding to establish interpersonal relationships must ensure they are free from the fear of rejection.

- *Pre-existing psychiatric/personality problems:* Individuals with pre-existing personality problems (schizotypal, schizoid, histrionic and narcissistic personality problems) and other psychiatric problems (anxiety, depression, manic-depressive psychosis, schizophrenia and obsessive compulsive disorder) may have problems in developing and maintaining interpersonal relationships. Therefore, people dealing with these individuals must have special skills of therapeutic communication so that a congruent interpersonal relationship may be established.
- *Other miscellaneous personal barriers:* Some miscellaneous factors which may block the development of positive interpersonal relationships are depicted in Box 2.6.

II. SITUATIONAL BARRIERS

Situational barriers play a major role in interpersonal relationship as well. Some major situational factors that influence interpersonal relationships are discussed below.

- *Complex interactional settings:* Interactional settings may play a significant role in interpersonal relationships. The depth of interpersonal relationships required by a situation depends on how complex the task is, whether the people involved possess expertise of different kinds, the frequency of interaction in the setting and the degree of certainty with which the task outcomes can be predicted. For example, two workers (A and B) working in a work situation that is very simple and familiar to both of them need minimal assistance from each other as both know their tasks very well. That is why their interaction will also be less and the situation will demand a less intimate relationship. If they have to work in a different work situation that is complex in nature and demands utilization of both of their knowledge then this situation will demand more interaction duration and an intense relationship.
- *Adverse environmental situations:* Environment is where the transition takes place. It can be a problem to maintain an interpersonal relationship if the environment is not cordial. Adverse environmental situations always play a crucial role in blocking interpersonal relationships.
- *Lack of territoriality:* Territoriality is the innate tendency to own space. All individuals lay claim to certain areas as their own and feel safer in their own area. Lack of territoriality leads to distortion in interpersonal relationships.

BOX 2.6 OTHER MISCELLANEOUS PERSONAL BARRIERS

- Lack of integrity
- Manipulative behaviour
- Inconsistency
- Past bad experiences
- Lack of courtesy
- Not meeting commitments
- Lack of respect for values
- Lack of compassion
- Unwillingness to accept reality
- Rude behaviour

- Arrogance
- Closed mind
- Suspiciousness
- Lack of discipline
- Impatience
- Selfishness
- Negative attitude
- Lack of listening
- Uncaring attitude
- Inconsiderate behaviour

- *High density of individuals:* Density refers to the number of people within a given environmental space. Prolonged exposure to high-density situations elicits certain behaviours, such as aggression, stress and hostility. These behaviours can stop a person from building effective interpersonal relationships.
- *Increased physical distance:* The means by which various cultures use space to communicate. If this distance is more than required, sometimes it can be a source of hindrance in interpersonal relationships. There are certain specifications about the distance to be kept in interpersonal relationships (e.g. *intimate distance:* the closest distance individuals allow between themselves and others is recommended at being about 0–18 inches; *personal distance:* distance in interactions that are personal in nature, such as close conversation with friends, is expected to be about 18–40 inches; *social distance:* the distance in conversations with strangers or acquaintances, carried out at places such as a cocktail party, is believed to be about 4–12 feet).
- *Lack of time:* Time plays an important role in relationships. Every relationship needs time and an individual's effort to grow. Frustrations arise when people do not have time to meet or interact with each other. Even in organizations, individuals must spend quality time with their co-workers to strengthen the bond between them. Married couples must take time out for each other for the magic to stay in the relationship forever.

III. SOCIOCULTURAL BARRIERS

Some common sociocultural barriers of interpersonal relationships are given below.

- *Cultural diversity:* Culture plays an important role in the development of interpersonal relationships as cultural mores, norms, ideas and customs provide the basis for our way of thinking. For example, a man and a woman who hug each other on the street give a different message in the Indian culture than they would in the American culture. Similarly, an organization's culture (which can be a hospital setting also) influences the general nature of employee relationships. There are some organizations whose culture discourages making intimate relationships by keeping distance from each other while some organization cultures encourage having family-like closeness to share one's feelings with each other regardless of work, for emotional balance which can increase work output. More cultures foster competitiveness, aggressiveness and hostility between the employees with a view to increase output, in spite of this employees become cautious and on guard with each other. For example in a hospital, when providing care to a patient, the nurse must be aware about the patient's cultural norms or ideas. A patient from American culture admitted in an Indian hospital might hold the nurse's hand while greeting her. The nurse must know that this is a cultural norm of the patient and should not take it in a wrong sense. The nurse while respecting the patient's cultural norms must make the patient understand the Indian cultural norms. This will help both of them establish a therapeutic relationship.
- *Ethnic diversity:* People with ethnic diversity have different values, attitude and beliefs that can influence the development of an interpersonal relationship. For example, certain attitudes of prejudice are expressed through negative stereotyping.
- *Social diversity:* People from a high-status often convey their power with gestures. For example, less eye contact, a more relaxed posture, higher voice pitch, frequent use of hands on hips, power dressing, greater height and more distance when communicating with individuals are considered gestures of being from a lower social status in some societies.
- *Language diversity:* Different languages are in use in different regions of the world. Language plays a significant role in interpersonal relationships. For example, individuals with different language abilities may fail to establish strong interpersonal relationships.

METHODS TO OVERCOME BARRIERS OF INTERPERSONAL RELATIONSHIPS

Several strategies or guidelines may be used to overcome the barriers of interpersonal relationships. The essential guidelines to overcome these barriers are given below and in Table 2.1.

I. STRATEGIES TO OVERCOME PERSONAL BARRIERS

- In interpersonal relationships, gender differences must be given due consideration.
- Honesty and trust must be maintained while establishing and building interpersonal relationships.
- Individuals involved in an interpersonal relationship must be compatible.
- Individuals must try and adapt according to the others' backgrounds and try to be compatible with their aims, attitudes and thought processes.
- A sense of security must be ensured between the people involved in an interpersonal relationship.
- Effective communication is a key aspect of efficient interpersonal relationships. Clarity of thought is also essential in interpersonal relationships.
- Individuals involved in an interpersonal relationship must have a sound self-concept and positive self-esteem.
- Individuals must try and improve self-concept by minimizing the use of misperception and selective interaction and evaluation of the other person. They must also avoid selective self-evaluation and response evocation.
- Flexibility in ideology and philosophy of the individuals in a relationship must be ensured for a more effective adaptation and the success of an interpersonal relationship.
- A mutual sense of respect must be ensured by the people involved in a personal and professional relationship.
- Fear of rejection must be eliminated between the individuals involved in an interpersonal relationship.
- Skilled therapeutic communication is required to interact with individuals suffering from psychiatric or personality problems.

II. STRATEGIES TO OVERCOME SITUATIONAL BARRIERS

- The interaction setting should be simple and familiar to the individuals and each individual should make the other feel as important.
- During interaction in adverse environmental situations or between individuals of diverse territories and high densities, special care must be taken.
- Even in organizations, individuals must spend quality time with their co-workers to strengthen the bond between them.

III. STRATEGIES TO OVERCOME SOCIOCULTURAL BARRIERS

- One can try to overcome the cultural diversity by trying to enhance the four primary factors that decide the interaction pattern such as openness, trust, owing and risk to experiment.
- In situations of social diversity between the people involved in a relationship, individuals should try to understand their social variations and make a sincere effort to adapt to these variations with flexibility.
- Individuals must try to enhance interpersonal communication skills such as maintaining good eye contact, appropriate body language and listening with patience.

JOHARI WINDOW

The Johari window model is a simple and useful tool for illustrating and improving self-awareness and mutual understanding between individuals within a group. The Johari window terminology refers to *self* and *others*. *Self* refers to the person subject to the Johari window analysis and *others* refers to other people in the person's group or team.

I. FACTS RELATED TO JOHARI WINDOW

- The Johari window model was devised by American psychologists, Joseph Luft and Harry Ingham, in 1955.
- The model was first published in *Proceedings of the Western Training Laboratory in Group Development* by UCLA Extension Office in 1955.
- The model was called *Johari* after combining the first names of the founders, *Joe* of Joseph Luft and *Harry* of Harry Ingham. In early publications, the model appeared as *JoHari*; it was later modified to *Johari*.
- The model was later expanded by Joseph Luft.
- The Johari window model represents *self-awareness* of an individual towards himself or herself, and later on became a widely used model for self-development by helping the person understand and learn about improvement of communication skills and interpersonal relationships.

II. THE CONCEPT OF JOHARI WINDOW

The word *window* in the Johari window model represents *an open area* or *quadrant* of one's personality (similar to a window in a house through which one can look inside or outside) which actually represents information especially feelings, views, attitudes, intentions, skills, etc., within or about a person from four different perspectives. These perspectives are also known as *regions, areas* or *quadrants*. Thus, the Johari window model can be referred to as a *disclosure/feedback model of self-awareness* because it helps a person analyse his or her feelings or behaviour and is an *information processing tool* for other people because they can process information about a person subjected to the Johari window analysis. Therefore, the terminology used in this model refers to *self* and *others*: *self* means oneself or a future group and *others* means other people in the person's group or other future groups who are subjected to the Johari window analysis. The Johari window's four regions (areas, quadrants or perspectives) are as follows (Fig. 2.6):

1. *Open area/open self/free area/free self:* This is the part of an individual's personality that is open for the individual himself or herself and for others also. It represents all that is known by the person about himself or herself and is also known by others.

2. *Blind area/blind self/blind spot:* As the quadrant's name implies, this is the area of one's personality about which the individual is totally unaware, i.e. the person does not know about his or her behaviour or feelings but other people are aware about those.

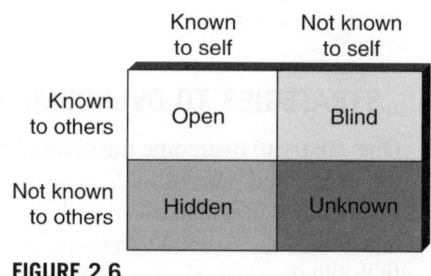

FIGURE 2.6

Johari window.

3. *Hidden area/hidden self/avoided area/avoided self:* This is the area that includes feelings, fears, etc., that are known to the person about himself or herself but are purposely hidden from others because of some reasons.
4. *Unknown area/unknown self:* This is the area that is not known to the person about himself or herself and others also do not know about the person.

III. FUNCTIONS OF JOHARI WINDOW MODEL

- It has become a widely used model for understanding and training self-awareness and personal development and improving communication, interpersonal relationships, group dynamics, team development and inter-group relationships.
- It puts emphasis on soft skills, behaviour, empathy, cooperation, inter-group development and interpersonal development.
- It can also be used to improve an individual's relationship with others or a group's relationship with other groups.
- The model is a simple and useful tool for illustrating and improving self-awareness and mutual understanding between individuals in a group.
- The Johari model can also be used to assess and improve a group's relationship with other groups.
- The Johari window actually represents information—feelings, experiences, views, attitudes, skills, intentions, motivation, etc.—within or about a person in relation to their group from four perspectives.
- Self-disclosure is a process of making internal revelations about oneself that others would be unlikely to know otherwise. Johari window provides a useful way to graphically visualize the process of self-disclosure. The four quadrants or panes represent the different ways information can be seen and observed, both by oneself and by others.

IV. DESCRIPTION OF JOHARI WINDOW AND ITS APPLICATION IN NURSING

The Johari window tool is used in nursing to assess and improve a patient's relationship with others as its major emphasis is on the development of soft skills, behaviour, empathy, cooperation, intergroup development and interpersonal development. It can help an individual gain an insight about the self and others from the four quadrants. Therefore, it will become easy for a nurse to improve unhealthy behaviour of an individual with the application of the Johari window model.

Johari window quadrant 1: Open area

- This is the part of an individual's personality that is open for the individual himself or herself and for others also. It means all that is known by the person about himself or herself is also known by others.
- An individual must develop an open area in his or her personality because through this free space there can be an exchange of good communication and cooperation between people. Because this open area helps everyone work in the most effective and productive manner. It can also lead to the development of good interpersonal relationships free from mistrust, confusion, conflict and misunderstanding.
- The members who are working together from a long time logically tend to have larger open areas than new members. Starting work with a new member in a team, either in a work situation or in general, both individuals will share a relatively small open area because relatively little knowledge

about each other will be shared. For example: when a nurse starts to develop a therapeutic relationship with a patient, the patient will share a relatively small open area.

- A process known as *feedback solicitation* can help to expand the size of the open area horizontally into the blind space by actively listening to feedback from other group members. Thus, it will help reduce the size of *blind space* from one's personality and offer a larger open space to others.
- To expand the size of the open area vertically downwards into the hidden or avoided space, one must disclose information, feelings, etc., about himself or herself to the group and group members.
- The dynamics of expanding the open area in the Johari window is depicted in Fig. 2.7.

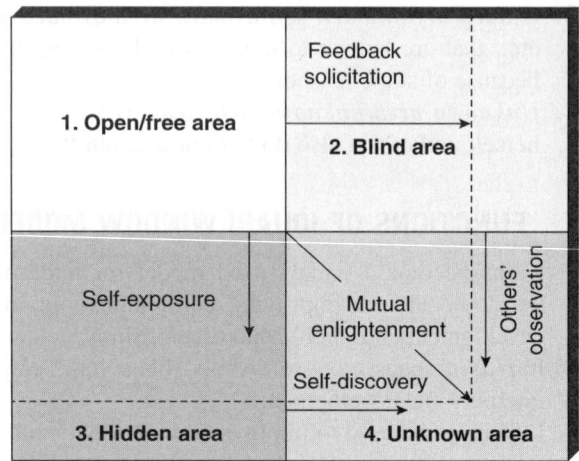

FIGURE 2.7

Dynamics of expanding the open area in the Johari window.

Johari window quadrant 2: Blind area

- This is the area of one's personality about which the individual is totally unaware, i.e. the person does not know about his or her behaviour or feelings but other people are aware of these.
- The blind area being a nonproductive space for individuals hinders open communication with each other because no one can work effectively when kept in the dark.
- In this quadrant, a person who is unaware of his feelings or behaviour might become a source of misinterpretation by others or sometimes others deliberately withhold disclosure about a person's behaviour to him or her to avoid issues in their relationship. Further, this can lead to the development of mistrust or fear in the relationship.
- The blind area will decrease the open area in a person if someone withhold a sensitive feedback related to the individual's behaviour to him or her. This will lead to a lack of development of self-awareness in individuals because they will always remain in the dark about their behaviour.
- While providing feedback to a person, one must take care that it is provided to that extent to which an individual seeks it and must be provided in a specific and sensitive way to avoid causing any emotional upset.

Johari window quadrant 3: Hidden area

- The hidden area includes the information that is sensitive enough to be shared with others—fears, manipulative intentions, hidden agendas, secrets, etc., that a person does not want to share with anyone because of some reason. This area is also known as *avoided self* because the person knows about his or her feelings but does not want to bring those in the open area.
- Most of the information and feelings that we want to keep in the hidden quadrant is usually not always personal, i.e. a lot of it is either related to our work or performance. But we don't want to share it with others because of some reason or fear.
- Self-disclosure can help a person move this hidden information and feelings into the open area by disclosing and exposing relevant information and feelings to others. It will help increase the open area

by telling others how we feel about ourselves and others which will enable a better understanding, cooperation and trust among individuals.

- One must increase the open area by bringing the hidden information or feelings into the open area through sharing the information with members in a group in order to reduce confusion, misunderstanding, poor communication, etc. But it should always be kept in mind that while encouraging the person to share their hidden feelings, the right must be preserved in the person to the extent to which an individual should disclose personal feelings and information and to whom it should be disclosed.
- Some people are more comfortable to disclose their hidden information or feelings in a single instance but some might like to disclose these at a slow pace and depth. One must provide appropriate feedback to encourage disclosure of the hidden information.

Johari window quadrant 4: Unknown area

- This is the area that includes information, feelings, attitudes, skills, aptitudes which are not known to the person about himself or herself and others also do not know about these.
- These feelings or capabilities can be positive and useful or they can be deeper aspects of a person's personality. But if the person is unaware about these, he or she might lack self-belief.
- One must uncover these aspects of one's personality by self-discovery or others can help a person by prompt observations or through collective or mutual discovery of those aspects.
- The unknown area may be uncovered by moving blind area through observations made by others or moving hidden area through self-discovery or moving open area through mutual enlightenment by self and others.
- Nurses can help patients by creating an environment that encourages self-discovery.

REVIEW QUESTIONS

Long-Answer Questions

1. Write how to establish effective interpersonal relations with patients in your clinical settings.
2. Explain phases of interpersonal relationship.
3. Explain Johari window and its use for improving IPR in nursing practices.
4. Explain barriers in developing interpersonal relationship.
5. Define interpersonal relationship; explain the phases of IPR and barriers of IPR.
6. Explain the methods for overcoming barriers in interpersonal relationship.
7. What is Johari window?
8. Describe IPR, its phases and therapeutic Impasse.
9. Define therapeutic IPR. Explain the phases of IPR.
10. Define therapeutic IPR. Describe the third phase of IPR and explain the therapeutic impasse.
11. Discuss the phases of interpersonal relationship.
12. What are the functions of interpersonal relationships in nursing?
13. What are the dynamics of interpersonal relationships?
14. Describe purposes of and types of interpersonal relationships.
15. How you will establish effective interpersonal relations with patients and coworkers? Explain.
16. Elaborate the following: (a) Principles of interpersonal relationship. (b) Phases of interpersonal relationship. (c) Explain about Johari Window model.

Short-Answer Questions

1. What is interpersonal relationship (IPR)? List down its four purposes.
2. Mention any four types of IPR.
3. Discuss briefly the phases of IPR.
4. List down four personal barriers of IPR.
5. Discuss briefly the purposes of Johari window.

Multiple-Choice Questions (MCQs)

1. Who gave the theory of interpersonal relations?
   (a) Dorothy Orem
   (b) Martha Rogers
   (c) Florence Nightingale
   (d) Hildegard Peplau
2. According to the theory of interpersonal relations, phases of nurse–patient relationship are
   (a) Identification, orientation, termination, exploitation
   (b) Orientation, identification, exploitation, termination
   (c) Exploitation, termination, identification, orientation
   (d) Identification, exploitation, orientation, termination
3. The nurse should make an effort towards building good interpersonal relationship with
   (a) Physician
   (b) Patient
   (c) Fellow nurses
   (d) All above
4. An important aspect of nurse–patient relationship is
   (a) Therapeutic
   (b) Personal
   (c) Social
   (d) Causal
5. The most stable form of relationship is
   (a) Dyad
   (b) Triad
   (c) Group
   (d) None of these
6. The most intimate form of relationship is
   (a) Dyad
   (b) Triad
   (c) Group
   (d) None of these
7. The most important purpose served by interpersonal relation for nurses is
   (a) Personal identity
   (b) Effective team building
   (c) Self-understanding
   (d) A sense of security

8. The most immediate relationship available to the patient is
   (a) Nurse
   (b) Doctor
   (c) Friends
   (d) Family
9. The orientation phase of nurse–patient relationship may be affected by which of the following factors except:
   (a) Gender, race
   (b) Culture, preconceptions
   (c) Beliefs, past experiences
   (d) Values, expectations
10. Problem of patient is usually defined in which of the following phase of interpersonal relationship:
    (a) Identification phase
    (b) Termination phase
    (c) Orientation phase
    (d) Exploitation phase
11. Which of the following is a socio-cultural barrier of interpersonal relationship?
    (a) Language diversity
    (b) Lack of time
    (c) Gender Variety
    (d) Preconceived beliefs
12. Which of the following statement depicts team work and effective collaborative relationship among nurse and physician?
    (a) "Doctor your prescribed dose of medicine is incorrect"
    (b) "I would like to like conform the dose of medicine which you have prescribed"
    (c) "Except me everybody is careless bout the this patient"
    (d) "Doctor you must reconsider your decision on prescribed dose of medicine"
13. An elderly migrant is not giving consent for blood transfusion. Which interpersonal barrier is best exhibited in this situation?
    (a) Age
    (b) Gender
    (c) Language
    (d) Culture
14. A nurse was collecting a history from a mother attending antenatal OPD; she gives very weird opinion regarding sex determination. Which of the following would be the best way so that the nurse will manage this situation:
    (a) Explain about the consequences of PNDT act
    (b) Stay nonjudgemental and explore further
    (c) Inform the physician
    (d) Continue with history taking
15. Johari window facilitates understanding of
    (a) One's own strengths and limitations
    (b) Implementation of nursing process
    (c) Learning theories
    (d) Feedback mechanism

Answers of the Multiple-Choice Questions

1. (d), 2. (b), 3. (d), 4. (a), 5. (c), 6. (a), 7. (b), 8. (d), 9. (a), 10. (c), 11. (a), 12. (b), 13. (d), 14. (b), 15. (a)

FURTHER READING

Alligood, M. R., & Tomey, A. M. (2006). *Nursing theory: Utilization and application* (3rd ed.). St. Louis, MO: Mosby, Elsevier.

Berscheid, E., & Peplau, L. A. (1983). The emerging science of relationships. In H. H. Kelley, E. Berscheid, A. Christensen, J. H. Harvey, T. L. Huston, G. Leaving, et al. (Eds.), *Close relationships*. New York: W. H. Freeman and Company.

Chinn, P. L., & Kramer, M. K. (1991). *Theory and nursing: A systematic approach* (3rd ed.). St. Louis, MO: Mosby Year Book.

Craven, R. F., & Hirnle, C. J. (2007). *Fundamentals of nursing: Human health and function* (5th ed.). Philadelphia, PA: Lippincott Williams & Wilkins.

Fincham, F. D., & Beach, S. R. H. (2010). Of memes and marriage: Toward a positive relationship science. *Journal of Family Theory & Review*, 2, 4–24.

Gable, S. L., & Reis, H. T. (2010). Good news! Capitalizing on positive events in an interpersonal context. *Advances in Experimental Social Psychology*, *42*, 195–257.

Gable, S. L., Reis, H. T., Impett, E. A., & Asher, E. R. (2004). What do you do when things go right? The intrapersonal and interpersonal benefits of sharing positive events. *Journal of Personality and Social Psychology*, *87*, 228–245.

George, J. B. (2002). *Nursing theories* (5th ed.). Upper Saddle River, NJ: Prentice Hall.

Harvey, J. H., & Pauwels, B. G. (2009). Relationship connection: A redux on the role of minding and the quality of feeling special in the enhancement of closeness. In C. D. Snyder, & S. J. Lopez (Eds.). *Oxford handbook of positive psychology* (2nd ed., pp. 385–392). Oxford, UK: Oxford University Press.

Levinger, G. (1983). Development and change. In H. H. Kelley, E. Berscheid, A. Christensen, J. H. Harvey, T. L. Huston, G. Leaving, et al. (Eds.). *Close relationships*. New York: W. H. Freeman and Company.

Maniaci, M. R., & Reis, H. T. (2010). The marriage of positive psychology and relationship science: A reply to Fincham and Beach. *Journal of Family Theory and Review*, 2, 47–53.

McCarmac B. Balancing engagement in caregiving. Image (IN), 1997;29(2):139-144.

McQuiston, C. M., & Webb, A. A. (1995). *Foundations of nursing theory: Contributions of 12 key theorists*. New Delhi: Sage Publications.

Richey, J. *"Confucius." Internet Encyclopedia of Philosophy*. Available from http//:www.iep.utm.edu. Retrieved November 12, 2011.

Snyder, C. R., & Lopez, S. J. (2007). *Positive psychology: The scientific and practical explorations of human strengths* (pp. 297–321). Thousand Oaks, CA: Sage Publications.

Human relations

3

Every human has four endowments—self awareness, conscience, independent will, and creative imagination. These give us the ultimate human freedom . . . the power to choose, to respond, and to change.
—**Stephen R. Covey**

LEARNING OBJECTIVES

This chapter is designed to enable the reader to

- Define human relations
- Understand the concept and dimensions of human relations in nursing
- Describe the strategies to promote the cardinal human relations
- Discuss the concept, importance and tools of understanding self
- Identify meaning, types of social behaviour and factors influencing it
- Define social attitude and appraise concept, importance and changes in social attitude
- Appraise meaning, concept and approaches of motivation
- Explore and compare the concepts of individual and groups
- Explain the concept of group dynamics, stages of group development and strategies to improve group functioning
- Recognize the concept and elements of the health team and team work
- Determine strategies to build a successful team and mention advantages and disadvantages of teamwork

KEY TERMS

INTRODUCTION

Human relations are fundamental in a civil society and in each profession (including psychology, social work and health care). Nurses are one of the largest groups in health care workforce and are constantly interacting with patients, their relatives, colleagues as well as other members of the multidisciplinary health care team inside and outside the health care organization. Moreover, nurses come from the same society and interact continuously with people in their personal and social life. Knowledge of human relations enables an individual understand human behaviour and develop a positive attitude towards his profession and the society. Nurses must, therefore, be well equipped and skilled in the science of human relationships to carry out their personal and professional responsibilities more efficiently.

DEFINITIONS OF HUMAN RELATIONS

Human relation is an area of management practice which is concerned with the integration of people into a work situation in a way that motivate them to work productively, cooperatively and with economic, psychological and social satisfaction.

—Keith Davis

Human relation refers to the science of applying principles of social psychology in improving the working of an organization to make it more productive and in making the worker happier to improve efficiency and satisfaction.

Human relations are the relations between human beings that are affected by many other factors and helps in the accomplishment of goals of an organization.

HUMAN RELATIONS IN NURSING

Human relations in nursing refer to the relationship of nurses with colleagues and other department personnel and of nurses with patient. In other words, it is intradepartmental, interdepartmental and interpersonal (nurse and patient/family) relationship to provide the quality care to their patients.

A nurse–patient relationship is the relationship between a nurse and a patient who interact with each other to face a health deviation, share and bring it to a resolution and discover ways of adapting to the situation. Human relations in nursing also develop when two health care personnel interact with each other to achieve the primary goal of maximum patient satisfaction and health promotion irrespective of their field of work.

Efficient patient care is a consequence of modern medical, nursing, paramedical skilled and unskilled personnel which acts as a motivation to work and execute the outlined plans to achieve desired objectives. It is believed that the real power of an organization stays in the hands of the personnel bearing good interpersonal relations established in their work environment.

I. DIMENSIONS OF HUMAN RELATIONS IN NURSING

Professional relationships are created through the nurse's application of knowledge and understanding of the human behaviour as well as his or her communication and commitment to ethical behaviour. Having a philosophy based on caring for and respecting others will help the nurse be more successful in

establishing such relationships. Some important dimensions of human relationships in
nursing are as discussed below (Fig. 3.1).

- ***Nurse–patient helping relationships:***
  Helping relationships are the foundations
  of clinical nursing practice. The nurse assumes the role of a professional helper in
  such relationships and comes to know the
  patient as an individual with unique health
  needs, human responses and patterns of
  living. The nurse's therapeutic use of
  communication helps patients overcome
  their problems by achieving optimum
  health.

  In therapeutic relationships, nurses often encourage patients to share personal
  stories, which are called *narrative interactions*. Through narrative interactions,
  nurses begin to understand the context of
  patients' lives and learn what is meaningful for them from their perspective.

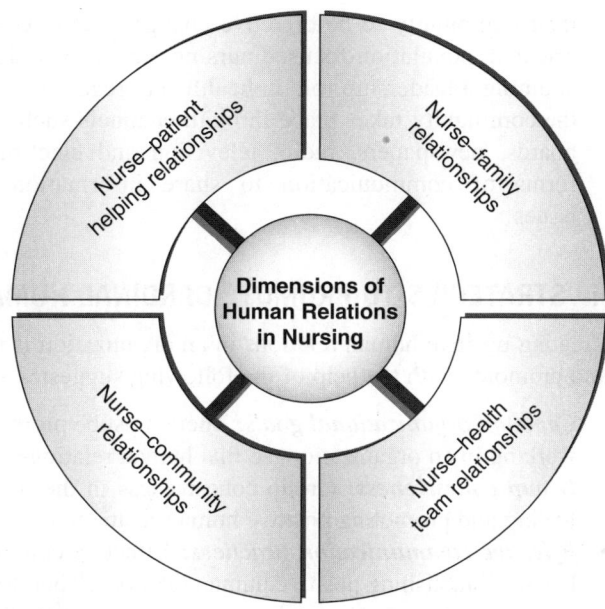

FIGURE 3.1

Dimensions of human relations in nursing.

- ***Nurse–family relationships:*** Many nursing situations, especially those in commu-
  nity and home care settings, require the nurse to form helping relationships with the patient's entire
  family. The same principles that guide one-to-one helping relationships also apply when the patient is
  a family unit, although communication within families requires additional understanding of the complexities of family dynamics, needs and relationships.
- ***Nurse–health team relationships:*** A nurse's functions or roles require interaction with multiple health team members. Many elements of nurse–patient helping relationships also apply
  in these collegial relationships focused on accomplishing the work and goals of the clinical
  setting. Communication in such relationships may be geared towards team building, facilitating the group process, collaboration, consultation, delegation, supervision, leadership and
  management. A range of communication skills are needed including presentational speaking
  persuasion, group problem solving, providing performance reviews and writing business
  reports.

  Both social and therapeutic interactions are needed between the nurse and health team members
  to build morale and strengthen relationships within the work setting. Everyone has interpersonal
  needs for acceptance, inclusion, identity, privacy, power, control and affection. Nurses need friendship, support, guidance and encouragement from each other to cope with the many stressors imposed
  by a nursing role and must extend the same caring communication they use with patients, to build
  positive relationships with their colleagues and co-workers.
- ***Nurse–community relationships:*** Many nurses form relationships with community groups by
  participating in local organizations, volunteering for community service or by becoming politically
  active nurses in a community-based practice. They must be able to establish relationships with

their community to be effective change agents. Understanding the importance of a community-oriented, population-focused nursing practice and developing the skills to practice it are critical in attaining a leadership role in health care regardless of the practice setting. Communication within the community takes place through channels such as neighbourhood, newsletters, public bulletin boards, newspapers, radio, television and electronic information sites. Nurses can use these forms of communication to share information and discuss important community health issues.

II. STRATEGIES TO PROMOTE CARDINAL HUMAN RELATIONS

Creating positive human relations in an organization is not an easy task. However, they can be created and promoted with the help of the following suggested strategies:

- *Common organizational goals:* There must be promotion of a common goal perception in personnel working in an organization, so that human relations can be strengthened further.
- *Group cohesiveness:* Group cohesiveness in the personnel may be helpful in generating the 'we' feeling and promoting positive human relations in a group of workers.
- *Effective communication practices:* Effective communication practices in an organization are the key for establishing positive human relations. Therefore, to create a positive human relation environment in an organization, it is essential to practice efficient communication practices.
- *Defined organizational structure:* A well-defined organizational structure can affect human relations in an organization. There should be a sound organizational structure mentioning duties, expectations and job responsibilities clearly for everyone.
- *Strengthening a sense of oneness:* Inculcating and strengthening a sense of oneness in employees in an organization helps establish positive human relations, which ultimately benefit the organization achieve organizational goals.
- *Training and skill building in human relations:* In the modern health care industry, it is believed that employees can be trained and their skills built pertaining to human relations to achieve a constructive organizational environment.
- *Policies to promote coordination and cooperation among employees:* Each institution must have policies and procedures to promote coordination and cooperation within their employees so that a positive human relation milieu can be created. To have effective human relations, the policy framer should keep in mind that human beings have emotions, drives, thoughts and feelings (the instinct of security and possession, etc.).

UNDERSTANDING SELF

Self-concept is a person's understanding of how and what someone thinks about him or her. An individual in not born with self-concept, rather, it evolves as the individual constantly interacts with people. Understanding the self is the ability to understand one's own thoughts and actions. It is a subjective sense of the self and a complex mixture of unconscious and conscious thoughts, attitudes and perceptions. An individual's interactions with these several factors have affected and continue to affect his or her self-concept. Past experiences make us what we are. They shape the way we feel about the self and the way we react to others. A child who is neglected and criticized at home may develop a negative self-concept. Experiences at home—with family members, relatives and friends—in school, college, work place, etc., contribute immensely to the development of our self-concept. Self-concept has four dimensions or components: body image, self-esteem, personal identity and role performance (Fig. 3.2).

I. DEFINITIONS OF UNDERSTANDING SELF

Understanding self represents the sum total of people's conscious perception of their identity as distinct from others. It is not a static phenomenon, but continues to develop and change throughout our lives.

—**George Herbert Head**

The understanding self is thinking about what is involved in being? What distinguish you from being an object, an animal or different person?

—**Richard Stevens**

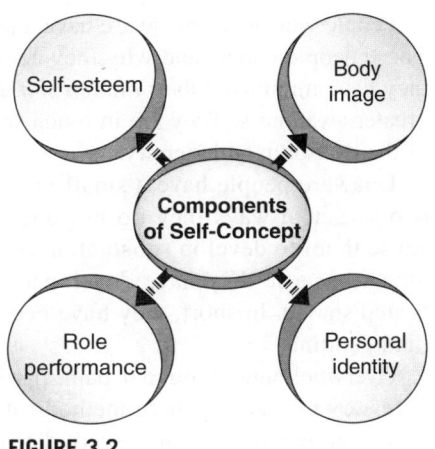

FIGURE 3.2

Dimensions or components of self-concept.

II. IMPORTANCE OF UNDERSTANDING SELF

Self-understanding has been recognized as a key competency for individuals to function the organizations efficiently. It influences an individual's ability to make key decisions about self, others around and organizations. As a result, it influences our effectiveness in work, the directions taken in our lives and our degree of fulfilment. Understanding the self equips individuals with making more effective career and life choices, the ability to strengthen relationships with others in their personal and professional life and their ability to lead, guide and inspire with authenticity resulting in significantly improved organizational productivity. Self-understanding can be accomplished by assessing an individual's personality preference, interests, values, skills, conflict style, learning style, leadership style and life experiences.

III. JOHARI WINDOW: A TOOL TO UNDERSTAND SELF

The Johari window, created by Joseph Luft and Harry Ingham, is a useful tool for providing self-explanation. The four *panes* of the Johari window represent the four parts of our *self*. The *public self* is what individuals show others about them. The *hidden self* is what individuals choose to hide from others. *Blind spots* are those parts of individuals others see but individuals themselves do not. The *unconscious self* is the part of individuals not seen by them and neither by others. All individuals have the four parts, as shown in the Johari window diagram, but their respective sizes vary for each individual (Fig. 3.3).

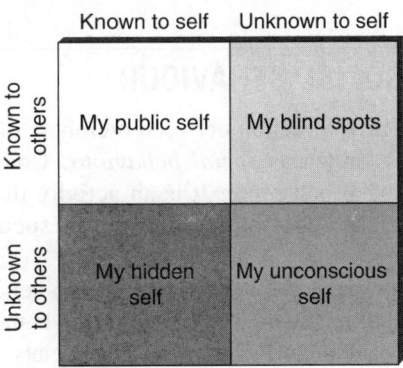

FIGURE 3.3

Johari window: A tool to understand self.

People who are more aware have a large *public self* with the other three areas smaller in comparison. These people understand why they act the way they do and are genuine and open with others because they have minimized their *hidden self* and *blind spots* while working to bring their *unconscious self* to greater awareness. They are in touch with their needs, feelings and values—their *true self*—the source of their wisdom and identity.

Unaware people have a small *public self* with the other three areas larger in comparison. These people act in ways they do not understand because outdated decisions and defence mechanisms cause them to develop substantial *blind spots*. In addition, they are guarded and less genuine with others because they have developed a significant *hidden self* as defence against their own deep-seated shame. In short, they have been disconnected from their *true self*, becoming more defensive than genuine.

Overwhelming emotional pain, particularly early in life, leads us to utilize methods and defences necessary to survive. These methods offer short-term relief but can create long-term problems because they often require us to repress or disconnect from our painful emotions. Thus, our *blind spots*, *hidden self* and *unconscious self* expand and our *public self* shrinks as we distance ourselves from our feelings and needs. In essence, we lose touch with our *true self* that is our real compass and the source of our wisdom and identity.

IV. STRATEGIES TO IMPROVE SELF-UNDERSTANDING

- To increase the size of the open window vertically downwards into the hidden space, one can disclose his or her personal information, feelings, etc., to the team members. This can also be increased by asking the person about himself or herself.
- The unknown area can be reduced by others' observation, self discovery or mutual enlightenment via group experiences and discussion.
- The blind self is not an effective space for individuals or groups, so it needs to be diminished. This can be done by seeking or soliciting feedback from others thereby increasing the open area. To increase self-awareness, a climate of nonjudgemental feedback and group response to individual disclosure should be maintained.
- The hidden window must always be at the individual's own discretion.

SOCIAL BEHAVIOUR

The interaction between members of the same species or the behaviour directed towards the society is known as *social behaviour*. Communication between members of two different species is not social behaviour. It is an activity that has a social meaning or context. In a sociological hierarchy, social behaviour is followed by social actions, is directed at other people and designed to provoke a response.

Antisocial behaviour refers to behaviour that may cause harm to the society. It is devoid of concern and consideration for others, whether deliberately or through negligence, in contrast to pro-social behaviour which benefits the society in some way. Lawsuits and legislations help in curbing antisocial behaviour in many countries. Social behaviour can be of several types: aggression, scapegoating, altruism, shyness, etc.

I. TYPES OF SOCIAL BEHAVIOUR

Some selected social behaviours manifested by individuals are discussed below:

- *Aggression:* It refers to the behaviour between members of the same species with an intention to hurt, ridicule or humiliate the other person. Ferguson and Beaver (2009) defined aggressive behaviour as behaviour which is intended to increase the social dominance of the organism relative to the dominance position of other organisms. Aggression can be displayed in many ways in humans and can be physical, psychological or verbal.
- *Altruism:* Altruism refers to a feeling of concern, sympathy and benevolence for others. It is a traditional virtue in some cultures or can be an inbuilt part of religious expectations that the followers feel motivated for. The virtue of altruism is opposite to selfishness. Altruism is differentiable from feelings of loyalty and duty. Pure altruism is an inconsideration for any reward or direct or indirect benefit with no expectation of any compensation. Philanthropism is somewhat parallel to altruism and refers to selfless service for mankind.
- *Scapegoating:* Scapegoating is the practice of isolation of any party for derogatory or negative treatment or blame. Anyone can be a prey to scapegoating, a child, peer, cultural or ethnic group, worker or a country. Scapegoating is the process where the mechanisms of projection or displacement are utilized in directing feelings of aggression, hostility, frustration, etc., upon another individual or group, with the amount of blame being unwarranted. Scapegoating is also practised to highlight a component's peculiar, absurd, unethical or immoral behaviour towards a group that has led to humiliation for the whole group.
- *Shyness:* Shyness is a feeling of discomfort, nervousness, lack of confidence or awkwardness when a person is in the proximity (especially in a situation where one has to deal with) of an unfamiliar person. Shyness can originate from genetic traits or the upbringing and personality type. It exists in various degrees. An unusually high feeling of shyness is referred to as social phobia.

Shyness is more likely to surface in unfamiliar situations but has a tendency to occur in familiar situations as well, where it hampers an individual's interaction in familiar situations. Shyness perpetuates as the person tries to escape from a situation, leading to apprehension. Shyness may fade with time as a shy child may interact with strangers, go out, tend to be social, learn to act like his or her counterparts, imitate them and learn to show confidence in such social scenarios.

II. FACTORS INFLUENCING SOCIAL BEHAVIOUR

The way men behave is largely determined by their relation to each other and by their membership in groups. Culture also plays a central role in determining the social behaviour of individuals. Culture determines an individual's rituals, traditions and values, way of talking to or greeting others and clothing. These rules and regulations differ from culture to culture and explain why the social behaviour of a particular group of people is distinct from others. Social behaviour is influenced by several factors such as social norms, customs, values and traditions that are passed from one generation to the next. Other than social norms and traditions, our motives, drives and ambitions are also reflected in our social behaviour (Fig. 3.4).

- *Social norms:* The behaviour of individuals is largely influenced by social norms. Different societies have different social norms that are primary influences on the behaviour of an individual. For example,

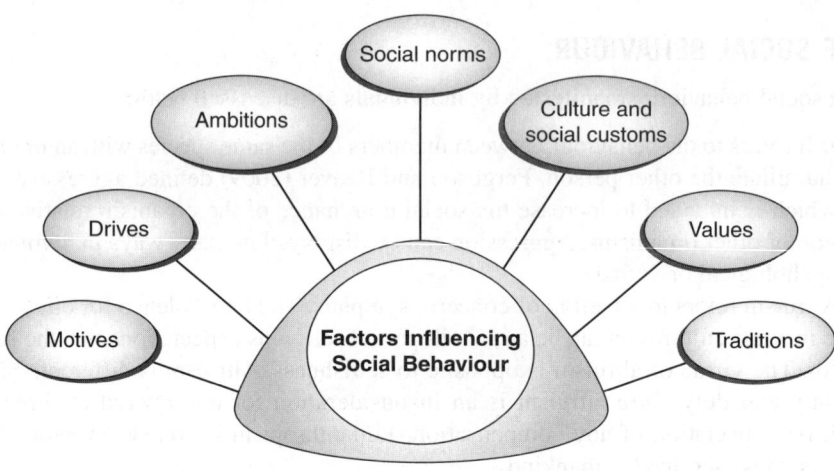

FIGURE 3.4

Factors influencing social behaviour.

a woman does not communicate freely in the presence of the father-in-law in North Indian societies; in other societies, however, this might not be the case. In another example, the social behaviour of Muslim women is defined by socioreligious leaders and they are expected to behave in the manner outlined by these leaders or face adverse consequences. It is clear from the above examples that social behaviour of individuals is influenced by the social norms of a particular group of people to a large extent.

- *Culture and social customs:* Culture and social customs are another important factors influencing an individual's social behaviour. For example, it is culturally not permitted to talk to elders with eye contact in the Indian society. In Western societies, however, talking to elders without maintaining proper eye contact is considered a sign of disrespect.
- *Values:* Individuals carry specific inherent values acquired from their parents, family, mentors and educational institutions. These inherent values significantly influence the social behaviour of individuals. For example, an individual having a value of not disobeying or arguing with anyone superior to him in hierarchy, either at work or community, is going to be governed by the values he or she owes.
- *Traditions:* Different societies have different traditions that are largely responsible for the overall social behaviour of individuals. For example, newly married women are expected to wear a particular type of dress and behave in a particular manner in some North Indian societies. Such traditions are certainly responsible for an individual's social behaviour.
- *Motives:* An individual's motive also significantly influences his or her social behaviour because motive governs the attitude as well as the psyche of an individual.
- *Drives:* Drive may be defined as an aroused awareness, tendency or a state of heightened tension in individuals that sets off reactions and sustains the reactions for increasing the general activity level of individuals. The drive starts from within the individuals and directs them to do things that may

bring about the satisfaction of that need. The strength of a drive depends upon the strength of the stimuli generated by the related need.

- *Ambitions:* An individual's ambition influences social behaviour as it gives a way to expect and respond to others. Unmotivated people exhibit sluggish social behaviour while ambitious people may display warm and proactive social behaviour.

SOCIAL ATTITUDE

Attitude is the state of consciousness within the individual human being. It refers to certain regularities of an individual's feelings, thoughts and predisposition to act towards some aspects of his environment.

Social attitude refers to how a group of people or individuals from a society perceive other objects, situations, people and phenomenon. For example, the social attitude of a selected group in a society may have a negative social attitude on the open expression of sexuality in women. Similarly, some individuals may have a negative social attitude about individuals diagnosed with HIV/AIDS. Social attitude is influenced by several factors such as social behaviour of other individuals in a society, ethnicity, culture, social milieu (parents, family and school), social customs and social dynamics. Lawrence K. Frank mentioned that attitude development begins in early childhood and continues to develop and change as it is a dynamic attribute. He further explained that young children strive to achieve tensional adjustment by reacting to objects and people when encountered in their environment. Each of these reactions results in a tensional change or attitudinal change children. This attitudinal change becomes relatively permanent with recurrent subsequent exposures to the same object or person in the environment.

Social attitude governs the psychosocial or health-related behaviour of an individual. Therefore, nurses must be equipped with understanding the magnitude of positive or negative social attitudes pertaining to selected health-related phenomenon in individuals from a particular society. This helps nurses take timely remedial measures to promote positive health-related social attitudes in vulnerable social groups.

I. DEFINITIONS OF SOCIAL ATTITUDE

Attitude is the sum total of a man's inclination and feelings, prejudices or bias, preconceived notions, ideas, fears, threats, and convictions about any specific topic.

—Thurstone

Attitude is a state of mind of the individual toward a value that may be love of money, desire for fame, appreciation for God.

—Thomas

An attitude is essentially an incompleted or potential adjustment behaviour process. It is the set of the organism toward the object or situation to which an adjustment is called for.

—Bernard

An attitude is a construct that forms notions, feelings and predispositions towards a value. It is a state of consciousness within a person to react to a particular situation or to hold considerations for any object or a norm.

II. CONCEPT OF SOCIAL ATTITUDE

The world is divided into many regions on the basis of climate, topography, life and environment. These factors put together impact the people living in these regions. As the living conditions differ everywhere, each group has a life experience that is peculiar and unique to their own region. These regional life experiences can be a core component of the group as it develops through stages of acceptance and rejection. Some groups may share the same values but they can vary from one group to another or even from one individual to another. An object or virtue can be pleasurable to one group, while it can be of displeasure to the other. Whatever the nature of the social values, the groups respond to them in their own individual way. This appreciation of social values is called *social attitude*.

Human behavioural tendencies appear to be natural and are an expression of the general human need or a common racial experience. Some behaviour appears to have their origin in inheritance. These attitudes attract the interest of sociologists because some of these attitudes constitute social behaviour. For instance, racial disparity is a cultural attitude. However, if the characteristic body odour of a specific ethnic group stimulates disgust in some other group, the natural attitude becomes a thing of social significance and plays a pivotal role in determining social behaviour, arousing the interest of sociologists.

Humans are social beings. They have to stay in social boundaries and so do their thoughts and beliefs. Being a part of the society, they have to conform to its norms. An individual's notions and attitudes are a mix of his individuality and societal forces, the latter being the dominating force. The code of behaviour prescribed by society demarcates the boundaries for an individual's personal expression.

III. IMPORTANCE OF SOCIAL ATTITUDE

- Social attitude determines the social behaviour of a person.
- Social attitude provides a mechanism of social control.
- Life organization demands membership in a group and attitudes are an expression of the desire for status.
- Approval or acceptance of an individual's behaviour reinforces social behaviour.
- Social rejection of an activity restrains the culprit from repeating the same activity in future, thus maintaining conformity.

IV. CHANGES IN SOCIAL ATTITUDE

- Attitude is a dynamic attribute that keeps on changing with new experiences. A change in social attitude could be positive or negative.
- Alterations in attitudes do not arrive alone; they come hand-in-hand with changed social values.
- A sudden change involving a radical modification of many attitudes is commonly known as a conversion. It is a sudden withdrawal from one's usual attitude to adjust to new needs. For example, on joining a new group, an individual develops habits of the new group over time if it is a permanent change. Acceptance of most attitudes is controlled by the unconscious mind.

MOTIVATION

Motivation is derived from the Latin word *movere* which means 'to move' or 'to energize' or 'to activate'. It is a process that produces energy or drive in the individual to proceed with an activity.

The activity is aroused, fulfills the need and reduces the drive of tension. Motivation is often used to refer to an individual's goals, needs, wants and intentions. For example, when one is hungry, the need is food and it induces drive. When the food is searched for, the hunger drive is reduced. All human behaviour is motivated by something. Very little human behaviour is completely random or instinctive. People do things for a reason, i.e. to get certain results, and thus, behaviour is relatively predictable.

I. DEFINITIONS OF MOTIVATION

Motivation is the process of arousing the action, sustaining the activity in process and regulating the pattern of activity.

—Young

Motivation refers to the states within a person or animal that drives behavior toward some goals.

—Morgan and King

Motivation can be defined as any idea, need, emotion or organic stage that prompts a man to action.

Motivation may be defined as the complex of forces inspiring a person at work in an organization to build his desire and willingness to use his potentialities for achievement of organizational objectives.

II. CONCEPT OF MOTIVATION

Motivation refers to sparking the personnel with zeal to perform a task for the achievement of established organizational goals. Motivation is not restricted to the sole achievement of a goal. In fact, it inculcates the spirit of working efficiently and wholeheartedly with grit to achieve desired objectives. To accomplish this level of working, the manager needs to give positive reinforcement to various personnel. The manager has to be consistent in figuring out areas of deficit and lack of infrastructure and provide incentives and perks with the desired appreciation to keep the personnel's morale high for a fruitful result.

Apart from providing incentives, making the personnel more decisive and giving exposure to best circumstances also prove to be lubricants for having a fruitful outcome. In addition, personnel's individuality cannot be neglected and they should be provided with freedom of expression and a chance to work the way they want.

III. MOTIVATIONAL APPROACH

The manager has to ponder over how to utilize the organization's personnel to their maximum potential and explore the lacunae that may cause a hindrance in the achievement of organizational goals. Some motivational approaches followed by managers to achieve organizational goals effectively are described below.

- *Be-strong approach:* Conventionally, the management resorted to being strong. According to this approach, the enterprise put a thrust on economic rewards. The assumption was that people work more efficiently if threatened with financial loss or penalty on failure to do their job. The higher the work efficiency, the better was the reward. This proved beneficial in the past because people believed in leading simple lives and had no other expectations from their job. In contrast, the expectations of personnel have risen beyond money these days. They expect good working conditions and many more incentives. Moreover, the growth of unions has made it difficult to fire personnel from their jobs.

- *Be-good/paternalistic approach:* The be-good approach refers to rewarding personnel to get productive work in return. Rewards may include job security, recreation, fair supervision and sound working conditions. This approach may prove futile in achieving its purpose because the personnel may take it as a load or a compulsion. Work is a way of paying back to the organization and hampers their freedom to work.

- *Effort reward approach:* This approach operates on the basis of the effort or endeavour on the part of personnel to achieve organizational objectives. The manager sets up standards of practice and observes adherence to these standards. Ultimately, the reward is decided on the basis of performance. This gives a sense of motivation and adherence to work. This approach makes the personnel more money-minded as they exploit their fullest potential to be promoted or receive higher remuneration. The pitfall of this approach is that it fails to provide the employees with job satisfaction.

IV. MASLOW'S PRIORITY MODEL OF MOTIVATION

Abraham Maslow developed the *Hierarchy of Needs* model in 1948 and it remains valid today for understanding human motivation, management training and personal development. Maslow proposed that human beings are driven by needs according to their priority, and that their behaviour is in accordance with the need with the highest priority.

According to Maslow, each of us is motivated by needs. Our most basic needs are inborn, having evolved over tens of thousands of years. The model helps explain how these needs motivate all of us. It states that we must satisfy each need, starting with the first need that deals with the most obvious need, for survival itself.

Only when the lower-order needs of physical and emotional well-being are satisfied are we concerned with the higher-order needs of influence and personal development. Conversely, if the things satisfying our lower-order needs are swept away, we are no longer concerned about the maintenance of our higher-order needs. The original version of this model consists of five needs discussed below (Fig. 3.5):

- *Basic physiological needs:* The needs related to the existence and maintenance of human life are our basic physiological needs. These include things such as food, clothing, shelter, air, water and other necessities of life.
- *Safety and security needs:* After being content with basic needs, there is a drift towards financial and personal security and insurance.
- *Social needs:* After the satisfaction of our security needs, our needs move towards being social. These needs include interaction, adoration, respect, belongingness, etc.
- *Esteem and status needs:* These needs include self-respect, reputation, confidence, self-reliance, achievement, finesse, etc., and take priority after our social needs are met.

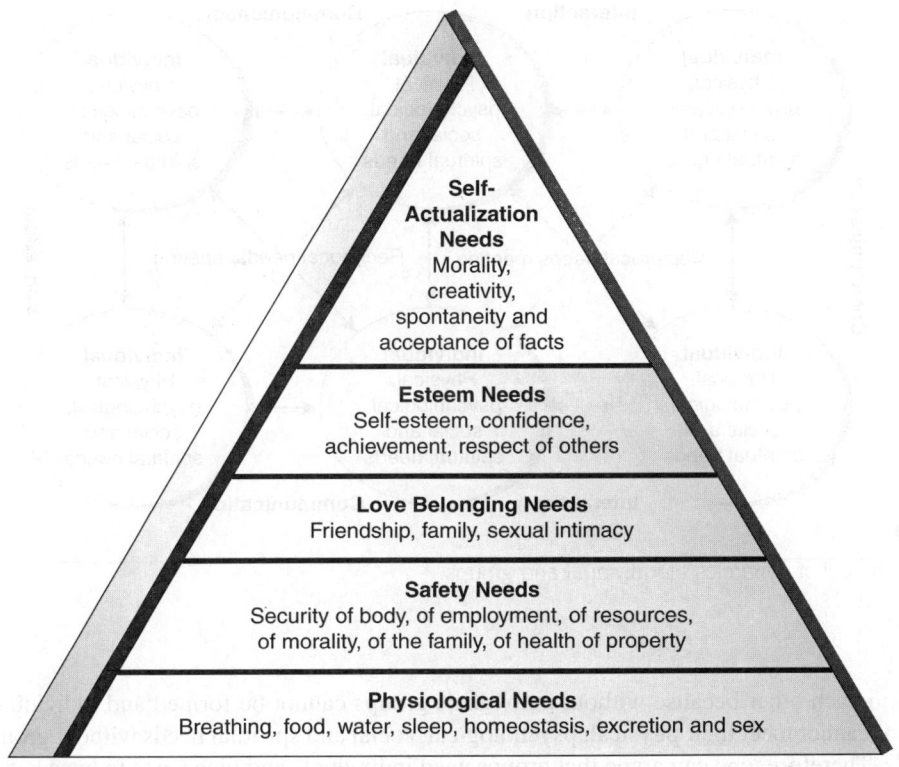

FIGURE 3.5

Maslow's Hierarchy of Needs model.

- *Self-realization:* Self-realization refers to the need for realizing personal potential, self-fulfilment, seeking personal growth and peak experiences. Achievement of these needs give a high degree of contentment, and complacency if they prove to be an uphill task to perform.

There are always people who place less priority on needs and are placed at more crucial levels. For instance, some people place self-esteem above love.

INDIVIDUAL AND GROUPS

An individual is a single unit in a group and a group is a collection of many individuals with a common purpose. In its elementary sense 'a group is a number of units of anything in close proximity to one another'. In the human field, by group we mean 'any collection of human beings who are brought into social relationships with one another'.

An individual is an emotional being who has inherent physical, physiological, psychological, spiritual and social dimensions of being and holds the values of a group to get an opportunity for the fulfilment of his physical, psychological, social and spiritual needs (Fig. 3.6). Individuals and groups are

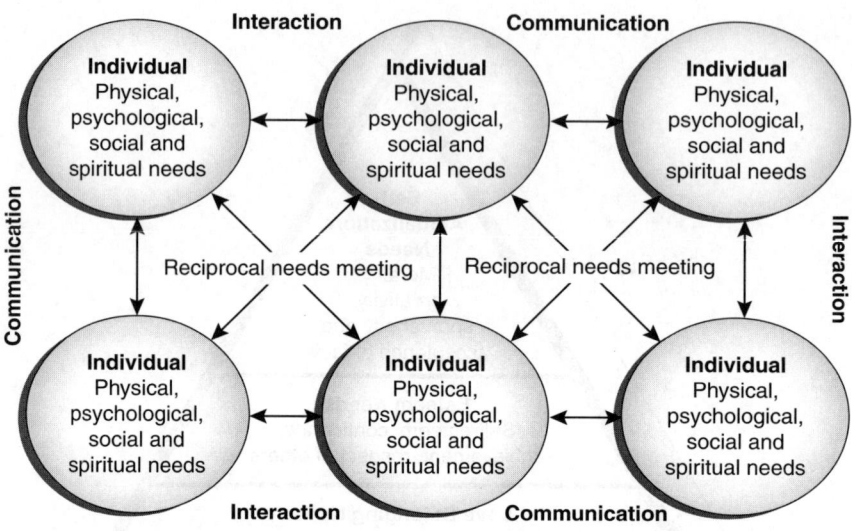

FIGURE 3.6

Conceptual model of dynamics of individual and groups.

reciprocal to each other because without individuals groups cannot be formed and individuals have no existence or cannot meet their physical, psychological, social and spiritual needs without groups of other individuals. Therefore, one can argue that groups need individuals and vice versa to have a valuable and purposeful existence.

I. DEFINITIONS OF GROUP

A social group is a given aggregate of people, playing inter-related roles and recognized by themselves or others as a unit of interaction.

—**Williams**

A group may be defined as two or more individuals interacting with one another for an identifiable purpose and who share at least one goal. The individuals concerned normally occupy roles and adhere to rules and norms implicitly or explicitly agreed between members.

—**Robert J. Gates**

A social group grows out of and requires a situation which permits meaningful interstimulation and meaningful response between the individuals involved, common focusing of attention, common stimuli and interest and the development of certain common drives, motivations or emotions.

—**Gillin and Gillin**

A group is a social unit which consists of a number of individuals who stand in definite status and rare relationships to one another and which possesses a set of values or norms of its own regulating the behavior of individual members at least in matters of consequence to the group.

—**Sheriff and Sheriff**

II. CHARACTERISTICS OF A GROUP

The common characteristics of groups are listed below.

- Each group has its own identity and structure.
- A group includes at least two or more people.
- Group members have a shared purpose or goal.
- Group members have a conscious identification with each other.
- Group members need each other's help to accomplish the purposes for which they have organized.
- Group members influence, interact and communicate with each other.
- Every group has its own rules and norms members are supposed to follow.

III. CLASSIFICATION OF GROUPS

Dwight Sanderson suggested a three-fold classification of social groups by structure. He classified them into involuntary, voluntary and delegate groups. An *involuntary group* is based on kinship such as family. Individual have no choice over the family they belong to. Individuals join *voluntary groups* of their own volition. They agree to be a member and are free to withdraw from its membership at any time. Individual joins a *delegate group* as a representative of a number of people, either elected by them or nominated by some power. The parliament is an example of a delegate group.

Charles Cooley classified groups into primary and secondary groups on the basis of the kind of contacts group members had with each other. In a *primary* group, there is face-to-face association and intimate relationships are indirect, *secondary* groups are impersonal.

George Hasen classified groups as unsocial, pseudosocial, antisocial and prosocial on the basis of their relationship with other groups. An *unsocial group* is one which largely lives to itself and for itself and does not participate in the larger society of which it is a part. It does not interact with other groups and remains aloof. A *pseudosocial group* participates in social life but largely for its own gain and not for the greater good. An *antisocial group* is one that acts against the interests of society. A trade union giving a call for a national strike is antisocial. Similarly, a political party planning to overthrow a popular government is antisocial. A *prosocial group* is the reverse of an antisocial group. It works for the larger interest of the society and is engaged in constructive tasks and concerned with people's welfare.

IV. TASKS OR ROLES OF AN INDIVIDUAL IN A GROUP

There are many tasks that each group performs and each member may perform several tasks. For the group's goal to be accomplished, all necessary tasks will either be carried out by a member or by the leader. These roles or tasks are given below.

- *Initiator:* The contributor who proposes or suggests group goals or defines the problem. There may be more than one initiator in the group's lifetime.
- *Information seeker:* Searches for a factual basis for the group's work.
- *Information giver:* Offers an opinion on what the group's view of pertinent values should be.
- *Opinion seeker:* Seeks an opinion that clarifies or reflects the value of other member's suggestions.
- *Elaborator:* Gives examples or extends meanings of suggestions given and how they could work.
- *Coordinator:* Clarifies and coordinates ideas, suggestions and activities of the group.
- *Orienteer:* Summarizes decisions, actions and identifies the questions and departures, and forms predetermined goals.

- *Evaluator:* Questions group accomplishments and compares them to a standard.
- *Energizer:* Stimulates and prods the group to act and raise the level of its actions.
- *Procedural technician:* Facilitates group action by arranging the environment.
- *Recorder:* Records group activities and accomplishments.
- *Group-building and maintenance roles:* The group task roles contribute to the work to be done; group-building roles provide for the care and maintenance of the group. Examples of group-building roles include:
  - *Encourager:* Accepts and praises all contributions, viewpoints and ideas with worth and solidarity.
  - *Harmonizer:* Mediates, harmonizes and resolves conflict.
  - *Compromiser:* Yields his or her position in a conflict situation.
  - *Facilitator:* Promotes open communication and facilitates participation of all members.
  - *Standard setter:* Expresses or evaluates standards to evaluate group process.
  - *Group commentator:* Records the group process and provides feedback to the group.
  - *Followers:* Accepts the group's ideas and listens to discussions and decisions.

GROUP DYNAMICS

Kurt Lewin, a social psychologist at the University of Iowa, USA, was the creator of the term group dynamics. Group dynamics is the study of groups and also a general term for a group process. Relevant to the fields of psychology, sociology and communication studies, a group is considered as two or more individuals connected to each other by a social relationship.

In organizational development or group dynamics, the phrase *group process* refers to an insight into the behaviour of group members and to incline their behaviours towards the achievement of group goals. An individual with capability, expertise and finesse assists in framing the objectives and ensures that the means to meet these objectives are followed. A group leader performs this task mends behaviour and endeavours to work with unified commitment.

On the basis of interaction between group members, each group holds a characteristic feature that sets it apart from the rest. The interaction is influenced by norms, roles, relations, need to belong, social influence and effects on behaviour.

I. MEANING OF GROUP DYNAMICS

Group dynamics is the study of activities or processes that are responsible for various group phenomena.

Group dynamics is the study of group interstimulation and invoking of response between individuals to perform various group phenomena.

II. ASPECTS OF GROUP DISCIPLINE

- Formation of group
- Group task
- Composition of group
- Communication between group members

- Mode of working relationships between members of a group
- Growth, downfall and resolution of the group
- Group dissolution
- Method to achieve oneness and building consensus
- Acclimatization to meet the needs of the group
- Task performance

III. STAGES OF GROUP DEVELOPMENT

Group formation is not a spontaneous phenomenon. It gradually progresses from a gathering to a goal-directed team. It has to muddle through a forming process where the group members interact, clash and ultimately gel into a common stream to work towards shared objectives.

The different group-forming stages are given below (Fig. 3.7).

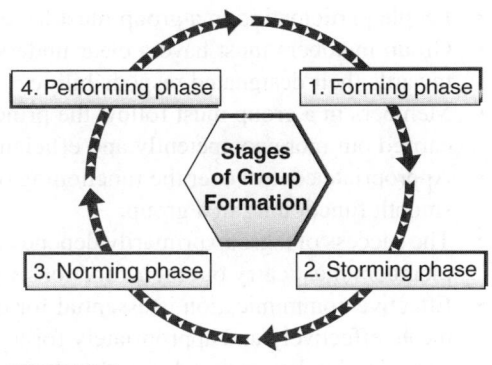

FIGURE 3.7

Stages of group development.

- *Forming phase:* The group members come together for a common purpose or motive and interact with each other to plan ahead for a joint venture in this phase. The interacting members may not be alike in their choices, decisiveness and notions, and individual roles and responsibilities are unclear.
- *Storming phase:* Individuals have a characteristic feature that gives them their identity. Individual differences are the factors leading to different beliefs imbibed by different people. In the storming phase, members voice out their differences and negotiate, bargain and assemble themselves into a unit. They strive to represent a particular position in the team/group. Amidst all the chaos arises a leader who achieves consensus on the purpose and objectives. Team members try hard for positions, as they attempt to establish themselves in relation to other team members and the leader. The team needs focus on its goals and avoid being distracted by relationships and emotional issues. Compromises may be required to facilitate the progress of the group.
- *Norming phase:* Members begin to realize a common commitment to achieve the common, defined goals in this stage. The team leader acts as a moderator and settles any dispute and maintains harmony and motivation in team members. Roles and responsibilities are clear and accepted. Commitment and unity is strong. The team may engage in fun and social activities.
- *Performing phase:* In this stage, the team realizes its efficiency and utilizes it to achieve established team goals. The members are motivated and inspired by each other. The team leader has a more indirect style of leadership and the members mingle together, share experiences and march ahead with grit and determination. Everyone has a shared vision and members are able to stand on their own feet with no interference or participation from the leader. The group members have a high degree of autonomy.

IV. STRATEGIES TO IMPROVE GROUP FUNCTIONING

The following basic strategies are followed to improve group functioning:

- Individuals participating in a group must have a clear understanding of individual goals as well as group objectives so that their interaction is goal oriented.

- People participating in a group must have a clear idea about expectations within a group.
- Group members must have a clear understanding of their responsibilities and should be committed towards their designated responsibilities.
- Members in a group must follow the principle of positive competence; so that assigned tasks can be carried out more competently and efficiently.
- Appropriate control over the functioning of group members must be maintained for cohesiveness and smooth functioning in a group.
- The success of a group primarily depends on the collaboration of the functions of its members. Group members must carry out their functions with a collaborative approach.
- Effective communication is essential for efficient group functioning. Group members must communicate effectively and appropriately for a group to function smoothly.
- Coordination between individual tasks is essential in achieving efficient group functioning. A group leader must coordinate individual tasks to obtain group objectives.

TEAMWORK

Teamwork divides the task and multiplies the success. It is also said that coming together is a beginning, keeping together is progress and working together is success. Teamwork is an action performed by a team towards a common goal. A team consists of more than one person, and each person typically has different responsibilities. The nurse leader can motivate practising nurses by encouraging teamwork. A team can be built from work groups to discuss and resolve work-related issues. Teams should have an identifiable output, inclusive membership, leaders with carefully circumscribed authority, agreement on purpose, rules of procedure and measurable goals, resources and feedback. Teams are successful because they pool interpersonal skills, knowledge and expertise to accomplish goals effectively and efficiently.

Teamwork leads to personal recognition, raises self-esteem and increases motivation and commitment. It is stimulated by trust, support, completion, acknowledgement, communication and agreement.

I. ELEMENTS OF A TEAM

A team comprises the following seven elements:

1. Common purpose
2. Interdependence
3. Clarity of roles and contribution
4. Satisfaction from working together
5. Mutual and individual accountability
6. Realization of synergies
7. Empowerment.

II. PRINCIPLES/STRATEGIES TO BUILD A SUCCESSFUL TEAM

The following principles are followed for building a successful team and are also illustrated in Fig. 3.8.

- *Clear expectations:* Members of a health team must be clear about their expectations to achieve the goals of teamwork. Roles and responsibilities must be clearly defined so that responsibility and accountability can be imposed on each member.

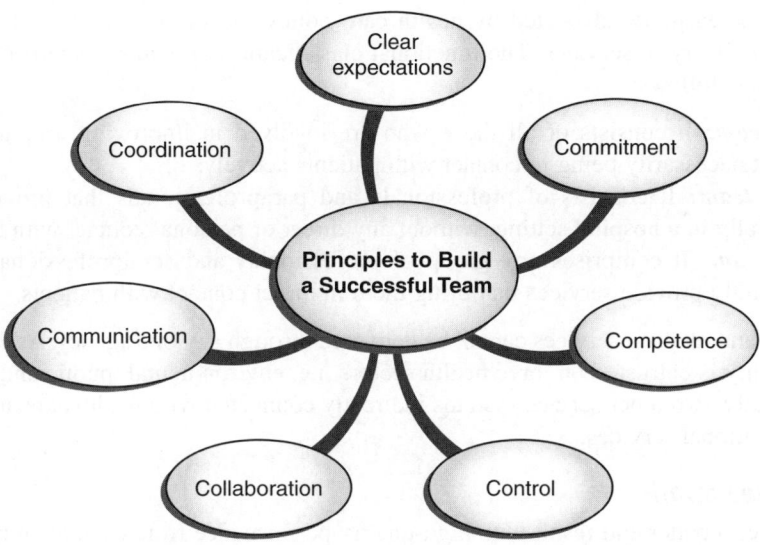

FIGURE 3.8

Principles to build a successful team.

- *Commitment:* All members should be committed to their work, roles and responsibility. The success of a teamwork is doubtful without commitment.
- *Competence:* Group members must be competent for tasks to be carried out smoothly and efficiently. A physiotherapist must be competent in providing physiotherapy.
- *Control:* The team leader should use effective control strategies to minimize conflict between team members, make sure of the availability of resources, smoothen the work, have a check on the performance of team members in relation to the objectives and should maintain discipline in the team.
- *Collaboration:* Collaboration is essential for the success of teamwork. Health care team members must collaborate with each other according to their competency and professional skills to achieve the patient's desired health care goals.
- *Communication:* Good interpersonal communication is essential for the smooth functioning of a team.
- *Coordination:* To enhance the effectiveness of teamwork, the team leader should coordinate with team members whenever required.

III. HEALTH TEAM

No single agency can deliver the entire range of health and medical care. The quality of health and medical care is best if professional groups such as physicians, nurses, paramedical workers, health educators, health visitors, public health engineers and many others share a common unifying goal. This joint effort materializes through teamwork.

Teamwork can be defined as a dynamic process involving two or more health care professionals with complementary backgrounds and skills, sharing common health goals and exercising concerted physical and mental effort in assessing, planning or evaluating patient care in health care.

Teamwork is increasingly advocated by health care policy makers as a means of assuring quality and safety in the delivery of services. The functional classification of teams concerned with group and personal health is as follows:

- *Health care team:* It consists of all those who are involved in improving a community's health setting without necessarily being in contact with patients actively.
- *Medical care team:* It consists of professionals and paraprofessionals that provide services for patients, generally in a hospital setting, without any direct or personal contact with them.
- *Patient care team:* It comprises any group of professionals and semiprofessionals in a hospital setting who jointly provide services that bring them in direct contact with patients.

Therefore, health and medical services cannot be delivered through any one agency. As discussed earlier, all the responsibility is entrusted on three health sectors, i.e. environmental, public and personal health sectors. Additionally, two other service systems indirectly connected with health care are social welfare services and educational services.

Advantages of teamwork

- Teamwork gives a better end result with high-quality performance from each team member.
- Teamwork involves every person and his expertise and responsibilities.
- The execution of new ideas can be more effective and efficient through teamwork.
- Teamwork increases ownership with wider communication.
- Teamwork leads to information sharing and increases learning in the team and the organization.
- Teamwork provides more security and develops personal relationships in the context of business operations.
- A particular problem can be easily solved in a team with more ideas at the same time.
- Teamwork helps provide a variety of solutions and the best solution from those possibilities can be selected.
- Teamwork increases the willingness of every member to take more risk.
- People can share common goals and interests with others in the team.
- It is easier to examine problems and identify various solutions in a team.
- A team can handle more difficult and complex problems in the workplace.
- A team increases the accuracy of problem solving.

Disadvantages of teamwork

- Teamwork may lead to *unequal participation* of members in a team.
- Some individuals may be good workers. However, they may not be good team players and may perform well at an individual level.
- Teamwork may also limit creative thinking because teamwork is everyone's work.
- A team can sometimes take longer to produce desired results. Teams typically need to go through a variety of processes such as member selection, organization and socialization on the way to completing the task at hand.
- Teams can also result in added expenses as they can tie up resources like money, manpower and equipment.
- Teamwork may face some inherent conflict because of contrasting personal styles and unwillingness to accept others' ideas.
- Peer pressure can also result in team members going against their better judgement to escape the wrath of other members or to facilitate a project's completion.

REVIEW QUESTIONS

Long-Answer Questions

1. Describe human relations in nursing.
2. What is an effective group? Explain briefly.
3. How can you improve group functioning?
4. What are the stages of group development? Explain briefly.
5. Explain the strategies to improve group functioning briefly.
6. Describe group dynamics.
7. Explain motivation.
8. Describe social behaviour.
9. Discuss the factors influencing behaviour.
10. Describe the importance of teamwork in nursing.
11. Explain the strategies to build a successful team.
12. What is learning and motivation? Explain with examples.
13. Explain the relationship between motivation and learning.
14. Discuss the methods of improving motivation of learners. Give examples wherever necessary.
15. Explain social behaviour. How will you develop effective human relations in context of nursing?
16. Describe how to understand the self.
17. Discuss team work.

Short-Answer Questions

1. Write two principles of group dynamics.
2. Enumerate the components of self.
3. List down the strategies to build a successful team.
4. Discuss briefly the stages of group development.
5. Mention the types of social behaviours.

Multiple-Choice Questions (MCQs)

1. The ultimate goal of effective human relations is
   (a) Mutual understanding
   (b) Conducive work culture
   (c) Civilized society
   (d) Self-understanding
2. Human relations in nursing encompass effective relationship with
   (a) Patient
   (b) Family
   (c) Community
   (d) All of these
3. Following are the strategies to promote effective human relations, except
   (a) Individualized goals
   (b) Common organizational goals
   (c) Group cohesiveness
   (d) Sense of oneness

4. Self-understanding is facilitated by the study of
   (a) Newman's window
   (b) Kothari window
   (c) Johari window
   (d) Bohari window

5. Nurse posted in geriatrics centre provides a dedicated selfless service. It is an example of
   (a) Aggression
   (b) Altruism
   (c) Scapegoating
   (d) Shyness

6. A ward in charge starts establishing 'Best Nurse' award on a monthly basis. She is appreciating the phenomenon of
   (a) Motivation
   (b) Persuasion
   (c) Communication
   (d) Information

7. Hierarchy of needs model was proposed by
   (a) George Marlow
   (b) Abraham Maslow
   (c) Thomas Malthus
   (d) Henry Mathew

8. As per Hierarchy of Needs model, there are _____ levels of needs.
   (a) Three
   (b) Four
   (c) Five
   (d) Six

9. As per Hierarchy of Needs model, the correct sequence is
   (a) Physiological, safety and security, love/belongingness, self-esteem, self-actualization
   (b) Safety and security, self-esteem, love/belongingness, self-actualization
   (c) Physiological, love/belongingness, self-esteem, self-actualization
   (d) Physiological, love/belongingness, safety and security, self-actualization

10. A nurse practitioner's behaviour of her keen interest in learning from evidences displays her need of
    (a) Safety
    (b) Belongingness
    (c) Self-esteem
    (d) Self-actualization

11. People prefer joining Facebook to
    (a) Have fun
    (b) Utilize time
    (c) Have social network
    (d) Learn internet

12. The correct sequence of group building is
    (a) Storming, norming, performing, forming
    (b) Forming, storming, norming, performing
    (c) Forming, norming, storming, performing
    (d) Storming, forming, norming, performing

13. Consensus of different viewpoints in group is achieved at
   (a) Forming phase
   (b) Storming phase
   (c) Norming phase
   (d) Performing phase
14. To build an effective team, the aspect of paramount importance is
   (a) Job specification
   (b) Competency
   (c) Dedication
   (d) Control
15. The main aim of health care team is
   (a) Communication and coordination
   (b) Creative solutions
   (c) Effective patient care
   (d) Security and relationships

Answers of the Multiple-Choice Questions

1. (c), 2. (d), 3. (a), 4. (c), 5. (b), 6. (a), 7. (b), 8. (c), 9. (a), 10. (d), 11. (c), 12. (b), 13. (c), 14. (d), 15. (c)

FURTHER READING

Bhushan, V., & Sachdeva, D. R. (2007). *An introduction to sociology*. Allahabad: KitabMahal.

Bruce, K. (2006). Henry S. Dennison, Elton Mayo, and human relations historiography. *Management & Organizational History*, 1, 177–199.

Bruce, K., & Nylan, C. (2011). Elton Mayo and the deification of human relations. *Organization Studies*, 32(3), 383–405.

Cooley, C. H. (1902). *Human nature and the social order*. New York Scribner's.

Donelson, R. F. (2010). *Group dynamics* (5th ed.). Belmont, CA: Wadsworth Cengage Learning.

DuBrin, A. J. (2007). *Human relations interpersonal job-oriented skills* (9th ed.). Upper Saddle River, NJ: Pearson Prentice Hall.

Ezzamel, M., & Willmott, H. (1998). Accounting for teamwork: A critical study of group-based systems of organizational control. *Administrative Science Quarterly*, 43, 358–396.

Faris, E. (1928). Attitudes and behavior. *American Journal of Sociology*, XXXIV, 271–281.

Ferguson, C. J., & Beaver, K. M. (2009). Natural born killers: The genetic origins of extreme violence. *Aggression and Violent Behavior*, 14(5), 286–294.

Frank, L. K. (1928). The management of tensions. *American Journal of Sociology*, XXXIII, 705–736.

Kohn, L., Corrigan, J., & Donaldson, M. (2000). *To err is human: Building a safer health system*. Washington, DC: National Academy Press.

Mcleod, M. (1983). Architecture or revolution: Taylorism, technocracy, and social change. *Art Journal*, 43(2), 132–147.

Messmer, M. (2001). *Motivating employees for dummies: A reference for the rest of us!* John Wiley & Sons: Indianapolis, IN.

Sheard, A. G., & Kakabadse, A. P. (2004). A process perspective on leadership and team development. *The Journal of Management*, 23(1), 7–11, 13–41, 43–79, 81–106.

Sullivan, E. J., & Decker P. J. (2003). *Effective leadership and management in nursing* (5th ed., pp. 156–169). Upper Saddle River, NJ: Pearson Prentice Hall.

Swansburg, R. C., & Swansburg R. J. (2002). *Introduction to management and leadership for nurse managers* (3rd ed., pp. 341–353). Boston, MA: Jones and Bartlett.

Taneja, S., Pryor, M. G., & Toombs, L. A. (2011). Frederick W. Taylor's scientific management principles: Relevance and validity. *Journal of Applied Management and Entrepreneurship*, 16(3), 60–78.

Taneja, S., Pryor, M. G., Humpheries, J. H., & Toombs, L. A. (2011). Where are the new organization theories? Evolution, development and theoretical debate. *International Journal of Management*, 28(3), 959–978.

Thurstone, L. L. (1928). Attitudes can be measured. *American Journal of Sociology*, XXXIII, 529–554.

Tyler, T. R. (2011). *Why people cooperate: The role of social motivations*. Princeton: Princeton University Press.

van Wormer, K. (2011). *Human behavior and the social environment, micro level: Individuals and families* (2nd ed.). Oxford University Press.

Wilson, D. C., & Rosenfeld, R. (2009). *Managing Organizations*. London, UK: McGraw Hill Book Company.

Wren, D. A., & Greenwood, R. G. (1998). *Management innovators: The people and ideas that have shaped modern business*. New York: Oxford University Press.

Xyrichis, A., & Ream, E. (2008). Teamwork: A concept analysis. *Journal of Advanced Nursing*, 61(2), 232–241.

Yoder-Wise, P. S. *Leading and managing in nursing* (5th ed., pp. 276–296). St. Louis, MO: Mosby.

Guidance and counselling

4

Just as treasures are uncovered from the earth, so virtue appears from good deeds, and wisdom appears from a pure and peaceful mind. To walk safely through the maze of human life, one needs the light of wisdom and the guidance of virtue.
—Gautama Buddha

LEARNING OBJECTIVES

This chapter is designed to enable the reader to

- Define guidance and counselling
- Distinguish between guidance and counselling
- Describe the purposes, needs, characteristics, scope and principles of guidance and counselling
- Classify the types of guidance services
- Demonstrate knowledge and skills of organization of counselling services
- Identify types of counselling approaches
- Explore the role and needed preparation of the counsellor
- Appraise the phases of counselling process
- Explain the tools and techniques used in counselling process
- Recognize the issues of counselling in nursing
- Discuss the strategies for management of disciplinary problem and crisis management
- Understand the concept of crisis intervention

KEY TERMS

INTRODUCTION

Everyone needs assistance at some time in his life; some will need it constantly and throughout their entire lives, while others need it at rare intervals at times of great crisis.

—Arthur J. Jones

Guidance and counselling are twin concepts and have emerged as essential elements of every educational activity. The much emphasized focus on a child's holistic development demands the education system be made comprehensive enough to foster all-round development. Professional guidance personnel can help students develop skills and competencies to facilitate their personal, social and career development. For a harmonious and integrated personality development of students in an institution, a healthy climate that fosters cognitive, behavioural, developmental and emotional growth is needed. Guidance and counselling plays an important role in education in this context.

Guidance and counselling are not synonymous terms. Counselling is a part of guidance. Guidance, in the educational context, means to indicate, point out, show the way, lead out and direct. Moreover, guidance means assisting students with selecting courses of study appropriate to their needs and interests, achieving academic excellence to the best possible extent, deriving the maximum benefit from institutional resources and facilities, inculcating proper study habits and their satisfactory participation in curricular and extracurricular activities.

Counselling is a specialized service of guidance. It is the process of helping individuals learn more about themselves and their present and possible future situations to make a substantial contribution to the society. It is also a process of solving one's own problems through a face-to-face relationship with the counsellor.

DEFINITIONS OF GUIDANCE AND COUNSELLING

I. DEFINITIONS OF GUIDANCE

Guidance is defined as assistance rendered by an expert to help an individual to manage his own point of view, make his own decisions and carry his own burdens.

Guidance is that aspect of educational programme which is concerned with helping the pupil to become adjusted to his present situation and plan his future in line with his interests, abilities and social needs.

—Hamrin and Erikson

Guidance is an assistance made available by a competent counselor to an individual of any age to help him direct his own life, develop his own point of view, make his own decision and carry his own burden.

—Crow and Crow

Guidance is a process of helping every individual, through his own efforts to discover and develop his potentialities for his personal happiness and social usefulness.

—Ruth Strang

Guidance is understanding a person and making himself, so that he may bring about in himself and in his environment such change through which his proper development becomes possible.

—Knapp

Guidance is a process which helps an individual to develop his personality fully and enables him to serve the society to the best of his capabilities and talents.

—Woodworth

Guidance is a continuous process of helping the individual for development in the maximum of their capacity in the direction most beneficial to himself and to society.

—Stoops and Wahlquist

Guidance is a process through which an individual is able to solve their problems and pursue a path suited to their abilities and aspirations.

—J.M. Brewer

Guidance involves personal help given by someone; it is designed to assist a person in deciding where he wants to go, what he wants to do, how he can best accomplish his purpose; it assists him in solving problems that arise in his life. It does not solve problems for the individual, but helps him to solve them. The focus of guidance is the individual, not the problem; its purpose is to promote the growth of the individual in self-direction.

—Jones

II. DEFINITIONS OF COUNSELLING

According to *Webster's Dictionary*, *counselling* is mutual consultation or deliberation. It involves a minimum of two people, the *counsellor* and the *counselee*. The counselee comes to the counsellor for counselling or consultation. In other words, counselling is talking to a professionally trained individual, who can help express pent-up feelings and emotions, provide an insight into these feelings and help the patient find solutions to problems.

Counselling, in the professional sense, is helping with counselee's problems, based on empirical studies and understanding of the individual, his interests, aptitudes and emotional maturity. Essentially, counselling is a one-to-one relationship where a professionally qualified individual tries to help another individual caught up in emotional conflict and difficult decision making.

Counseling is a helping process where one person purposefully gives his/her time, attention and skills to assist a client in exploring the situation, identifying and acting upon the solutions within the limitation of their given environment.

Counseling is a series of direct contacts with the individual which aims to offer him assistance in changing his attitude and behaviors.

—Carl Rogers

Counseling is essentially a process in which the counselor assists the counselee to make interpretations of facts relating to a choice, plan or adjustment which he needs to make.

—Glenn F. Smith

Counseling is an interactive process that facilitate meaningful understanding of self and environment and results in the establishment and or clarification of goals and values for future behaviour.

—Stone and Sherzes

Counseling is a dynamic and purposeful relationship between two people, who approach a mutually defined problem with mutual consideration of each other to the end that the troubled one or less mature is aided to a self-determined resolution of his problem.

—C. Gilbert Wrenn

Counseling is a process which takes place in a one-to-one relationship between an individual beset by problems with which he cannot cope alone and a professional worker whose training and experience have qualified him to help others reach solutions to various types of personal difficulties.
                                                                                        —Hahu and Maclean

Counseling is a personal and dynamic relationship between two individuals (one of whom is older, or more experienced, wiser than other), who altogether approaches a more or less well-defined problem of the younger or less experienced or less wise, with mutual consideration for each other to the end that the problem may be clearly defined and that the one who has the problem may be helped to a self-determined solution of it.
                                                                                                 —A.J. Jones

DIFFERENCE BETWEEN GUIDANCE AND COUNSELLING

Guidance and counselling are generally used interchangeably or synonymously. However, they are not synonyms. The following points are presented to illuminate the differences between the basic concepts of guidance and counselling:

- Guidance is broader and comprehensive whereas counselling is in-depth and narrows down the problems until patients are able to understand their own problems.
- Counselling helps people understand themselves and is an inward analysis. Alternative solutions are proposed to help understand the problem at hand. The focus of counselling is not on solution but on understanding the problem. The counsellor may be able to bring about an emotional change or a change in feelings. Guidance, on the other hand, is more external, helps a person understand alternative solutions available to him and makes him understand his personality and choose the right solution. The focus here is on finding solutions. Guidance may bring about an attitude change in the patient.
- Guidance is mainly preventive and developmental whereas counselling is remedial as well as preventive and developmental.
- Intellectual attitudes are the raw material of guidance whereas emotional rather than pure intellectual attitude are the raw materials of the counselling process.
- Decision making is operable at an intellectual level in guidance, whereas it operates at an emotional level in counselling.
- In the educational context, counselling is among the various services offered by the guidance programme.
- Guidance is generally education and career related, and may also include personal problems. It is usually impersonal whereas counselling is mostly offered for personal and social issues.

PURPOSES OF GUIDANCE AND COUNSELLING

Guidance and counselling services are an essential part of making proper use of human capabilities. Each of us finds ourselves at crossroads at some time in life; this is why guidance and counselling are an integral part of our lives. The main purposes of guidance and counselling are discussed in detail below (Fig. 4.1):

- ***Providing the needed information and assistance:*** Guidance and counselling is directed at providing and seeking information between two individuals as well as offering the desired assistance to an individual who requires help.

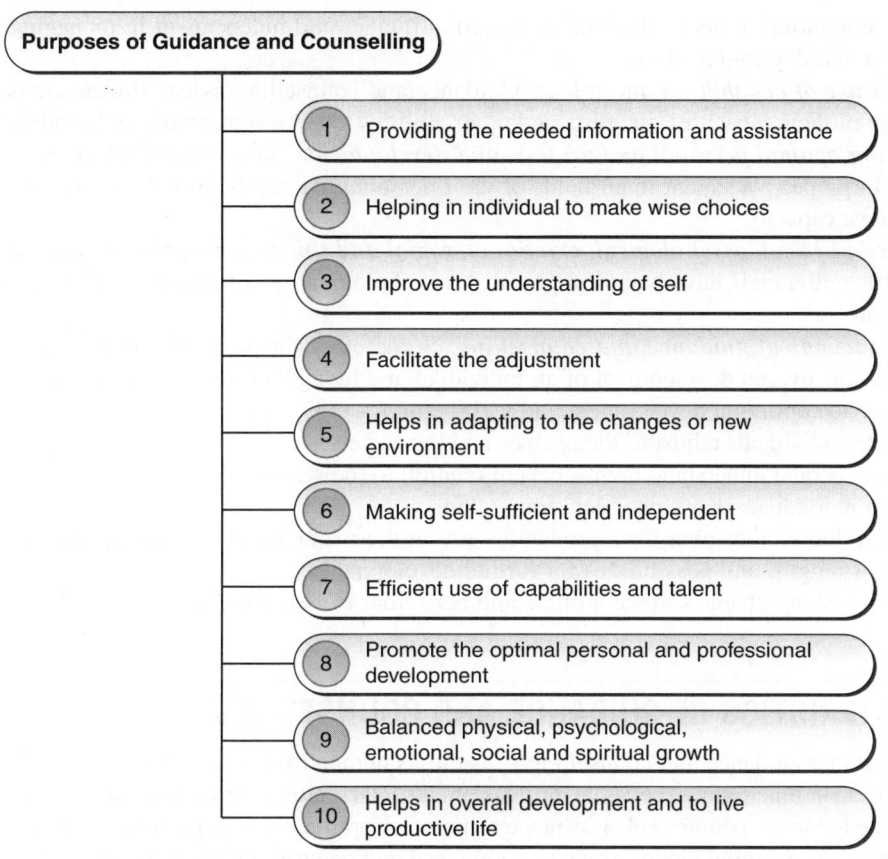

Purposes of Guidance and Counselling

1. Providing the needed information and assistance
2. Helping in individual to make wise choices
3. Improve the understanding of self
4. Facilitate the adjustment
5. Helps in adapting to the changes or new environment
6. Making self-sufficient and independent
7. Efficient use of capabilities and talent
8. Promote the optimal personal and professional development
9. Balanced physical, psychological, emotional, social and spiritual growth
10. Helps in overall development and to live productive life

FIGURE 4.1

Purposes of guidance and counselling.

- *Helping an individual make wise choices:* Guidance and counselling is primarily offered to make an individual capable of judging each aspect (strength and weakness) of a situation and finally making a wise decision to use the available opportunities efficiently.
- *Improve the understanding of self:* Guidance and counselling helps the individual get a true understanding of self, where he becomes capable of evaluating each situation with full intellectual capabilities leading to holistic development.
- *Facilitate adjustment:* Adjustment is one of the most fundamental essentiality of an individual in personal and professional life. Guidance and counselling is the most efficient tool for facilitating the assessment and management of adjustment problems of individuals in demanding situations.
- *Helping to adapt to changes or new environment:* Guidance and counselling assists or helps students adapt according to tradition and the rules and regulations in a particular situation. It also helps in creating a feeling of cooperation in individuals that finally helps them adapt to new and challenging situations.
- *Making self-sufficient and independent:* Guidance and counselling provide opportunities for learning the essentials of self-direction with respect to educational, vocational and personal–social aspects

of life. In addition, it also helps one to be self-sufficient and independent in managing demanding situations and day-to-day affairs.

- *Efficient use of capabilities and talent:* Guidance and counselling assists students make the maximum use of their capacities, interests and other abilities to achieve personal and academic goals.
- *Promoting optimal personal and professional development:* Guidance and counselling helps individuals in proper placement in all fields of their personal life and helps them in the development to their fullest capacity.
- *Balanced physical, psychological, emotional, social and spiritual growth:* Guidance and counselling helps individuals have balanced physical, psychological, emotional and social growth and development.
- *Other functions of guidance and counselling:* Some other functions of guidance and counselling helpful in the overall development of an individual and living a productive life are as follows:
  - To provide optimum development and well-being for individuals.
  - To help individuals adjust to themselves and the society.
  - To help people understand themselves in relation to the world.
  - To aid individuals in efficient decision making.
  - To help individuals plan for a productive life in their social context by focusing on their assets, skills, strengths and possibilities for further development.
  - To bring about changes in the attitude and behaviour of individuals.

CHARACTERISTICS OF GUIDANCE AND COUNSELLING

It is believed that guidance and counselling is as old as human existence and is found in each area and domain of human functioning (personal, professional, social, cultural and spiritual). Guidance and counselling is needed when people seek assistance to function optimally, both personally and professionally. Some of the most essential characteristics of guidance and counselling are as follows (Fig. 4.2):

- *Continuous process:* It is a continuous process starting in childhood and continuing through adolescence, adulthood and old age. Guidance and counselling is a dynamic process that helps individuals understand themselves and use their capacities, interests and other abilities to a maximum. Individuals continue to struggle for adjustment in different life situations to develop their capacity for effective decision making.
- *Process of mutual interaction:* Guidance and counselling is a process of mutual interaction where a trained person helps another person who needs his help for a general or specific problem.
- *Definite purpose-oriented processes:* Guidance and counselling is a well-planned, purpose-oriented process where two individuals, the person who is offering guidance and counselling and the person who is receiving guidance and counselling, interact keeping in mind the specific purpose to be achieved.
- *Self-realization and self-direction:* During the process of guidance and counselling, individuals are assisted in a way such that they are able to develop their capacities to the maximum extent. It helps individuals become familiar with their real self.
- *Individual assistance:* Guidance and counselling is the process of assisting individuals identify where to go, what to do and how to do, to accomplish their goals. An individual's personal development is promoted through guidance and counselling.

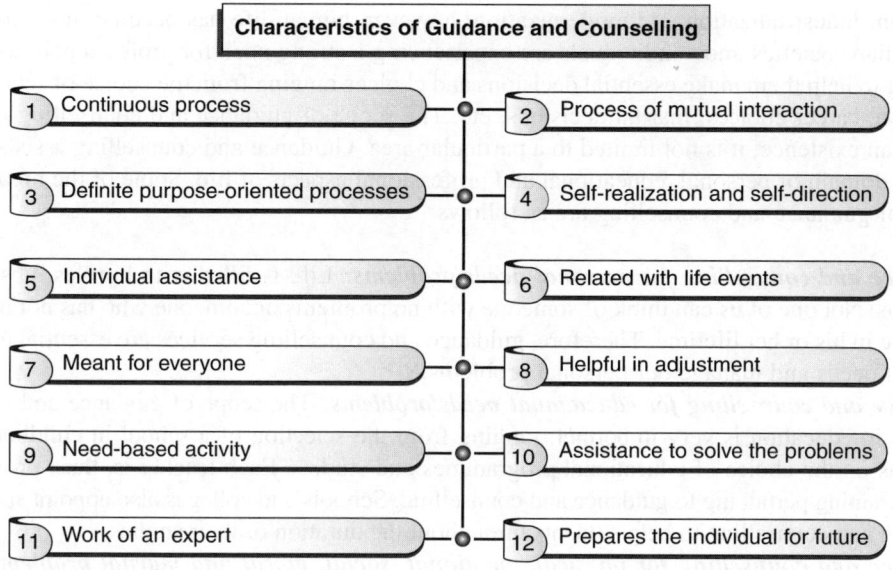

FIGURE 4.2

Characteristics of guidance and counselling.

- *Related with life events:* The process of guidance and counselling is related with life events as individuals get both formal and informal guidance and counselling in their lifetime.
- *Meant for everyone:* All individuals need guidance and counselling to reach their maximum potential.
- *Helpful in adjustment:* Guidance and counselling helps individuals adjust in different life situations.
- *Need-based activity:* Guidance and counselling is centred on the needs and aspirations of students. Guidance empowers individuals to discover their natural strengths so that they can use them to their best advantage making the maximum out of life.
- *Assistance to solve problems:* Guidance and counselling involves more than offering assistance in finding a solution to an immediate problem. Its function is to bring about changes in individuals and enabling them to deal with difficulties in a more productive and independent manner.
- *Work of an expert:* Providing guidance and counselling is the job of an expert. The person offering guidance and counselling services must be fully equipped with the skills to provide effective guidance and counselling services.
- *Prepares the individual for future:* It is well known that prevention is better than cure; therefore, individuals must be prepared and equipped to deal with future problems as quickly and efficiently as possible so that the problems can be assessed and managed before they become difficult to handle.

SCOPE OF GUIDANCE AND COUNSELLING

In ancient Indian societies, the scope of professional guidance and counselling was limited specifically because of the supportive social and joint family system. In this system, family members or people in close social proximity were considered an appropriate source of guidance and counselling. With rapid urbanization, industrialization and modernization, however, human life has become more complex. In modern Indian societies, most individuals are experiencing a strong need for professional guidance and counselling to help them make essential decisions and choices ranging from the choice of school, stream of education, career choices, marital decisions, etc. The scope of guidance and counselling is as broad as the human existence; it is not limited to a particular area. Guidance and counselling assists individuals in each domain of personal, educational and professional aspects of life. Some of the broad areas of the scope of guidance and counselling are as follows:

- *Guidance and counselling for personal needs/problems:* Life is filled with hurdles, obstacles and problems. Not one of us can think of someone with no problems or someone who has not needed any guidance in his or her lifetime. Therefore, guidance and counselling services are essential to meet our personal needs and manage our personal problems.
- *Guidance and counselling for educational needs/problems:* The scope of guidance and counselling services in education is very important; ranging from the selection of a school in childhood to later decisions on the choice of educational programmes and studies. Each teacher is, thus, provided with special training pertaining to guidance and counselling. Schools and colleges also appoint specialists in guidance and counselling to help students throughout the duration of their studies.
- *Guidance and counselling for physical, emotional, social, moral and marital problems:* Human beings are complex, social animals who have special physical, emotional, moral, social and marital needs and problems that need to be managed through professional guidance and counselling services. Appropriate guidance and counselling services help individuals maintain an optimal level of physical, emotional, moral, social and marital well-being and balance in his or her life.
- *Guidance and counselling for vocational, occupational and professional needs:* Vocational, occupational and professional guidance and counselling has a wide range of scope. Every individual has different potentialities, capabilities and abilities; through efficient guidance and counselling, individuals may be directed towards the right path at the right time so that they can achieve effective occupational and professional adjustment. Each institution imposes significantly different professional demands on individuals and has a wide scope of guidance and counselling services for their employees for better adjustment and work output.
- *Guidance and counselling for career advancement:* In ancient Indian societies, career options were available by chance and not by choices because individuals usually followed their family business/ work. In modern societies, career is opted by choice so each one of us requires professional guidance and counselling to make a right career choice. Guidance and counselling has a very wide scope in this area.
- *Guidance and counselling for holistic individual development:* The main purpose of guidance and counselling is the holistic and all-round development of an individual. Guidance and counselling services have a very wide and essential scope towards optimum development of an individual.
- *Guidance and counselling for situational problems:* Individuals may experience adverse situations at any point in life; they may require professional assistance in the form of guidance and counselling. Some of the most critical situations that may require guidance and counselling services are given below:
  - Disease and disability
  - Discharge from hospital
  - Death of loved ones
  - Disaster and crisis

- Divorce and marital disharmony
- Debt and economic crisis

NEED OF GUIDANCE AND COUNSELLING

Guidance and counselling is an essential source for making effective use of human interest, values and capabilities. Problems are a part of everyone's personal and professional life and each individual needs guidance and counselling at some time in life for one reason or another. It is generally observed that individuals joining the nursing profession have several professional adjustment problems initially and they simply waste their time and energy if timely guidance and counselling services are not offered. It is evident that guidance and counselling is important in each sphere of human existence including nursing and nursing education so that its professionals and patients can benefit the most. The main needs of guidance and counselling in nursing and nursing education are discussed below (Fig. 4.3).

I. NEEDS FOR PERSONAL AND SOCIAL DOMAIN

- *Personal and social development of individual:* For the personal and social development of an individual, self-understanding and an adjustment with the self and society is necessary. It helps students adjust to their current situation at home, educational institution or community in the best possible way. Guidance and counselling helps students with their problems related to career planning and educational programming and gives them a direction in long-term personal aims and values. It is concerned with helping people achieve self-development and self-realization.
- *To adapt in different stages of development:* Every individual has passed through specific stages of development: infancy, childhood, preadolescence, adolescence and adulthood. On various occasions, there are interpersonal and intrapersonal clashes of interests for which guidance is needed. Without proper guidance, individuals may experience stress and strain. Guidance and counselling is essential to adapt to life's different developmental stages.
- *Offering art of better living:* Well-planned guidance and counselling services help individuals develop a proper attitude towards life and equip them to live a meaningful life with self-esteem and effective interpersonal relationships.
- *Proper use of leisure time:* These days, many people either indulge in drugs or gambling due to a lack of proper guidance. To keep them from such situations, individuals need to be guided to make use of their leisure time to enhance their education, status or adjustments in life.
- *Holistic personality development:* Guidance and counselling can help students understand the self and have a better understanding of their own abilities, aptitudes, intelligence and personalities so that they can choose their own path with ease and comfort.
- *Best use of available opportunities:* With the expansion of education, career opportunities have expanded as well. Guidance is needed to provide the youth with information regarding training, educational facilities, availability of jobs, avenues for promotion, etc., that will ultimately help him make the best use of possible opportunities.
- *Motivates for effective utilization and development of self:* Every individual needs a catalyst or spark to initiate movement in a particular direction. Guidance and counselling services are essential for effective self-utilization and development in individuals for the achievement of personal and professional goals.

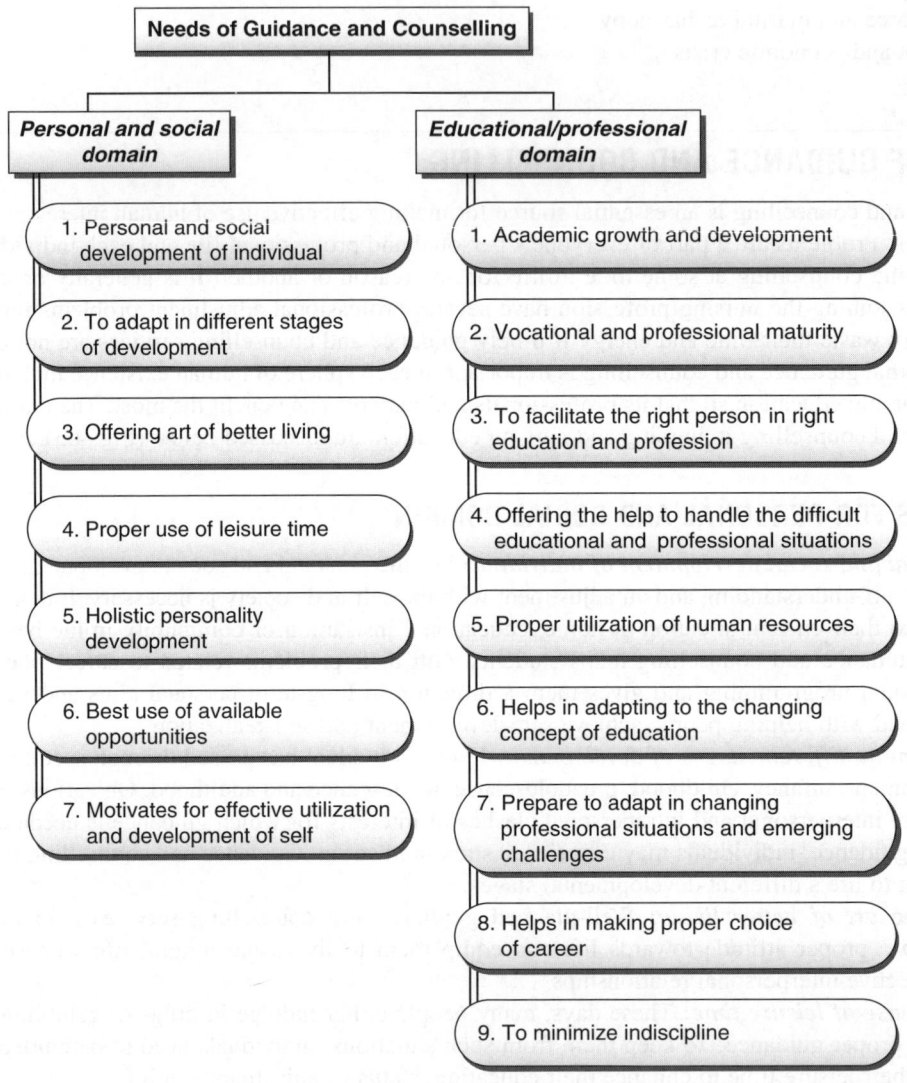

FIGURE 4.3

Need of guidance and counselling.

II. NEEDS FOR EDUCATIONAL/PROFESSIONAL DOMAIN

- *Helps in academic growth and development:* Guidance and counselling is needed to help with the academic growth and development of individuals. It helps by eliminating problems related to the subject matter and developing abilities and skills according to changing situations.
- *Helps in vocational and professional maturity:* With the society getting industrialized so rapidly, young students need help with information about various jobs available to them and the

requirements, responsibilities and nature of work involved in a particular job or career. Guidance and counselling services may help individuals attain the much needed vocational and professional maturity.

- *Facilitates an individual in the right education and profession:* Advancement in science and technology, rapid industrialization, global phenomenon and fast changing socioeconomic situations are imposing dilemmas in individuals to choose the right educational programme or professional stream choice. In such situations, guidance and counselling services can play an important role so that the individual can make the right choice of educational and professional options. This will ultimately lead to better socioeconomic growth of a country and satisfaction of the individuals.
- *Offers help to handle difficult educational and professional situations:* Individuals face many ups and downs in their personal and professional lives. Individuals must possess the qualities to handle positive and negative situations with the same strength and attitude. Guidance and counselling services may equip the individuals to respond positively to difficult situations in educational and professional pursuit.
- *Helps in the proper utilization of human resources:* With the help of guidance and counselling services, students can make the right choice of educational programmes or professions saving a lot of energy. When individuals make the right choice in education and profession at the right time, human resources may be used more efficiently without a waste of undue time and energy.
- *Helps in adapting to the changing concept of education:* The concept of education is changing with a rapid pace because of constant changing socioeconomic situations, science and technological development, cultural transformation and political and global interest. Efficient guidance and counselling services are needed to adapt to the changing concepts and demands of education in the current scenario.
- *Prepares to adapt in changing professional situations and emerging challenges:* In today's world, professions or occupations have become so varied and complex that everyone has to undergo training for adapting to the new emerging challenges of a particular profession. Hence, guidance is needed to equip individuals with the desired capabilities so that they can optimally adjust to the changing professional situations and emerging professional challenges.
- *Helps in making proper career choice:* Our educational system is very complex and competitive these days. Parents expect more from their children without caring for their abilities and aptitude leading to wrong career choices, which can ultimately affect their whole life. Therefore, well-planned, efficient guidance and counselling services must be offered to help individuals so that they can choose the right career option based on their abilities, interests, capabilities and aptitude.
- *Helps to minimize indiscipline:* Each individual has ample energy that needs to be channelized, otherwise individuals may engage themselves in nonproductive and destructive activities. Timely guidance and counselling services are needed for proper and optimum utilization of energy in productive and constructive activities.

BASIC PRINCIPLES OF GUIDANCE

Guidance is an essential and integral part of every educational programme to help students achieve the maximum self-understanding, self-insight and productive actions to be an intellectual and a useful member of the civilian society. For a better understanding of guidance, one must learn its basic principles. A few eminent educationists and philosophers gave their views on guidance which were later recognized as the principles of guidance. These principles are discussed below.

I. ACCORDING TO CROW AND CROW

Crow and Crow gave the following principles of guidance:

- *All-round development of individuals:* Every aspect of a person's complex personality pattern constitutes a significant factor of his or her total displayed attitudes and forms of behaviour. Guidance services aimed at bringing about desirable adjustments in a particular area of experience must take into account the all-round development of the individual.
- *Principle of individual differences:* No two individuals are alike. Although all human beings are similar in many respects, individual differences must be recognized and considered in any effort aimed at providing help or guidance to a particular student.
- *Guidance is related to every aspect of life:* The guidance programme should be related to all aspects of life, study an individual's physical and mental hygiene, his or her family and school and social and vocational needs.
- *Cooperation among persons:* The existing social, economic and political unrest gives rise to many maladaptive factors that require the cooperation of experienced and thoroughly trained guidance workers and the individuals with the problem.
- *Guidance is a continuous and lifelong process:* The guidance process is continuous and goes on lifelong from childhood to adulthood. The occurrence of problems in life and efforts for their solution are natural and, hence, the need for guidance always persists.
- *Guidance for all:* The main principle of guidance is that it is not for a specific person but for everyone. A person may need guidance at every step of life. Guidance services should not be limited to the few who give observable evidence of its need, but should be extended to people of all ages who can be benefited either directly or indirectly.
- *Principle of elaboration:* Curriculum materials and teaching procedures should evidence a guidance point of view. In addition, guidance services should be as elaborative as possible so that the beneficiaries can take its best possible advantage.
- *Responsibility of teachers and parents:* Parents and teachers have guidance-appointed responsibilities. The responsibilities for administration of the guidance programme should be centred by a personally qualified and adequately trained person, working cooperatively with his or her assistance and other community welfare and guidance agencies.
- *Flexibility:* In view of the ever-changing needs of the society and community, flexibility in the guidance programme is a must. An organized guidance programme should be flexible according to individual and social needs.
- *Principle of evaluation:* To administer guidance intelligently and with as thorough knowledge of the individual as possible, programmes of individual evaluation should be conducted and accurate consultative records of progress should be made accessible to guidance workers.
- *Guidance by a trained person:* Specific guidance problems at any age should be referred to people who are trained to deal with particular areas of adjustment so that the individual seeking guidance can benefit to the maximum extent.
- *Principle of periodic appraisal:* Periodical appraisals should be planned for existing guidance programmes. The success of any programme can be evaluated from the outcomes reflected in the periodic appraisal.

II. ACCORDING TO HOLLIES AND HOLLIES

Hollies and Hollies gave eight principles on which any guidance programme should be based. These principles are as follows:

- The dignity of the individual is supreme.
- Each individual is different from every other individual.
- The primary concern of guidance is the individual, in his or her social setting.
- The attitude and personal perceptions of the individual are the basis on which he acts.
- The individual generally acts to enhance his or her perceived self.
- The individual has the innate ability to learn and can be helped to make choices that will lead to self-direction consistently with social improvement.
- The individual needs a continuous guidance process from early childhood through adulthood.
- Each individual may need the information and personalized assistance given by competent professional personnel at some time.

TYPES/AREAS OF GUIDANCE SERVICES

Guidance services can be used in almost every sphere of human existence. Each individual needs help and guidance in some or other phase of life to cope and adjust with personal, social and professional needs and challenges. Guidance promotes proper adjustment of students with the educational environment in which they live and learn so that the purpose of education is achieved to an optimal level. Some of the most essential types or areas of guidance that may benefit students/individuals are discussed next (Table 4.1 and Fig. 4.4). The microscopic details of guidance services can be seen in Fig. 4.5.

- *Personal guidance:* Each student is different in personal, physical, psychological, social, cultural, economic and spiritual dimensions of life and development. He/she may experience unique personal problems in the educational environment. Therefore, guidance services should be directed towards offering personal guidance whenever required.
- *Social guidance:* The main purpose of education is to make students efficient citizens. Therefore, social guidance services are essential for students to assume social leadership, conform to social

Table 4.1 Description of Types/Areas of Guidance Services

Types/Areas of Guidance	Description
1. Personal guidance	This deals with a student's personal and family life, marriage and economic and emotional problems.
2. Social guidance	This helps the individual deal with social and cultural problems.
3. Educational guidance	This helps the individual adjust in institutions, in the selection of curriculum, identification of future possibilities, and involves meeting the educational needs of pupils and creating favourable conditions.
4. Vocational guidance	This helps in the selection of a vocation, vocational adjustment, knowing about essential attributes and qualifications for vocations.
5. Health guidance	This helps the individual maintain positive physical development, sound health and emotional behaviour.
6. Avocational guidance	This helps to efficiently use their leisure time to enjoy life and promote creativity.

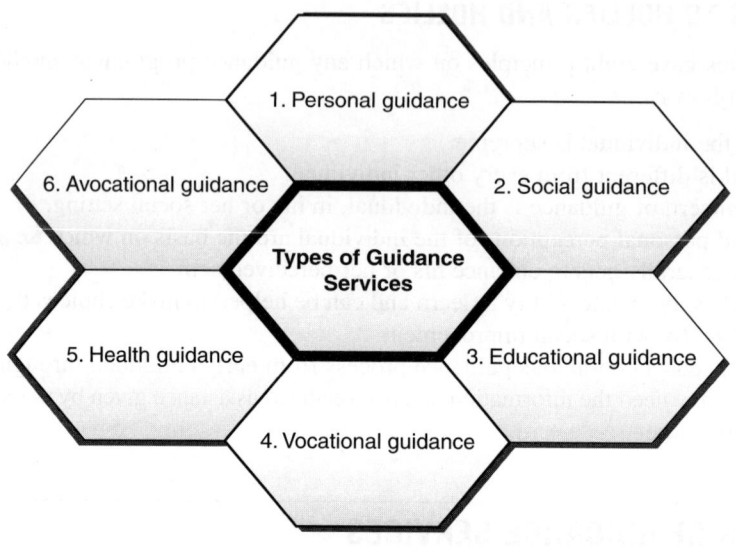

FIGURE 4.4

Types/areas of guidance services.

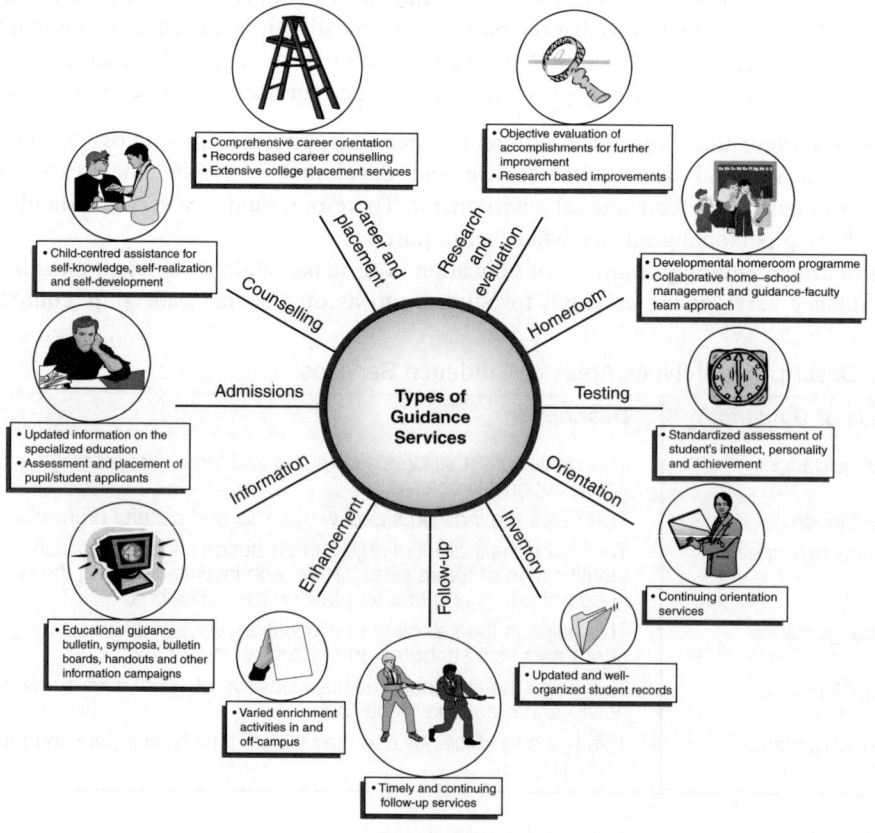

FIGURE 4.5

Types of guidance services.

norms, work as team members, develop healthy and positive attitudes, appreciate the problems of society, respect the opinions and sentiments of fellow beings and acquire traits of patience, perseverance, fraternity and friendship.

- *Educational guidance:* Educational guidance includes support offered to students in each and every aspect of the learning process. The purpose of educational guidance is to optimize the capabilities and satisfaction of the learner in academic work including the selection of programme, managing difficulties encountered in learning, promoting academic creativity and efficient utilization of institutional resources (classroom, faculty, library, learning material, books, etc.).
- *Vocational guidance:* It is generally observed that in the absence of efficient vocational counselling, individuals usually land in the wrong place. Therefore, vocational guidance is essential in making right and appropriate choice of occupation from the available options. In addition, individuals acquire information about career opportunities, career growth and career advancement facilities.
- *Health guidance:* Maintenance of sound health of the learners is an essential responsibility of educational institutions. In addition to curricular activities, students must receive guidance on the promotion of sound health, prevention of illness, early recognition of illnesses and seeking appropriate treatment at the right time so that physical and psychological health can be ensured. A sound mind exists in a sound body; therefore, sound health is a principle prerequisite of effective learning.
- *Avocational guidance:* Avocational guidance refers to the efficient use of leisure time by individuals leading to refreshment. It boosts the brain for creative and innovative learning. Avocational guidance helps individuals choose the right recreational activities, such as games, photography, drama and fine arts, so that they enjoy life as well as have a holistic all-round development for the achievement of personal and professional objectives.

ORGANIZATION OF COUNSELLING SERVICES

Organization means planning, coordinating and performing certain activities systematically within the policy framework of the institution. The level and size of the educational institution, student needs, community interests, faculty attitude and budgetary provisions are some factors that determine the nature of the guidance and counselling service in any institution. The major types or forms of the organization of counselling services in an educational institution are given below:

I. *Centralized counselling services:* In centralized counselling, the entire responsibility of the guidance and counselling service is vested upon a group of trained personnel or the department of guidance and counselling service. Counselling activities are carried out by selected members of the teaching staff under the direction and supervision of the guidance staff. They conduct and control most of the guidance activities from the central guidance office. All teachers or faculty members also perform their duties under the supervision of the central guidance bureau and its orders.

II. *Decentralized counselling services:* The responsibility of the counselling service is vested upon teachers in decentralized counselling services. The teachers may give excellent and timely assistance to their students. As the teachers remain in close contact with pupils in their class, they understand the needs and problems of their pupils. Because of this reason, teachers can help students in a better way. Absence of trained personnel to give professional assistance to students is the drawback of this type of service.

III. *Combination of centralized and decentralized counselling services:* In this mixed form, guidance and counselling services are provided by teachers and experts collectively. Adopting the midway between centralization and decentralization is the best way to organize an effective guidance and counselling service. Crow and Crow supported the mixed form. The school guidance programme includes the coordinated services of administrators, teachers, employees and social institutions. The counselling department headed by the counsellor and the faculty cooperates with each other for students' welfare. Teachers provide counselling services and refer students who need specialized services to the counsellor.

I. PURPOSES OF ORGANIZING COUNSELLING SERVICES

The purposes of organizing counselling services in an educational institution so that optimum learning, growth and development of an individual can be achieved are discussed below:

- To help individuals with normal developmental problems.
- To help individuals through a temporary crisis during the different stages of life.
- To identify signs of disturbed/problem behaviour at the earliest possible time so that timely management can be obtained.
- To refer critical cases to specialists for the best possible management of problems.
- To facilitate communication within and between nursing institutions, homes, communities and resources.
- To support not only the tutors/nursing faculty who are helping individuals but also who themselves want guidance and reassurance at times.

II. INGREDIENTS OF GUIDANCE AND COUNSELLING SERVICES

The main ingredients of guidance and counselling services that may be offered to students in an educational institution for effective adaptation to the new educational environment and promote the best possible learning are given below:

- *Planning service:* It is meant to help students overcome their hostel, mess and financial problems. Help is also rendered to enable foreign students adjust to new situations. A school can organize programmes for securing scholarships for students, for getting funds from different sources and arrange different cocurricular activities, educational tours and cultural programmes with the help of the student adviser.
- *Placement service:* It refers to assistance offered to an individual in taking the next step, whether towards further training or a job. A strong emphasis is laid on placing students in jobs suitable for them. This can be done through coordination with employment exchanges and different employment agencies.
- *Follow-up service:* It involves keeping in touch with students who have graduated from the school and the school dropouts. This is done to find opportunities to help these students and to evaluate the programme. The common tools used for conducting follow-up services consist of questionnaires, interviews, letters and telephone calls.
- *Research and evaluation:* It is a service meant to evaluate the school counselling programme. The counsellor acts as a researcher and conducts surveys. He also carries out follow-up as well as formative and summative evaluation to assess the ultimate effect of the counselling programmes.

III. BASIC COMPONENTS OF COUNSELLING SERVICES

The principle components of counselling services (such as organizational set-up for counselling services, counselling committee, tools for counselling services and the basic requirements for counselling services) are discussed in the following section.

A. Organizational set-up

A sound organizational set-up is required to provide effective guidance and counselling services. A different organizational set-up is recommended for different levels of educational institutions (university, constituent college of university and affiliated colleges). These set-ups are briefly discussed below:

- *At universities:* Deans are assisted by the head of departments (HODs) of psychology and education, the guidance committee and the counselling officer.
- *For constituent colleges:* A counselling officer assisted by the guidance committee in cooperation with the deputy chief and academic advisor can plan according to their needs and number of students (<1000 students need a liaison officer while >1000 students need an assistant counselling officer).
- *For affiliated colleges:* A counselling officer assisted by the guidance committee and a vocational guidance officer are needed for ≥1000 students while a liaison officer only can manage the counselling services for <1000 students.

B. Counselling centre

All universities and large colleges should have a counselling centre headed by a trained professional, i.e. a counselling officer with PhD or a master's degree in psychology and counselling, with considerable experience. The counselling centre generally provides assistance, offers psychological testing, helps in training, conducts special clinics, maintains integrity and confidentiality, arranges orientation talks and gives information about the course and facilities, holds career talks and career conferences, maintains cumulative records, identifies students with problems and arranges personality counselling. In addition, it also performs the following functions:

- Selection, registration and orientation of students
- Educational and vocational counselling
- Personal adjustment counselling
- Physical and psychological services
- Remedial services
- Residence and food services
- Activities programme

C. Counselling committee

The main purpose of the guidance committee is to carry forward the total guidance programme through the united efforts of management, dean, counselling/liaison officer, deputy chief counselling officer, vocational guidance officer, peer group, librarian, warden, medical staff, principal, guidance personnel, teachers, parents and student. To this end, the committee should be a representative of all these groups, with the possible exception of parents and students. The guidance committee serves the following additional purposes:

- It establishes and maintains policies related to guidance and counselling services.
- It articulates the programme between the institution and the community.
- It acts in a planning capacity to ensure that the various functions of guidance are properly coordinated.
- It helps to clarify particular roles and offers support when these roles are challenged.
- It paves the way for the guidance personnel to function in cooperation with community agencies such as business organizations, employer groups and voluntary agencies.
- It serves as a source of ideas and recommendations to be submitted to appropriate bodies (such as curriculum committees, professional associations of teachers and the department of education).

D. Members of the counselling committee

Generally, the counselling committee constitutes the following members:

- Administrator
- Principal/Dean
- Counselling/Liaison officer
- Deputy chief of counselling section
- Counselling personnel/Counsellor
- Vocational guidance officer
- Teacher/Faculty from different departments/Specialities
- Hostel warden/Librarian (co-opted members in special situations)
- Student representatives
- Parents

E. Assigning responsibilities for counselling services

The guidance abilities and interests of individual members of the staff have to be assessed so that specific functions can be assigned according their personal capacity. Establishing clear-cut lines of authority will help everyone distinguish their duties from those of others. This will prevent misguidance to the students. The following pattern may be followed for the assignment of responsibilities for counselling services:

- Formation of the guidance and counselling committee.
- The committee lists problems requiring group solution.
- Plans monthly, quarterly and yearly programme.
- Coordinates guidance activities and assesses the work done.

IV. TOOLS FOR COUNSELLING SERVICES

Counselling services impose a special need to use specific tools for collecting primary information from students. The tools for collection of information for counselling are divided into two broad categories:

A. Nontesting tools

These types of tools are usually used for individual assessment without any intention of testing the individual. These tools are generally developed by the counsellor and/or teachers themselves. Some nontesting tools are as follows:

- *Interview:* Interviews are the basic tools of counselling. An interview can be described as an interaction between the counsellor and counselee with a definite objective in mind. Interviews help the counsellor obtain desired information from students, their family members, friends or teachers, etc., or prove the same to them. This flexible tool of counselling helps the counsellor customize the interaction with a student for a specific purpose.
- *Observation:* It is the careful watching or monitoring of the counselee by the counsellor with a specific objective in mind. Observation could be participatory or nonparticipatory based on the specific purpose of counselling. Further, observation could be overt (where counselee knows he is being observed) or covert (counselee does not know he is being observed and the counsellor is concealed).

Observation is a very useful tool of counselling in situations where gathering information from the counselee is not possible through an interview or other methods such as the behaviour of students in a specific situation or circumstances.

- *Anecdotal record:* It consists of recording an important incident that happened and is a carefully recorded snapshot of the incident. Anecdotal recording must be recorded with specific care so that the incident is recorded as it happened. Further, the counsellor must involve the people who directly observed the incident such as teachers, faculty and peer group.
- *Cumulative record:* It is a method of recording and providing meaningful, significant and comprehensive information about an individual, over the years. It is useful in organizing and integrating information collected through the use of different tools. Besides recording attendance and achievement, it also registers students' social adjustment in school, their behaviour with other pupils and their attitude towards the school and teachers. It also records the estimate of qualities like hard work, tolerance, sociability, etc. Cumulative records can be maintained in folders, files or in a card form.
- *Checklist:* Generally, a checklist is used to identify the presence or absence of specific attributes or skills of a particular expected behaviour in students. A checklist is a very commonly used tool to assess the skills of communication or nursing tasks in nursing students.
- *Rating scale:* Rating scales are better tools to assess the degree or extent of the performance of a particular task or the possession of a trait (truthfulness, honesty, initiative, responsibility and attitude of cooperation, etc.).
- *Sociometry:* It is used to measure sociability or the social distance between students or members of a group.
- *Autobiography and diary:* Autobiographies or diaries may also provide useful information about students. Students should be encouraged to keep diaries or a life autobiography.

B. Psychological tests

Psychological tests provide information about an individual's psychological characteristics such as intelligence, aptitude, interests, abilities and personality. Before the selection and use of these tests, their reliability, validity and practicability must be clearly assessed. Psychological tests are generally classified as follows:

- *Personality tests:* There are several personality tests available to assess the personality types of people. For instance, *The Rorschach* and *The Minnesota* are examples of personality measurement tests.
- *Aptitude tests:* These tests are used to estimate the extent to which an individual would profit from a specific course or training to predict the quality of his achievement in a given situation. Two types of aptitude tests usually employed are specialized aptitude test and general aptitude test.
- *Achievement tests:* These are used to assess academic performance devices rather than being used as selection instruments. Some achievement tests are cooperative test, College Board series, test of educational development, English reading test, etc.
- *Interest inventory tests:* These tests are used to assess the interests of an individual in specific disciplines such as specific vocational or occupational interests. Blank and Kuder preference inventory is one of the most commonly used tests for this purpose.
- *Study habit inventory tests:* These tests are used to assess study habits in students. The Brown–Holtzman survey of study habits is the most commonly used study habit test.

V. SPECIFIC REQUIREMENTS FOR THE ORGANIZATION OF COUNSELLING SERVICES

Some of the main requirements for organizing guidance and counselling services are discussed below:

- Presence of physical facilities, i.e. rooms, furniture and other equipment needed for the guidance and counselling department
- Provision of private offices as well as general counselling rooms
- Trained counsellors and guidance personnel
- Planned programmes to meet objectives
- Consultation services
- Evaluation instruments like psychological tests, inventories, etc.
- Student data bank
- Educational and vocational information service
- Programmes for cooperation between home and school
- Programmes for integrating community services with guidance services
- Educational programmes for teachers, counsellors and other personnel to provide knowledge of current trends in guidance
- Budgetary provisions

VI. APPRAISAL OF COUNSELLING SERVICES

Appraisal of the guidance programme is essential to maintain its relevance. The efficiency of the programme should be tested against the changing needs of students and the society. Appropriate measures should be taken to rectify any noted defects to keep the programme student friendly.

VII. ORGANIZATION OF COUNSELLING SERVICES IN NURSING INSTITUTIONS

In recent years, a number of nursing institutes have mushroomed without proper and adequate provision for guidance and counselling services to nursing students. These institutions offer a basic diploma in doctoral nursing programmes such as Diploma in General Nursing & Midwifery, Bachelor of Science in Nursing, Master of Science in Nursing and PhD in Nursing. There is a strong need for efficient guidance and counselling services in these institutions because of reasons like rapid social changes, changing roles of nurses, more demanding patients, changes in the health care system, complexity of modern life and the global demand for qualified nurses, etc.

A. Importance of counselling services in nursing education

An increasing global demand for qualified nurses and the emergence of various specialties in nursing to meet the challenges of the modern health care system has given a facelift to the area of guidance in nursing education. A large number of students opt for the nursing profession without prior knowledge about the profession. Guidance and counselling services are needed to provide a clear picture of the latest trends and the emerging new specialties. The main functions of counselling services in nursing education are as follow:

- *Help students adjust in the new educational environment:* A well-planned guidance and counselling programme will help the nursing students adjust to the new educational atmosphere and make them feel more comfortable and reduce home sickness.
- *Protection from ragging:* Guidance and counselling services in the institution help students gain information about the preventive measures of ragging. An antiragging committee can be constituted in

the institute in coordination with the counselling service to help newly admitted students against ragging. There should be active participation of senior students to report any ragging incident so that disciplinary action can be taken by the administration.

- *Assist students adjust with new learning experiences and overcome learning difficulties:* Personal guidance and counselling is needed to help students adjust with new learning experiences especially those provided in clinical areas.
- *Help students develop emotional maturity:* In the clinical area, nursing students have to face many situations, which may cause emotional distress especially in the newly admitted students. Helping students develop empathy rather than sympathy, teaching them to analyse events in the clinical area and to ventilate their emotions through efficient counselling services may help them develop strong emotional maturity.
- *Assist students cope with stress:* Sometimes nursing students are utilized to replace the staff nurses for patient care in situations of acute staff shortage, which create additional stress in student nurses. Teaching relaxation techniques, ensuring availability of teachers to help students in crisis situations, constituting peer groups and assigning senior students to look after juniors are some ways to deal with stress in nursing students.
- *Help students achieve balance between personal and professional life:* Students should be taught from the very beginning about how to maintain balance between personal and professional life. They should be instructed to concentrate on other responsibilities after returning from clinical areas instead of being preoccupied with matters related to patient care.
- *Help students develop a healthy interpersonal relationship with other members of the health care team:* Success of any health team is determined by how well the nurses render their services. Special attention should be given to inculcate a sense of accountability and responsibility in nursing students along with health care team cohesiveness which helps in improving the quality of patient care.
- *Train students for leadership qualities:* Leadership development programmes should be conducted under a guidance and counselling service to promote leadership qualities in nursing students.
- *Assist students acquire desirable set of values and develop a positive life philosophy:* Value-based nursing education is the need of the time. Through well-planned guidance and counselling services emphasis must be placed on inculcating basic moral values in nursing students so they can be good human beings, citizens and nurses.
- *Motivate students contribute towards bridging the gap between nursing education and nursing service:* In the Indian scenario, there is still a large existing gap between nursing education and nursing practice, what is taught to nursing students in the classroom is not practised in organizations. Therefore, nursing students must be motivated through guidance and counselling services to practice what is taught to them in the classroom or the simulation laboratory.
- *Financial guidance:* Financial guidance can be given to help needy students determine the financial assistance they need in light of expected expenses. They need to be guided on fee concessions, scholarships and available stipends in the institution or those offered by other welfare agencies.

B. Strategies to organize counselling services in nursing education

The following strategies may be used to offer guidance and counselling services in nursing institutions:

- A combined centralization and decentralization approach of counselling may be used to organize guidance and counselling services in the nursing institution.
- The department of guidance and counselling is headed by a qualified counsellor and is assisted by one or two clerical staff.

- Faculty members are trained to provide nonspecialist guidance and counselling to students with the help of the counsellor.
- Any student in need of specialized services is referred to the counsellor, who provides counselling with the help of the faculty members.
- Many nursing institutions have successfully implemented teacher guardian programmes. In a teacher guardian programme, each faculty member is given full responsibility of a group of ten students. In addition, the class coordinator also looks after all students in the class. Thus, a student is looked after by a teacher guardian at the ground level and the class coordinator at the next level. The teacher guardian has to conduct periodic meetings with the assigned group of students to assess their performance and send the filled *proforma* to the counselling department for further verification and filing through the principal. During the meeting, the teacher guardian also has to fix a date for the next follow-up session. Students can approach the teacher guardian as needed to seek help in academic and personal matters. Further,
  - when the teacher guardian feels that a student needs specialized help, he reports the students details to the student's class coordinator, counsellor and principal. The counsellor then takes over the student and with the help of faculty members and other concerned personnel (like parents and peers) renders help as needed.
  - a number of student problems are solved at the teacher guardian or class coordinator level and students who need a specialized service are referred to the counsellor.
  - the counsellor is not overloaded and can concentrate on other areas/services of guidance and counselling this way.
  - the proforma sent to the counselling department through the principal is verified by the counsellor before filing.
- To review the functioning of the guidance and counselling services, a monthly meeting is held under the chairmanship of the principal. In this meeting, teacher guardians, class coordinators and the counsellor present a brief report.

TYPES OF COUNSELLING APPROACHES

Counselling is a continuous, mutual and interactive process between the counsellor and the counselee for definite objectives. Three basic types of counselling approaches, i.e. directive, nondirective and eclectic, may be used based on the nature of the counselling procedure and the role of the counsellor.

I. DIRECTIVE COUNSELLING APPROACH

The directive counselling approach is also known as *prescriptive counselling* or *counsellor-centred approach of counselling*. In directive counselling, the counsellor is the central figure and plays a more active role. This approach of counselling is advocated by E.G. Williamson, a professor at University of Minnesota. In directive counselling, the counsellor plays a leading role and uses a variety of techniques to suggest appropriate solutions to the counselee's problems. This approach is also called an *authoritarian* or *psychoanalytic approach*. The counsellor is active and helps individuals in making decisions and finding solutions to their problems. The counsellor believes in the limited capacity of the patient. This approach emphasizes on the cognitive and intellectual aspects of the problem. The patient makes the decision but the counsellor does all he can to get the patient make a decision keeping with his diagnosis. The counsellor tries to direct the patient's thinking by informing, explaining, interpreting and advising. The basic assumptions related to directive counselling approach are discussed below:

- *A need-based approach:* It is assumed that the directive counselling approach is a need-based approach. Whenever a patient has problems and is incapable of handling them himself, the counsellor helps solve these problems.
- *Problem focused rather than patient focused approach:* The major focus is placed on the patient's existing problems rather than the patient himself. The existing problems of the individual are targeted in this approach. It is solely a remedial measure to solve an individual's acute problems.
- *Used for patients incapable of solving their problems:* It is assumed that directive counselling is used in situations where the individual is not capable of solving his problems and desires help from a competent person. The counsellor uses his intellectual abilities to solve these problems by offering the best possible solutions.
- *Task of a competent counsellor:* Directive counselling is a counsellor-centred task; it requires a competent counsellor to minutely analyse an individual's problems and offer the best possible solutions using his intellectual and counselling competence.
- *Making the best possible use of counselee's intellectual abilities and resources:* Although directive counselling approach is counsellor-centred, it is still assumed that the counsellor must make the best possible use of the counselee's intellectual abilities, strengths and resources.

A. Steps of the directive counselling approach

E.G. Williamson has given the following six steps in providing directive counselling to individuals:

- *Information gathering and analysis:* In this step, the counsellor tries to elicit relevant details from the counselee. The data or detailed information is gathered that helps in focusing on the current problem. Information may be collected using different tools such as interview, questioning, observation, case history and psychological tests.
- *Synthesis:* Synthesis is the process of summarizing and organizing data from the analysis to reveal the counselee's assets, liabilities, adjustments and maladjustments. Initially, collected data is retained in a nonsystematic manner. The data is organized under specific heads to establish the status of the counselee as well as his problem.
- *Diagnosis:* In this stage, the actual problem is identified, defined and focused upon. The synthesized data leads to identification of the problem. The problem is identified in terms of assets and liabilities of the counselee. It also identifies the root cause of the problem.
- *Prognosis:* This step may or may not be a part of the diagnosis step. The problem is identified and the counsellor determines what has to be offered to help the counselee mange his problem at the best possible level.
- *Counselling:* This is the most important step of the whole procedure. The counsellor asks the counselee questions and offers the best possible solutions to manage the present problems. Alternatively, the counsellor also makes the best possible use of the counselee's strengths and resources to manage the identified problems.
- *Follow-up:* In this stage, the effectiveness of the counselling process is evaluated. The counsellor assesses how far the planned objectives of the counselling session are achieved. In certain cases, follow-up may be required to give a few counselling sessions to the counselee.

B. Advantages of the directive counselling approach

The advantages of the directive counselling approach are listed below:

- Directive counselling approach saves time.
- It emphasizes the problem and not the individual. The counsellor can see the patient more objectively than the patient himself.
- Directive counselling lays more emphasis on the intellectual rather than the emotional aspects of an individual's personality. The counselee is helped to solve the intellectual problem rather than emotional problems.
- The methods used in directive counselling are direct, persuasive and explanatory.

C. Limitations of the directive counselling approach

The limitations of the directive counselling approach are listed below:

- The patient does not gain any liability for self-analysis or solve new problems of adjustment by counselling.
- Counselling serves to make the counselee overdependent on the counsellor. He never becomes independent of the counsellor and this kills his initiative.
- Problems regarding emotional maladjustment may be better solved by nondirective counselling.
- Sometimes the counselee lacks information regarding the counselee. This lack of information leads to wrong counselling.
- Directive counselling does not guarantee that the counselee will be able to solve the same problems on his own in future.

II. NONDIRECTIVE COUNSELLING APPROACH

The chief exponent of this counselling approach, Carp R. Rogers, originally referred to it as the *patient-centred counselling approach*. It is also known as the *permissive counselling approach* where the counsellor's role is passive and the counselee's role is active. It is a counselee-centred or patient-centred humanistic approach. The counselee makes the final decisions as individuals are thought to have full right to make final decisions for the self and solve their problems. The counsellor has to accept the counselee's capacity to make adjustments and adapt. The principles of acceptance and tolerance are extremely important in this approach.

The basic assumptions related to nondirective counselling approach are given below:

- Patient is given more importance than the counselling directions and interventions.
- Emotional aspects are more significant than intellectual aspects.
- Creation of an atmosphere where patients can work out their understanding is more important than cultivating self-understanding in the patient.
- Counselling leads to a voluntary choice of goals and a conscious selection of courses of action.

A. Steps of the nondirective counselling approach

Carp R. Rogers has given the following five steps in the nondirective counselling approach:

- *Defining the problem situation:* This is the first stage of counselling where the counselee and counsellor collectively identify and define the actual problem. So that counselling can be focused to help the individual to solve that particular problem.

- *Counselee given freedom to express his feelings:* The counselee is given freedom to express his feelings so that the counsellor can help manage his problem in this stage.
- *Identifying counselee's feelings:* The counsellor carefully records the positive as well as negative feelings of the counselee. This helps the counsellor estimate the gravity of the present problem and the counselee's available resources to manage the problem.
- *Developing counselee's insight:* The counsellor helps the counselee develop insight into problems as well as available resources to manage the problems. This insight helps the counselee set realistic goals to solve the problem.
- *Termination of counselling:* In the final stage, the counsellor and the counselee mutually agree to end the counselling relationship because either the problem is managed or the counselee is now capable of solving his problem with insight if it recurs.

B. Advantages of nondirective counselling approach

The advantages of the nondirective counselling approach are listed below:

- It is a slow but sure process to make an individual capable of making adjustments.
- No tests are used so one avoids all that is laborious and difficult.
- It removes emotional block and helps an individual bring repressed thoughts on a conscious level thereby reducing tension.

C. Limitations of nondirective counselling approach

The limitations of the nondirective counselling approach are discussed below:

- It is a slow and time-consuming process. It is not easily possible because a counsellor has to attend to many patients.
- One cannot rely upon one's resources, judgement and wisdom as the patient is immature in making the decision himself.
- It depends too much on the ability and initiative of the patient. The patient is already under stress and inexperienced.
- There are likely to arise occasions when it becomes difficult to control the pace of the interview discussion.
- As this approach to counselling is individual centric, it may not be possible for the counsellor to attend to every patient equally well.
- It requires a high degree of motivation in the patient. The counsellor's passiveness is likely to prove a hurdle in the way.

III. ECLECTIC COUNSELLING APPROACH

This approach is based on the fact that all individuals are different from one another. No single approach can, therefore, be applied to each and every problem. The counsellor makes use of both directive and nondirective counselling that may be considered useful for the purpose of modifying the patient's ideas and attitudes. The techniques are elective in nature because they have been derived from all sources of counselling. This approach is based on selecting the best and leaving out what is least required.

The assumption of this nondirective counselling approach is that every individual is capable of solving his or her own problem. The counsellor should assist the counselee in seeing the nature of the problem. The goal of this approach is independence and integration of the patient. The counsellor creates an atmosphere in which the patient can work out his own understanding. It leads to a voluntary choice of action. This counselling approach rests on fundamental respect for an individual and the belief in a person's ability to solve personal problems with the aid of a sympathetic listener. This method is useful in solving educational, vocational and marital problems. In this approach, the counsellor respects the personal autonomy of the patient. This means the patient has to make the final decision. The basic assumptions related to the eclectic counselling approach are given below:

- There is objectivity and co-ordination between the counsellor and the patient during the counselling experience.
- The patient is active and the counsellor remains passive in the beginning.
- The principle of low expenditure is adopted.
- The counsellor makes use of all the tools and methods in his armour. His professional skills are an important factor in the successful completion of the counselling experience.
- The counsellor enjoys the freedom to resort to directive and nondirective counselling methods.
- The counselling relationship is built during the counselling interview. This helps the patient gain reassurance and confidence.

A. Steps of the eclectic counselling approach

The following six steps are recommended in the eclectic counselling approach:

- *Establishing rapport:* In the first stage of the eclectic counselling approach, the counsellor tries to establish intimate rapport with the counselee so that interaction between the counsellor and the counselee is smooth. Rapport establishment helps the counsellor understand the counselee's problems, strengths and weaknesses more deeply and extensively.
- *Diagnosing the problem:* After establishing rapport with the counselee, the counsellor tries to assess and diagnose the counselee's problem. During this stage, the counsellor asks the counselee a few essential questions to understand problems accurately and establish a prompt diagnosis of the problem.
- *Analysing the case:* During this stage of counselling, the counsellor obtains more information related to the counselee's problem from other sources, so that he can get detailed information about the counselee's problems and resources to plan for suitable and best possible solutions so the counselee may acquire better self-understanding.
- *Preparing a tentative plan for modifying behaviour:* At this stage, the counsellor is in a position to prepare a tentative plan for the patient's modification of behaviour. This also requires emotional release and a change in the patient's perception and attitude about himself.
- *Counselling:* Eclectic counselling approach believes that effective counselling uses one-to-one interview, stimulates the counselee to develop his own resources and assumes responsibilities for finding solutions to his problems.
- *Follow-up:* This is the final stage of counselling and is carried out to either assess the effectiveness of the counselling process or to provide a few more follow-up sessions if more help is required by the counselee.

B. Advantages of eclectic counselling approach

The advantages of eclectic counselling approach are as follows:

- It is a more cost effective and practical approach of counselling as it includes features of both directive and nondirective counselling based on the needs, abilities and resources of the counselee.

- It is a more flexible approach of counselling, where the counsellor and the counselee may assume active and passive roles based on the needs and nature of the problem.
- It is a more objective and coordinated approach of counselling and is more suitable to handle complex problems of the modern era.

C. Limitations of eclectic counselling approach

The disadvantages of eclectic counselling approach are as follows:

- The roles of counsellor and the counselee are not predetermined so they may experience dilemma about their roles at a particular phase of counselling.
- It requires more skilled counsellors to handle the dynamic feature of this counselling approach.

IV. OTHER TYPES OF COUNSELLING

Counselling may be further classified based on the length of the counselling session, the number of counselees involved and the purpose of counselling as follows.

A. Based on length of the counselling session

- *Short-term counselling:* This type of counselling service is used in situational crisis where disruption of life occurs. It focuses mainly on concerns of the patient or family. The counsellor assists the patient and guides him in problem solving or decision making in a systematic and logical manner.
- *Long-term counselling:* It can be on a daily, weekly or monthly basis, and extends over a prolonged period of time. It is focused on patients experiencing a developmental crisis.

B. Based on number of counselees involved

- *Individual counselling:* It is a process of mutual one-to-one interchange of opinions to get and give information. The counsellor tries to establish rapport and structures counselling plan so that the patient understands what to expect during counselling.
- *Group counselling:* It is a technique where a group of people are counselled by applying the group interaction method to arrive at a solution to the problem. All group members are provided with an opportunity to discuss their problems together in a free environment. In group counselling, group work helps the group members in understanding and finding solutions to their problems. Some components like knowledge of reality, self-understanding and self-realization can be achieved through the group interaction process.

C. Counselling for educational and professional purposes

- *Student counselling:* Students are considered to be capable of setting goals, making decisions and generally assuming responsibility for their own behaviour and future. Student counselling is mainly concerned with helping students solve their problems pertaining to the selection of educational institution, course, method of study and adjustment.
- *Educational counselling:* This type of counselling helps the students get the maximum benefit out of education and solve their problems related to education. Students understand or orient themselves to the new purpose or philosophy of education. Educational counselling also assists the students in identifying the need of educational planning. Students develop study habits and choose specializations according to their need and interest.

- *Vocational counselling:* For any problem within a specific vocation, advice is sought to solve those problems through vocational counselling. The counsellor helps the patient improve his all-round personality development and helps him develop skills, efficiency and mastery over the vocation so that the counselee is best among his colleagues.
- *Career counselling:* Career choice is one of the most difficult tasks. Therefore, career counselling is needed for individuals so that they can make a wise choice in choosing careers that suit them best according to their interests, abilities and capabilities.
- *Placement counselling:* The counsellor gives advice to the counselee regarding jobs and posts suitable for the patient depending on his abilities, attitude, aptitude and interest.

D. Counselling for health-related purposes

- *Psychotherapeutic counselling:* Individuals trained in providing psychological counselling consciously attempt to assist the person verbally to modify his or her maladaptive behaviour. There are various methods of psychotherapy like the following:
  - Behaviour counselling
  - Transaction analysis
  - Gestalt therapy
  - Psychoanalytic psychotherapy
- *Crisis counselling:* It helps individuals overcome the effects of a crisis such as loss of a family member and family conflict. These situations may affect the normal behaviour of an individual and he/she may develop feelings of anxiety or guilt. The counsellor helps the individual understand the situation and develop a new pattern of behaviour.
- *Health counselling:* It involves helping an individual learn more about health and healthy habits. This helps the person become more aware of the role of exercise, nutrition and healthy habits to maintain good health.
- *Genetic counselling:* This is a specialized type of health counselling, where individual or families with genetics problems are guided to receive the best possible genetic diagnostic and therapeutic interventions.

E. Counselling for personal/social purposes

- *Personal counselling:* Student face certain problems about which they may be very anxious. They generally try to cope with these problems. The counsellor helps students understand and solve these problems. The counsellor helps students by providing advice on personal problems. The counsellor also helps students develop interpersonal skills, improve study habits and accept themselves and others.
- *Marriage counselling:* Marriage counselling is directed at improving a disturbed marital relationship. It is a centred effort to change the psychodynamics and behaviour of the partner. Two partners meet the therapist in joint sessions. Marital counselling may be conducted on a problem-solving level. It focuses on the need of each partner to understand the other's point of view and feelings.
- *Motivational counselling:* Motivational counselling involves discussing feelings and incentives with the patient. The counsellor can encourage an individual by establishing a helping relationship to avoid feelings of despair and work towards developing feelings of motivation.
- *Developmental counselling:* Different stages of development in life impose a need for specialized counselling services such as child counselling, adolescent counselling, premarital counselling, preconception counselling, child-rearing counselling and geriatric counselling. All these stages in life require guidance and counselling, collectively known as *developmental counselling.*

ROLE AND PREPARATION OF THE COUNSELLOR

A counsellor is the key player in the counselling process. The success of the counselling process primarily depends on the vision and planning of the counsellor. A counsellor is not from another world, however, he must possess some special qualities and attributes (Table 4.2). He is one who has the right understanding of the relation between what counselee thinks, wants and do and say. The word *counsellor* is derived from *counselling* and means a 'person who performs counselling'. D.W. Lefeuer states that a counsellor will be one who devotes half or more of his time to guidance; *a teacher–counsellor* is one who has been relieved of at least one class for guidance work but who will not denote as much as half the time to counselling.

I. ROLE OF THE COUNSELLOR

The major role of a counsellor is to help all students with growth in self-understanding, developing interpersonal, problem-solving and decision-making skills and occupational awareness. This is accomplished through classroom guidance, large and small group sessions and individual counselling. The counsellor must understand and fulfil a number of his patient's needs. A counsellor is expected to perform the following main roles and responsibilities:

- Arrange orientation programmes for the other support staff to enlist their cooperation.
- Prepare an up-to-date list of resources, information, referral and energy available to him.
- Organize the guidance committee.
- Set up an educational and occupational information centre.
- Display the information collected in an attractive way.
- Disseminate information through educational and career talks, group discussions and so on.
- Arrange talks by experts from different fields.
- Organize career days, career weeks, career conferences, parents day and so on.
- Educate students regarding proper study habits and assist them in their development.
- Arrange individual discussions with students and their parents for giving them educational and occupational information.
- Arrange visits to places of work like industries, business establishments, offices, higher education institutions and other important educational places.

Table 4.2 Qualities of a Good Counsellor

G – Good technical knowledge	C – Confidentiality maintenance
O – Obtaining appropriate information from the patient	O – Observant
O – Objectively answering questions	U – Unbiased
D – Demonstrating professionalism	N – Nonjudgemental
	S – Sensitive to the needs of the patient
	E – Empathetic
	L – Listens carefully
	L – Lets the patient make decisions
	O – Open minded
	R – Respects the rights of the patients

- Maintain an active relationship with schools, colleges, universities and other regional, national and social agencies.
- Maintain an active liaison with clubs like Lions Club and Rotary Club.
- Refer serious mental cases to clinical psychologists or psychiatrists.
- Maintain complete secrecy of the discussion between him and the patient.
- Administer psychological tests.
- Provide counselling services to students.
- Help in the student placements.
- Take up research projects relating to the fields of educational, vocational, personal and social guidance in the colleges.
- Prepare guidance leaflets, brochures and monographs and get them printed for distribution to the students.

II. PREPARATION OF COUNSELLOR

Preparation of a counsellor must include the following components so that he can impart efficient counselling services.

- *Educational background:* Master's or bachelor's degree in teaching and education. Counsellors should have completed basic courses in the principles and practices of guidance programmes and additional areas of training in behavioural science (such as psychology, sociality or community health). Essentially, the counsellor must be trained in the areas of counselling process, understanding individual, educational and occupational information, administrative and occupational information, and research and evaluation procedures used in counselling.
- *Experience:* A practising counsellor must have at least 2 years of counselling experience. Further, one year of cumulative work experience in the field of school programmes and 3–6 months of supervised counselling experience. The counsellor must have significant experience in social activities, e.g. working within the community, volunteer work and participating in community training programmes to reveal interest.
- *Personal fitness and attributes:* A good counsellor should show positive interest in working with others and indicate a leadership ability to work for the people. The characteristics or qualities of a counsellor are discussed below:
  - *Personal characteristics:* The following personal characteristics must be enhanced in a person to act as an efficient counsellor:
    - Should be imbibed with basic human qualities.
    - Should be a person with cultural values and awareness.
    - Should have a deep interest in helping people.
    - Should patiently listen to others.
    - Should be sensitive to other's attitude and reactions.
    - Should have a capability for being trusted by others.
    - Should have respect for the personal autonomy of the patients.
    - Should be tolerant of and accept the patient's point of view.
    - Should have ability to understand himself and his emotional limitations.
  - *Interpersonal relationships:* Some interpersonal qualities a counsellor must possess are as follows:
    - Friendly nature
    - Sympathetic understanding

- Sincerity
- Tactfulness
- Patience
- Ability to maintain confidentiality
- Attentive listener
- Show concern
- *Personal adjustment:* Some personal adjustment qualities a counsellor must possess are as follows:
  - Maintain emotional stability
  - Emotionally sound and healthy
  - Able to accept criticism
  - Knowledge of self
- *Scholastic potentialities:* Some of the scholastic potentialities a counsellor must possess are as follows:
  - Relevant knowledge and efficient skills
  - Motivated and committed
  - Aware of policies, beliefs, misconceptions and rumours in the community
  - Possess common sense and use good judgement while tackling issues
  - Experience in teaching and follow-up services
- *Health and personal appearance:* Some health and personal appearance related qualities a counsellor must possess are as follows:
  - Pleasing voice and appearance
  - Vitality and endurance
  - Free from any mannerism
- *Leadership skills:* Some leadership qualities a counsellor must possess are as follows:
  - Ability to stimulate and lead others
  - Reinforce important information
  - Direct the counselee to ways to solve the problem
- *Philosophy of life:* A counsellor must have the following ingredients in his philosophy of life:
  - Good character
  - Integrated personality
  - Faith in human values and human nature
  - Show significant human values and religious belief
- *Professional dedication:* The type of professional dedication a counsellor must possess are as follows:
  - Show enthusiasm in providing services
  - Maintain helping relationship
  - Have a high sense of morality

COUNSELLING PROCESS

The counselling process takes place through a series of phases, which are interrelated, interconnected and overlap such as the nursing process. The process is not a rigid entity; it is flexible and can be modified based on the nature of problems and person to be counselled. The basic phases of a counselling process are as discussed below (Fig. 4.6).

I. PHASE I: ESTABLISHING RELATIONSHIP

This is the first and main phase of the counselling process, and is considered as the foundation to the counselling process. It is an ice-breaking session during which the counsellor and the counselee introduce each other and establish a primary rapport that continues building further in the following phases of the counselling process. Good rapport building provides the respect, trust and sense of psychological comfort to the counsellor–counselee relationship for progression to the counselling process. Establishing a relationship may not be possible in a single session but may require multiple sessions before the next phases of counselling begin, so that the counsellor and the counselee interact with ease. The following strategies may be used by a counsellor to establish an effective relationship:

- Introduce yourself.
- Begin the phase with adequate social skills.
- Always address the individual by his or her name and remember the patient's name.
- Ensure physical comfort of the counselee and self.
- Do not interrupt the individual when he/she is talking.
- Listen attentively.
- Observe nonverbal communication.

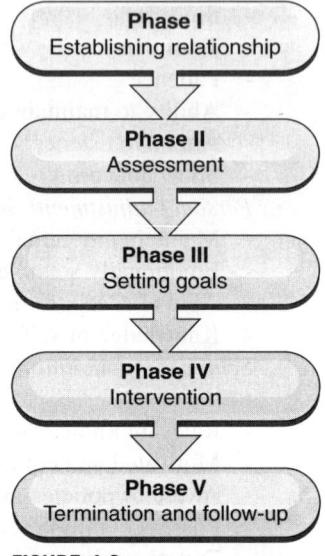

FIGURE 4.6

Phases of the counselling process.

II. PHASE II: ASSESSMENT

The second phase of counselling is basically a data collection phase, where the counsellor motivates the counselee to provide complete information about the problem. During this phase, the counsellor's job is to motivate the counselee to speak about the problems and listen to him patiently. The counselee's job is to provide all the relevant information pertaining to the present problem for which he is seeking counselling. During this phase, detailed information is collected from the counselee. The type of information collected from the counselee during this phase is depicted in Table 4.3. After the collection of information, diagnosis related to the counselee's behaviour is made. Diagnosis in a counselling situation refers to the concise statement of the patient's problems in his present condition. It tries to identify possible causes of difficulty to predict future patient behaviour. Diagnosis thus may be considered as a hypothesis of the counsellor regarding a counselee's present attitudes, thoughts and possible future behaviour (as presented in Table 4.4). Various tools may be used in the collection of information during the assessment phase as illustrated in Box 4.1.

III. PHASE III: SETTING GOALS

During this third phase of the counselling process, goals are set co-operatively by both the counsellor and the counselee. While setting goals, the counselee's strengths, weaknesses, constraints and available resources must be kept under consideration. The goal could be immediate and ultimate which directs the counsellor and the counselee to further progress in the counselling process and finally help in evaluation of the counselling outcome. Goals set during counselling are not fixed, but are dynamic, which may

Table 4.3 Types of Information Collected from the Counselee During the Assessment Phase

Type of Data	Description
General data	Information that is helpful in locating an individual and establishing contact.
Physical data	Information about an individual's health and physical characteristics.
Psychological data	Information about an individual's mental characteristics such as intelligence and special aptitude and personality traits.
Social/environment data	It includes social and environmental conditions and factors that influence the individual and his vocational plans.
Achievement data	It includes information of what an individual has achieved in school and outside.
Data and educational and vocational plans	It includes information about an individual's plans regarding educational and vocational progress.

Table 4.4 Types of Problems Diagnosed During Assessment Phase of Counselling

Type of Problem	Description
Personality problems	Difficulties pertaining to adjustment, family conflicts, personal problems, etc.
Educational problems	Unwise choice of courses of study, differential scholastic achievement, inadequate general scholastic aptitude, ineffective study habits, reading difficulties, lack of motivation, under achievement and the like. The patient is primarily concerned with adjustment to current academic situations rather than planning for the future.
Vocational problems	Deals with career choice and planning, choice of college and educational planning that would ultimately be implemented and lead to a career plan. It includes unwise vocational choice, differences between interest and attitudes, etc.
Financial problems	Problems related to financial support needed for school or college education.
Health problems	Inability to go about one's routine activities owing to problems of health.

Williamson and Darley (1937) proposed the above classifications.

BOX 4.1 TOOLS AND TECHNIQUES USED FOR DATA COLLECTION DURING COUNSELLING

Standardized	Nonstandardized	
Intelligence tests	Questionnaires	Rating scale
Achievement tests	Interview	Cumulative record charts
Aptitude tests	Observation	Case studies
Interest tests	Autobiography	Sociometric techniques
Personality tests	Anecdotal records	Informal collection of information
		Systematic recording

change based on needs and new information. Effective and reliable goal setting requires the following skills in counsellors:

- Multifaceted knowledge related to the problems of the counselee
- Ability to think critically and inference-drawing skills
- Judgement, planning and management skills
- Skills to segregate and differentiate the provided information
- Ability to teach individuals to think critically and realistically
- Help the counselee set feasible, reliable and achievable goals

IV. PHASE IV: INTERVENTION

This stage of counselling is an operational phase where the counselee is suggested the best possible options for the management of the present problem. This phase is affected by the counsellor's own thoughts about the counselling process. The intervention will depend on the approach used by the counsellor, the problem and the individual. The choice of intervention is a process of adaptation and the counsellor should be prepared to change the intervention when the selected intervention does not work.

V. PHASE V: TERMINATION AND FOLLOW-UP

This is the final stage of the counselling process, where counselling comes to an end. Termination must be planned well ahead so that the counselee may feel comfortable at the departure and gradually able to handle the problem independently. Some follow-up sessions may be required to help the counselee further to handle the problem independently.

TOOLS AND TECHNIQUES FOR THE COUNSELLING PROCESS

A number of tools and techniques are used in a guidance and counselling programme. With the help of these tools and techniques, data pertaining to all aspects of an individual's life is collected. These tools and techniques can be divided into two categories.

I. STANDARDIZED TOOLS AND TECHNIQUES

Standardized tools are also known as *testing techniques* and are more widely used than nonstandardized techniques to collect information about an individual as they are objective and reliable. They are developed by special agencies or institutions with the help of psychologists. The various types of standardized tools/tests generally used to collect information about an individual are as follows:

- *Intelligence tests:* Intelligence tests are used to measure the intelligence of an individual keeping in view the different dimensions of intelligence.
- *Achievement tests:* These are used to evaluate the achievement of an individual in different subjects of study.
- *Aptitude tests:* These tests are also called *special ability tests*. They are meant to judge the capacity of an individual to be skilled in some work or some subject of study after receiving formal or informal education.

- *Interest tests:* These tests are used to know the tendency of an individual to become absorbed in an experience and to continue it for a long time.
- *Personality tests:* These tests are meant to find out the traits, aptitudes, areas of interest, potentialities and behaviour of an individual at all times.

II. NONSTANDARDIZED TESTS

There are certain nonstandardized tests/techniques for collection of information about an individual. They are used to supplement other information available concerning the patient. Some nonstandardized techniques commonly used in counselling are as follows:

- *Autobiography:* An autobiography is an introspective report of one's own experience. It is designed to provide answers to specific questions put up by the counsellor. Structured autobiographies are asked to be written along a suggested outline consisting of topics such as my family, my childhood, my years before school, places I have lived, trips I have taken, my experiences in high school, my teachers and my class fellows, my ambitions and my aspirations.
- *Anecdotal records:* Froehlich and Hoyt (1959) define anecdotal records as 'an anecdotal record consists of an objective description of pupil behaviour in a particular environmental setting, an interpretation of the behaviour by the observer, writing the description and recommendation for future action based on the incident and its interpretation'.
- *Questionnaire:* A list of questions is prepared pertaining to information about the individual. He is asked to give answers. The questionnaire consists of items regarding the student's home, family, health, educational and vocational plans, out of school and in school activities, study habits, etc. They are used to obtain comprehensive information dealing with the student, employing both his idiographic and normative data and serve to supplement incomplete information available about a student and improve the collection of data in an efficient manner.
- *Interview:* An interview is a face-to-face contact between the individual and the counsellor. The counsellor can get direct information from the individual through this technique.
- *Observation:* In this technique, the counsellor observes the counselee without letting him know he is being observed. Hence, his natural behaviour is observed through this technique under natural circumstances.
- *Cumulative record chart:* A cumulative record chart contains a record of all the important aspects of an individual. It provides an organized, progressive record of information regarding the student which distinguishes him from all other individuals. The cumulative folder includes information such as personal data and family background, medical and health condition, date of admission, academic attendance, academic performance, grades, test results, personality and behaviour trait ratings and performance in other curricular and cocurricular activities, etc.
- *Case study:* A case study is the full study of an individual, about the various aspects of his life to bring about an adjustment with society and life at large. It is an analysis and documentation of data collected in the case history. It comprises the information gathered about a patient, including the family history, physical development, etc. Educational, social and vocational history is also covered in a case study. It presents a cumulative picture of an individual's personality. The information is gathered from sources such as cumulative records, observations, interviews, autobiographies, self reports, tests and other school records. The case study provides an opportunity for the person to be understood and treated as an individual. It helps in the prediction of behaviour. One of the disadvantages of the case history

method is that it leads to a delay in providing assistance to the individual. Another limitation is that the case study may not be sufficient as a basis for drawing conclusions and formulating diagnosis for a patient.

- *Rating scale:* Rating scales are used for evaluating the characteristics of an individual. The student's characteristics such as dependability, honesty, cooperativeness, self-reliance and leadership are rated by teachers and counsellors. The rating scales are subject to bias and halo effect.
- *Sociometric technique:* It is a technique to discover the nature of an individual's relationships within a group. It measures the interpersonal preferences among the members of the group in reference to a criterion. The purpose of this technique is to measure each individual's social worth or personal value as viewed by his peers.
- *Informal collection of information:* Information about an individual can be collected informally. There are social and cultural functions/events the individual may participate in. Information about his behaviour can be collected in such functions.

ISSUES OF COUNSELLING IN NURSING

Counselling services in nursing education are quite essential but generally neglected, especially in the Indian scenario. The several pertinent issues of counselling in nursing, which need immediate attention, are discussed below:

- **Scarcity of qualified and competent counsellors:** In our own scenario, there is great scarcity of qualified and competent counsellors, either in nursing education or nursing services. One can hardly find a qualified and competent counsellor working for nurses in educational institutions or practice settings. It is generally observed that newly selected student nurses are found in great need of guidance and counselling services for better adjustment with the new demanding and challenging environment of their college and hospital. Therefore, the Indian Nursing Council must ensure that each college has at least one part-time counsellor who is qualified and competent.
- **Lack of awareness about needs and resources of counselling:** It is generally observed that there is a lack of awareness in nursing students and nurses about the need and importance of counselling services for a better future. Most of the student nurses join nursing education without any formal preadmission counselling and face difficulties adjusting with this demanding professional education, which leads to quite a stressful time for them. In spite of all the odds, nursing students and nurses are found to be quite unaware about the need and importance of counselling services. In addition, in situations where they feel a need for counselling services, they are not aware about the available resources, which adds to their problems. Therefore, nursing institutions must be proactive in improving the awareness in nursing students about the need and importance of counselling services as well as the availability of best resources.
- **Minimal procounselling environment:** Nursing institutions or hospitals do not give much importance to counselling services for nursing students and practising nurses. Very few health care institutions realize the importance of counselling for nurses or students nurses. In the absence of such procounselling environment, one cannot expect nurses or student nurses to receive standardized counselling services. It is high time the institutions realize the importance of counselling services for nurses and nursing students so that they can adjust to the new environment or their stressful job better for better learning and job performance, which is most essential for quality patient care.

- **Lack of counselling training for nurses/nursing faculty:** The nursing faculty or teachers could act as good counselling resources in nursing institutions, but there is a lack of adequate training for the nursing faculty and nursing teachers. The same is observed in the hospital setting, where nurses could act as a good counsellor for their patients. It is therefore recommended that there must be adequate curriculum related to counselling in the basic as well-advanced level of nursing education. In addition, there must be regular continuing education related to counselling for nurses and nursing faculty so that they can be updated with new aspects of counselling to benefit their patients.
- **Poor organizational set-up for counselling services:** A good organizational set-up is required for the efficient implementation of counselling services such as infrastructure, money and manpower. There is very poor attention towards building a competent and quality organization set-up for counselling services in health care institutions of either nursing education or nursing services.
- **Lack of interest and initiatives for counselling services:** There is poor interest and initiative for establishing counselling services among the nursing faculty, nursing teachers, nurses and management in India. Interest brings about the motivation to act and one can achieve initiatives. Therefore, nursing faculty, nursing teachers and nurses must be motivated to spark an interest in establishing counselling services for their patients so that the standard and quality of nursing services and nursing education can be ensured.
- **Poor counsellor–counselee ratio:** There are few initiatives to establish counselling services in Indian institutions. There is very poor counsellor–counselee ratio that has created a poor image and outcome of the counselling services. An adequate counsellor–counselee ratio must be ensured to achieve a better counselling outcome.
- **Lack of funds for counselling services:** There is a scarcity of funds for providing counselling services (including to nursing students and practising nurses) in Indian health care institutions. In the absence of adequate funds for counselling services, one cannot imagine anything positive happening in the field of counselling services for nursing students and practising nurses. Therefore, the government and management must realize the importance of counselling services and dedicate adequate funds for these services for nursing students and practising nurses, so that the actual objective of nursing services and nursing education can be achieved.
- **Noncompliance with counselling interventions:** The other most crucial issue in the field of counselling services in nursing and nursing education is the problem of noncompliance with counselling interventions. This nonadherence or noncompliance is because of several reasons such as lack of interest, incompetent counsellors, poor access to qualified counsellors, lack of time and inadequate funds.
- **Ethical and moral issues:** This is also one of the most crucial issues of counselling services in nursing because the absence or poor practice of ethical and moral principles in counselling services may cause several serious problems. There are some critically essential ethical principles in counselling services that must be followed by counsellors such as autonomy of practice, anonymity of subjects and confidentiality of information so that ethical, moral and legal problems pertaining to counselling can be prevented.

MANAGING DISCIPLINARY PROBLEMS

Disciplinary problems are not only observed in Indian institutions but may also be seen in institutions around the world. Common disciplinary problems seen in Indian students are absenteeism, nonsubmission or late submission of assignments, disturbing classroom atmosphere, threatening strikes, damaging or spoiling institutional property, picking quarrels over small matters, using mobile phones in the classroom and so on. Disciplinary problems have increased many folds in Indian schools, colleges and universities. According to the Indian Education Commission, 'briefly there have been many ugly strikes and demonstrations often without any justifications, leading to violence, walk out from classrooms and examination halls, ticketless travel, clashes with police, burning of buses and cinemas, houses and sometimes even manhandling of teachers'. Reports of student trouble and indefinite closure of schools, colleges and even universities are pouring in from all over the country. Naturally this state of affairs has attracted the attention of educationists, leaders, social scientists and general public to seriously manage this problem so that the image and objectives of education can be optimally achieved.

I. STRATEGIES FOR MANAGEMENT OF DISCIPLINARY PROBLEMS

Disciplinary problems may arise because of several factors such as complex educational system, incompetence of teachers in handling students, student's personal and professional stress, lack of adequate cocurricular and extracurricular activities, inappropriate selection and use of disciplinary standards, neglecting the importance of positive reinforcement, poor teacher–student relationship, inadequate parent–teacher–student contacts and lack of efficient guidance and counselling services. The following strategies may be quite helpful in the prevention and management of disciplinary problems in students:

- *Appropriate training of faculty and teachers:* Adequate education and updated training is required to maintain the effective competence of practice including disciplinary management. There must be a provision of adequate training for principals, faculty and teachers to handle the disciplinary problems of students efficiently.
- *Adequate practice of cocurricular and extracurricular activities:* It is sometimes observed that exclusive intense curricular activities become a source of boredom and stress and may trigger an episode of indiscipline in students. Therefore, adequate incorporation of co-curricular and extracurricular activities is required in routine academic schedule. So the boredom of the students can be minimized and academic activities made more interesting.
- *Appropriate selection and use of disciplinary standards:* In the selection and use of disciplinary rules and standards, the following guidelines must be followed:
  - Identify the specific behaviours that are necessary to maintain a conducive learning environment in the institution.
  - Simplify disciplinary standards to three or four general classroom rules. They should be broad enough to cover the spectrum of appropriate expected behaviour.
  - Determine the positive and negative consequences of the disciplinary standards based on inputs received from teachers, parents and student.
  - Display standards in the classroom with a list of approved consequences from which effective consequences can be selected to fit the needs of each student.
  - Review the discipline plan daily with the class during the first two weeks of admission in the institution.
  - Meet with parents individually or collectively during the first two weeks of admission in the institution. Obtain parents' written approval for the discipline plan.
  - Implement the discipline plan. Be consistent, focus on praise and encouragement. Address infractions firmly, fairly and consistently.

- *Use reward and punishment:* Positive reinforcement is a tool often absent in the majority of educational institutions. Often, only the negative consequences are placed on the wall; there is no visual display for consequences for positive behaviour. Overemphasis of the negative and minimization of the positive is detrimental in maintaining strong classroom discipline. Therefore, there must be adequate use of reward and punishment so that students are inclined towards positive behaviour and refrain from negative behaviour.
- *Promoting better teacher–student relationship:* An intimate teacher–student relationship always helps in the early identification and management of problems related to indiscipline. In addition, because of good teacher–student relationships, disciplinary problems may be prevented in time.
- *Cultivation of ethical, moral and spiritual values:* Values are the foundation to discipline in life. They guide the person on right path and act as a preventive measure for indiscipline. There must be significant stress on the cultivation of ethical, moral and spiritual values in students so that indiscipline can be prevented.
- A *close teacher–parent–student contact:* Parents are the first teachers and teachers are the second parents for students in their life. Both parents and teachers have a significant impact and influence on a student's life. Teachers must regularly communicate to students and their parents about their progress. A close loop of contact between the teacher, parents and students must be maintained and may be very helpful in the prevention and management of disciplinary problems.
- *Effective use of guidance and counselling programmes:* Guidance and counselling services may help students resolve their problems and they may feel comfortable and satisfied with their stay in the institution. In addition, regular guidance and counselling programmes can be helpful in the assessment and management of disciplinary problems in time.

MANAGEMENT OF CRISIS AND REFERRAL

A sudden, generally unanticipated event can profoundly and negatively affect a significant segment of the institution population and often involves serious injury or death. Crisis events like an incidence of suicide, school bus crashes, natural disasters or multiple injuries, deaths can quickly escalate all over the educational institution. Crisis must be managed promptly and skilfully to minimize chaos, rumours and the impact of the crisis on the victims and other students.

I. STRATEGIES OF EFFECTIVE CRISIS MANAGEMENT

The five essential elements of effective crisis management in educational institutions are as follows:

- *Policy and leadership:* Policy provides both a foundation and a framework for action. The chances of effectively managing a crisis are increased with a district level plan and individual building plans that operate within the framework of the district plan but are tailored to the conditions and resources of the individual school. Leadership is necessary to ensure effective implementation of plans and maintenance of preparedness.
- *Crisis response team:* A school crisis response team can be a highly effective organizational unit for dealing with a variety of crisis. Such teams can operate at three levels: individual school, district and community. Well-functioning teams at each level provide a network that can support action whenever crisis arise.

- ***Institution's crisis management plan:*** The plan should be in writing, updated as often as necessary and given to every staff member. The plan should identify clearly what response is needed in each emergency situation so that staff members know in advance how to react in times of crisis. (The safety/security assessment report found later in the booklet is a good starting point for crisis plan development and review.)
- ***Communications:*** When a crisis occurs, effective communication is essential within the building and the district, with parents and the community and with the news media, which is often the fastest conduit to the public. Effective communication can speed the restoration of equilibrium; conversely, poor communication can make a bad situation even worse. Every crisis management plan should include provisions for a sensitive and professional communication plan.
- ***Training and maintenance:*** Preparation for and response to crisis relies on people understanding policies and procedures and knowing what they are supposed to do at such times. This preparedness is achieved through training. Maintaining preparedness is an ongoing process that involves debriefing following a crisis, periodic review and updation and ongoing training.

II. CRISIS MANAGEMENT PLANNING CHECKLIST

(Check off each item as you complete it during your crisis management planning)

- Define crisis for your school and district.
- Decide who will be in charge during a crisis.
- Select your crisis response team.
- Develop appropriate policies and procedures for handling crisis situations (what to do before a crisis happens, when a crisis happens and during postcrisis follow-up).
- Train the crisis response team.
- Establish law enforcement, fire department and emergency management team liaisons.
- Establish a media liaison and a plan for communicating with the media.
- Establish a working relationship with community service providers and develop a list of telephone numbers and contact persons.
- Set up phone number trees, which are adequately and appropriately displayed.
- Create or reserve space for service providers involved in crisis management and for community meetings.
- Develop and print forms to assist in crisis management.
- Develop a plan for emergency coverage of classes.
- Establish a code to alert staff.
- Develop a collection of readings and sample letters to parents.
- Obtain a legal review of crisis response procedures and forms.
- Practice crisis alerts periodically through the year.
- Establish procedures for annual in-service of new staff and update/review for all staff.
- Periodic districtwide training of all substitute staff.

CRISIS INTERVENTIONS

An individual or a group of people who have been through a crisis may require crisis interventions. Stressful events or crisis are a common part of life. They may be social, psychological or biological in nature and there is often little a person can do to prevent them. As the largest group of health care providers, nurses are in N excellent position to help promote a healthy outcome for people in times of crisis. Crisis experienced by students in educational institutions are quite often managed by the school health nurse or the counsellor.

Gail W. Stuart defines crisis as a sudden disturbance generally caused by unanticipated social, psychological or biological stressful event or perceived threat that profoundly and negatively affects the person and could have a serious health and life impact. A person's usual way of coping becomes ineffective in dealing with the threat causing anxiety. The threat or precipitating can usually be identified.

Crisis interventions is a brief, focused and time-limited treatment strategy that has been shown to be effective in helping people adaptively cope with stressful events. Knowledge of crisis management is an important clinical skill of all nurses, regardless of clinical setting or practice of setting.

I. TYPES OF CRISIS FOR INDIVIDUALS

Crisis can be maturational and situational. Sometimes they may come simultaneously. For example, an adolescent having difficulty to a change in role and body image (maturational crisis) may at the same time undergo stress of failure in the first year nursing university examination (situational crisis).

- *Maturational crisis:* Maturational crisis are developmental events requiring role changes. For example, successfully moving from early childhood to middle childhood requires the child to become socially involved with people outside the family. With the move from adolescence to adulthood, a financial responsibility is expected. Both social and biological pressure to change can precipitate a crisis. The transitional periods during adolescence, parenthood, marriage, midlife and retirement are key times for the onset of maturational crisis.

  The nature and extent of maturational crisis can be influenced by a role model, interpersonal resources and others response. Positive role models show the person how to act in the new role. Interpersonal resources encourage trying out new behaviours to achieve role changes. Other people's acceptance of the new role is also important. The greater the resistance of others, the more stress a person may face in making the changes.
- *Situational crisis:* Situational crisis occurs when a life event upsets an individual's or group's psychological equilibrium. Examples of situational crisis include loss of a job, loss of loved one, unwanted pregnancy, onset or worsening of a medical illness, divorce, school problems and witnessing a terrorist attack, crime and disaster.

II. FEATURES OF CRISIS SITUATION

- Crisis is complex and not very easy to resolve.
- It threatens psychological integrity and personal safety.
- It may cause disorganized feelings and emotions.
- It may distort routine life and psychological, social and spiritual well-being.
- It may have serious short-term as well as long-term psychological, physical, social and spiritual impact.
- It requires additional support from family, friends, peer groups and counsellors.

III. CRISIS RESPONSES OF AN INDIVIDUAL

After the precipitating event, a person's anxiety begins to rise and the following three phases of a crisis response emerge:

- *Phase I:* In the first phase, the anxiety activates the person's usual methods of coping. If these do not bring relief, anxiety increases because the coping mechanism has failed.
- *Phase II:* In the second phase, new coping mechanisms are tried or the threat is redefined so that old ones can work. Resolution of the problem can occur in this phase. However, if resolution does not occur, the person goes on to the last phase of crisis.
- *Phase III:* In the third phase, the continuation of severe and/or panic levels of anxiety may lead to psychological disorganization and individuals may experience the following manifestations (also other manifestations exhibited after a crisis in Box 4.2):
  - Being over conscious, watchful and extra sensitive
  - Doubtful and inability to trust others
  - Tiredness and insomnia
  - Lack of concentration and confidence
  - Change in appetite, sleep pattern and bowel movements
  - Depression, distorted thought process and suicidal tendencies
  - Irritability, anxiety and fear of unknown causes
  - Hopelessness, helplessness and decreased self-esteem
  - Headache and poor general well-being

IV. CRISIS INTERVENTIONS FOR A PATIENT

Crisis intervention is a short-term therapy to solve immediate problems. It is usually limited to 6 weeks. The goal of crisis intervention is for the individual to return to a precrisis level of functioning. The person often advances to a level of growth that is higher than the precrisis level because new ways of problem solving have been learned.

It is important for a nurse to remember that culture strongly influences the crisis intervention process, including the communication and response style of the crisis workers. Cultural attitudes are deeply

BOX 4.2 MANIFESTATIONS COMMONLY EXHIBITED AFTER CRISIS		
Anger	Headache	Poor concentration
Apathy	Helplessness	Sadness
Backache	Hopelessness	School problems
Boredom	Insomnia	Self-doubt
Crying spells	Intrusive thoughts	Shock
Diminished sexual drive	Irritability	Social withdrawal
Disbelief	Liability	Substance abuse
Fatigue	Nightmares	Suicidal thought
Fear	Numbness	Survivors guilt
Flashbacks	Over-or under-eating	Work difficulties
Forgetfulness		

ingrained in the processes of asking for giving and receiving help. They also affect the victimization experience; so it is essential to understand and respect the sociocultural context of crisis care. Specific cultural factors to be considered in crisis intervention include the following:

- Migration and citizenship status
- Gender and family roles
- Religious belief system
- Use of extended family and support system
- Housing and living conditions
- Socioeconomic status

In addition, age is also important because response to the stressor differs at different ages. For example, 4-year-old children may best express themselves through play whereas adolescents may work through crisis issues through peer-group discussion. Crisis intervention includes the following stages:

- *Assessment:* The first step of crisis intervention is assessment. Data about the nature of crisis and its effect on the person must be collected at this stage. People with crisis may manifest many symptoms as depicted Box 4.2. Sometimes these symptoms can cause further problems. For example, terminal illness may lead to loss of job, financial problems and low self-esteem. During this phase the nurse establishes a positive relationship with the patient. A number of balancing factors are important in the development and resolution of a crisis and should be assessed:
  - Precipitating events or stressors
  - Patient's perception of the event or stressor
  - Nature and strength of the patient's support systems and coping resources
  - Patient's previous strength and coping mechanisms
- *Planning and implementation:* The next step of crisis intervention is planning. The previously collected data is analysed and specific interventions are proposed. Dynamics underlying the present crisis are formulated from the information about the precipitating events. Alternative solutions for the problems are explored and steps for achieving solutions are identified. Four basic levels of crisis interventions may be used to resolve the crisis, i.e. environmental manipulations, general support, generic approach and individual approach and represent a hierarchy most basic to most complex (Shields, 1975) (Fig. 4.7).
  - *Environmental manipulation* includes interventions that directly change the patient's physical or interpersonal situations. These interventions provide situational support or remove stress.
  - *General support* includes interventions that convey the feeling that the nurse is on the patient's side and will be a helping hand. The nurse uses warmth, acceptance, empathy, caring and reassurance to provide this type of support.
  - *Generic approach* is designed to reach high risk individuals and large groups as quickly possible. It applies a specific method to all people faced with a similar type of crisis. An intervention used after acute stress is called *debriefing*, where people are asked to recall events and clarify traumatic experiences, ventilate feelings within

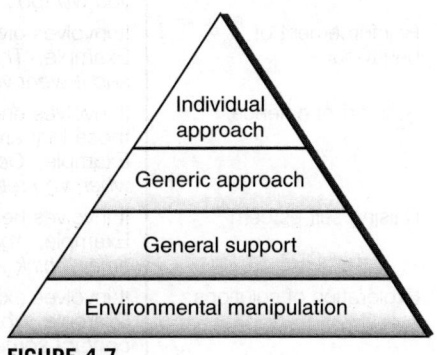

FIGURE 4.7

Levels of crisis intervention.

a context of group support. It also provides normalization of responses and education about psychological reactions to traumatic events.

- *Individual approach* is a type of crisis intervention similar to diagnosis and treatment of a specific problem in a specific patient. This approach is used when the patient has not responded to generic approaches and/or has symptoms of homicide/suicide. The nurse understands the specific patient's characteristics and interventions are aimed to facilitate cognitive and emotional processing of the traumatic event and improve coping. The five core interventions to assist patients of acute stress are as follows:
  - Restore psychological safety
  - Provide information
  - Correct and support effective coping
  - Ensure social support
- ***Techniques of crisis intervention.*** The nurse should be creative, flexible and willing to try different techniques. These should be active, focused and explorative techniques that can facilitate achieving the target interventions. Some of these techniques include catharsis, clarification, suggestion, reinforcement of behaviour, support of defences, raising self-esteem and the exploration of solutions. Interventions must be aimed at achieving quick resolution. The nurse must also be active in guiding the crisis intervention through its various steps. A passive approach is not appropriate because of the time limitations of crisis situations. A brief description of these techniques is shown in Table 4.5.

Table 4.5 Techniques of Crisis Intervention

Type of Technique	Description of Technique with Example
Catharsis	Catharsis is the release of feelings that takes place as the patient talks about emotionally charged areas. Example, *'Tell me how you have been feeling since you failed in your final examination'.*
Clarification	It involves encouraging the patient to express the relationship between certain events more clearly. Example, *'I have noticed that after being scolded by the principal you have become sick and are not coming to school regularly'.*
Suggestions	It involves influencing a person to accept an idea or belief, particularly the belief that the nurse can help and the person will feel better in time. Example, *'Many other people have found it helpful to talk about this and I think you will too'.*
Reinforcement of behaviour	It involves giving the patient positive responses to adaptive behaviour. Example, *'That is the first time you were able to defend yourself with your boss and it went very well. I am so pleased that you were able to do it'.*
Support of defence	It involves encouraging the use of healthy, adaptive defences and discouraging those that are unhappy or maladaptive. Example, *'Going for exercise when you were so angry was very helpful because when you returned, you and your husband were able to talk things through'.*
Raising self-esteem	It involves helping the patient regain feelings of self-worth. Example, *'You are a very strong person to be able to manage the family all this time. I think you will be able to handle this situation too'.*
Exploration of solutions	It involves examining alternative ways of solving immediate problems. Example, *'You seem to know many people in the nursing field. Could you contact some of them to see whether they might know of available jobs?'*

• *Evaluation:* The last phase of crisis intervention is evaluation where the nurse and patient evaluate the intervention that resulted in a positive resolution of the crisis. Specific questions the nurse might ask include the following:

  • Has the expected outcome been achieved and patient returned to the precrisis level of functioning?
  • Have the needs of the patient that were threatened by the event been met?
  • Have the patient's symptoms decreased or been resolved?
  • Does the patient have an adequate support system and coping resources on which to rely?
  • Is the patient using a constructive coping mechanism?
  • Is the patient demonstrating adaptive crisis responses?
  • Does the patient need to be refereed for additional treatment?

The nurse and the patient should also review the changes that have occurred. Nurses should give patients credit for successful changes so they can realize their effectiveness and understand that they learned from a crisis and this may help in coping with further crisis situations. If the goals have not been met, the patient and the nurse can return to the first stage of assessment and progress through the phases again. At the end the evaluation process, if the nurse and the patient believe that referral for additional professional help would be useful; referral should be made as quickly as possible.

REVIEW QUESTIONS

Long-Answer Questions

1. List down the purpose of guidance and counselling.
2. Describe how you will organize counselling services.
3. Explain the differences between guidance and counselling.
4. What are the objectives of guidance and counselling services in a college of nursing?
5. Explain the steps of the counselling process.
6. What is the importance of guidance and counselling for nursing students?
7. Discuss the basic principles of counselling.
8. Describe the approaches of counselling and steps of the counselling process.
9. Explain the organization of counselling services for first year B.Sc. (N) students.
10. Describe the issues of counselling services in nursing.
11. What are the different types of counselling, and how will you differentiate counselling from guidance?
12. Discuss the principles of counselling. How will you organize a counselling programme for students in your college of nursing?
13. Discuss the scope of guidance and counselling in nursing education.
14. Discuss the needs and purposes of guidance and counselling.

Short-Answer Questions

1. Discuss the terms guidance and counselling.
2. List down four issues for counselling nursing students.
3. Mention four principles of counselling.

Multiple-Choice Questions (MCQs)

1. An elder sibling helps his younger one to make the right career choice. The approach used in this situation is best called as
   (a) Guidance
   (b) Counselling
   (c) Motivation
   (d) Appreciation
2. A teacher advises a student to face the sudden death of her mother with courage. The approach used in this situation is best called as
   (a) Guidance
   (b) Counselling
   (c) Motivation
   (d) Appreciation
3. At which one of the following levels does counselling operate?
   (a) Intellectual
   (b) Cognitive
   (c) Emotional
   (d) Social
4. Guidance and counselling is offered in which of the following situation(s)?
   (a) Personal
   (b) Educational
   (c) Social
   (d) All of these
5. The ultimate purpose of guidance and counselling is
   (a) Facilitating the adjustment
   (b) All-round development of personality
   (c) Self-understanding
   (d) Adjustment of the environment
6. Following are the characteristics of counselling except
   (a) Required in childhood
   (b) Self-realization
   (c) Professional activity
   (d) Need-based assistance
7. Which of the following plays an important role in delivering guidance and counselling services?
   (a) Teachers
   (b) Parents
   (c) Counsellors
   (d) All of these
8. While counselling an individual, an important principle to follow is
   (a) Cooperation with patient
   (b) Continuity of interaction
   (c) Individual differences
   (d) Joint responsibility

9. Which of the following approaches should be used while counselling an individual?
   (a) Firm
   (b) Flexible
   (c) Manipulative
   (d) Rigid
10. Organization of counselling services can be
    (a) Centralized and decentralized
    (b) Commanding and discommending
    (c) Reciprocal and mutual
    (d) Coordination and cooperation
11. Checklist and rating scales as tools of counselling are
    (a) Testing tools
    (b) Nontesting tools
    (c) Standardized tools
    (d) Personality tools
12. For counselling services at an affiliated college of the university having more than 1000 students, there should be provision of
    (a) HOD of psychology and team
    (b) Liaison officer and team
    (c) Counselling officer and team
    (d) Team of teachers
13. Following are the types of counselling types, except
    (a) Directive
    (b) Nondirective
    (c) Eclectic
    (d) Impersonal
14. Directive counselling is also called
    (a) Patient oriented
    (b) Problem oriented
    (c) Goal oriented
    (d) Counsellor oriented
15. Who evolved the concept of nondirective counselling?
    (a) Carl Rogers
    (b) E.G. Williamson
    (c) A.J. Jones
    (d) Gilbret Wrenn

Answers of the Multiple-Choice Questions

1. (a), 2. (b), 3. (c), 4. (d), 5. (b), 6. (a), 7. (d), 8. (c), 9. (b), 10. (a), 11. (b), 12. (c), 13. (d), 14. (b), 15. (a)

FURTHER READING

Aguileta, D. C. (1998). *Crisis intervention: Theory and methodology* (8th ed.). St. Louis, MO: Mosby.

Bhatia, K. K. (2002). *Principles of guidance & counselling* (1st ed.). Ludhiana: Kalyani Publishers.

Blanco, P. J., & Ray, D. C. (2011). Play therapy in elementary schools: A best practice for improving academic achievement. *Journal of Counseling & Development*, 89, 235–243.

Bodenhorn, N., Wolfe, E. W., & Airen, O. E. (2010). School counselor program choice and self-efficacy: Relationship to achievement gap and equity. *Professional School Counseling*, 13, 165–174.

Brigman, G. A., & Campbell, C. (2003). Helping students improve academic achievement and school success behavior. *Professional School Counseling*, 7, 91–98.

Brigman, G. A., Webb, L. D., & Campbell, C. (2007). Building skills for school success: Improving the academic and social competence of students. *Professional School Counseling*, 10, 279–288.

Bruce, A. M., Getch, Y. Q., & Ziomek-Daigle, J. (2009). Closing the gap: A group counseling approach to improve test performance of African-American students. *Professional School Counseling*, 12, 450–457.

Buser, J. K. (2010). American Indian adolescents and disordered eating. *Professional School Counseling*, 14, 146–155.

Cholewa, B., & West-Olatunji, C. (2008). Exploring the relationship among cultural discontinuity, psychological distress, and academic achievement outcomes for low-income, culturally diverse students. *Professional School Counseling*, 12, 54–61.

Froehlich, C. P., & Hoyt, K. B. (1959). *Guidance testing* (p. 34). Chicago: Science Research Associates.

Holcomb-McCoy, C. (2007). *School counseling to close the achievement gap: A social justice framework for success*. Thousand Oaks, CA: Corwin Press.

Holcomb-McCoy, C. (2007). Transitioning to high school: Issues and challenges for African American students. *Professional School Counseling*, 10, 253–260.

IGNOU, (2000). *Guidance and counselling in nursing education.*

Ivey, A. E., Ivey, M. B., & Simek, D. L. (1996). *Counselling and psychotherapy: Integrating skills theory and practice* (3rd ed.). New Jersey: Prentice Hall International.

Jeynes, W. (2007). The relationship between parental involvement and urban secondary school student academic achievement: A meta-analysis. *Urban Education*, 42, 82–110.

Johnson, R. S. (2002). *Using data to close the achievement gap: How to measure equity in our schools*. Thousand Oaks, CA: Corwin.

Jones, A. J. (1963). *Principles of guidance* (5th ed.). New York: McGraw Hill Company Inc.

Kochhar, S. K. (1984). *Guidance & counseling in colleges & universities*. New Delhi: Sterling Publishers Pvt. Ltd.

Miranda, A., Webb, L., Brigman, G., & Peluso, P. (2007). Student success skills: A promising program to close the academic achievement gaps of African American and Latino Students. *Professional School Counseling*, 10, 490–497.

Nanda S. K. (1985). *Educational psychology*. Jalandhar: New Academics Publishing Co.

Newman, B. M., Lohman B. J., Myers, M. C., & Newman P. R. (2000). Experiences of urban youth navigating the transition to ninth grade. *Journal of Youth and Society*, 31, 387–416.

Newman, B. M., Myers, M. C., Newman, P. R., Lohman, B. J., & Smith, V. L. (2000). The transition to high school for academically promising, urban, low-income African American youth. *Adolescence*, 35, 45–66.

Pasricha P. (1976). *Guidance and counseling in Indian education*. National Council of Educational Research and Training.

Poynton, T. A., Carlson, M. W., Hopper, J. A., & Carey, J. C. (2006). Evaluating the impact of an innovative approach to integrate conflict resolution into the academic curriculum on middle school students' academic achievement. *Professional School Counseling*, 9, 190–196.

Rosatl, G., & Marianmett, M. (2001). *Introduction to guidance and counselling* (6th ed.). New York: Publishers.

Schellenberg, R. (2008). *The new school counselor: Strategies for universal academic achievement*. Lanham, MD: Rowman Littlefield Education.

Schellenberg, R., & Grothaus, T. (2009). Promoting cultural responsiveness and closing the achievement gap with standards blending. *Professional School Counseling*, 12, 440–449.

Schellenberg, R., & Grothaus, T. (2011). Using culturally competent responsive services to improve student achievement and behavior. *Professional School Counseling*, 14, 222–230.

Sciarra, D. T. (2010). Predictive factors in intensive math course-taking in high school. *Professional School Counseling*, 13, 196–207.

Shields, L. (1975). Crisis intervention: Implications for the nurses. *Journal of Psychiatric Nurses*, 13, 37.

Sink, C. A. (2009). School counselors as accountability leaders: Another call for action. *Professional School Counseling*, 13, 68–74.

Stuart, G. W. (2009). *Principles and practice of psychiatric nursing* (9th ed.). (pp. 184–193). St. Louis, MO: Saunders Elsevier.

Stone, C. B., & Dahir, C. A. (2011). *School counselor accountability: A measure of student success* (3rd ed.). Boston, MA: Pearson.

Suri S. P., & Sodhi, T. S. (2006). *Guidance and counseling* (3rd ed.). Patiala: Bawa publications Pvt. Ltd.

Trusty, J., Mellin, E. A., & Herbert, J. T. (2008). Closing achievement gaps: Roles and tasks of elementary school counselors. *Elementary School Journal*, 108, 407–421.

Tucker, C., Dixon, A., & Griddine, K. (2010). Academically successful African American male urban high school students' experiences of mattering to others at school. *Professional School Counseling*, 14, 135–145.

Villalba, J. A., Akos, P., Keeter, K., & Ames, A. (2007). Promoting Latino student achievement and development through the ASCA National Model. *Professional School Counseling*, 12, 272–279.

Walia, J. S. (1982). *Foundations of educational psychology*. Jalandhar: Paul Publishers.

Webb, L. D., & Brigman, G. A. (2006). Student success skills: Tools and strategies for improved academic and social outcomes. *Professional School Counseling*, 10, 112–120.

Weinbaum, A. T., Allen, D., Blythe, T., Simon, K., Seidel, S., & Rubin, C. (2004). *Teaching as inquiry: Asking hard questions to improve student achievement*. New York: Teachers College Press.

West-Olatunji, C., Shure, L, Pringle, R., Adams, T., Lewis, D., & Cholewa, B. (2010). Exploring how school counselors position low-income African American girls as mathematics and science learners. *Professional School Counseling*, 13, 184–195.

Young, A., & Kaffenberger, C. J. (2011). The beliefs and practices of school counselors who use data to implement comprehensive school counseling programs. *Professional School Counseling*, 15, 67–76.

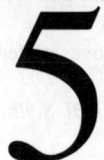
Principles and philosophies of education

Since philosophy is the art which teaches us how to live, and since children need to learn it as much as we do at other ages, why do we not instruct them in it?
—De Montaigne

LEARNING OBJECTIVES

This chapter is designed to enable the reader to:

- Understand the Indian and international concept of education.
- Identify the aims and functions of education and nursing education.
- Define philosophies of education.
- Explain the interdependence of philosophy and education.
- Classify the traditional and modern philosophies of education.
- Describe traditional and modern philosophies of education.

KEY TERMS

INTRODUCTION

According to Albert Einstein, education is what remains after one has forgotten what one learned in school. Education may be looked upon as the process of providing desirable knowledge and experience to a child to develop his inner powers to the maximum possible extent which helps the child lead a full and worthy life. It is a process of training the individual through various experiences of life, so as to draw out the best in him.

MEANING OF EDUCATION

The term *education* has its origin in the Latin words *educo, educare* and *educatum*. Etymologically, the word *education* is derived from the Latin words *educo* where *e* means 'out of' and *duco* means 'I lead.' According to this view, *education* means 'I lead out of darkness into brightness'.

In another perspective, the word education is derived from the Latin word *educare* which refers to breed, to bring up and to rear.

Also, *educatum* denotes education that means 'an act of teaching or training'.

Therefore, education means to lead, to lead forth or to unfold the hidden talents of man. It is very much the art of developing and cultivating the various powers of mind, physical, mental and moral.

I. INDIAN CONCEPT OF EDUCATION

In India, disciplining the mind and imparting knowledge have always been the foremost priorities. There are various synonyms prevailing in the Indian society for the word *education*.

- One of them is *shiksha* which is derived from the Sanskrit root *shas* referring to 'discipline', 'control', instruct' or 'teach'.
- Another synonym of the word *education* is *vidya*, which is derived from the Sanskrit root *vid*, which means 'to know'. Vidya is thus the subject matter of knowledge.
- It is mentioned in the Upanishads that the end product of education is salvation. Also, it is stated in the *Bhagwad Gita* that nothing is more purifying on the earth than knowledge.

II. DEFINITIONS OF EDUCATION BY INDIAN PHILOSOPHERS

Famous Indian philosophers or educationists have given the following concepts of education with their own meanings:

Education means the training for the country and love for the nation.

—Chanakya

Education is realization of self.

—Shankaracharya

Education is self-realization and service of the people.

—Guru Nanak Dev

Education is the manifestation of divine perfection already existing in man; education means the exposition of man's complete individuality.

—Swami Vivekananda

Education means enabling the mind to find out that ultimate truth which emancipates us from the bondage of dust and gives us the wealth not of things but of inner light, not of power but of love, making the truth its own and giving expression to it.

—Rabindranath Tagore

Education is an all-round drawing out of the best in child and man—body, mind and spirit.

—**Mahatma Gandhi**

III. DEFINITIONS OF EDUCATION BY INTERNATIONAL PHILOSOPHERS

Education has been viewed in various ways by philosophers or educationists internationally as given below:

Education is the capacity to feel pleasure and pain at right moment. It develops in the body and in the soul of the pupil all beauty and all perfection which he is capable of.

—**Plato**

Education is the process of living through a continuous reconstruction of experiences. It is the development of all those capacities in the individual which will enable him to control his environment and fulfil his possibilities.

—**John Dewey**

Education is the natural, harmonious and progressive development of man's innate power.

—**Pestalozzi**

Education is the deliberate and systematic influence, exerted by the mature person upon the immature through instruction, discipline and harmonious development of physical, intellectual, aesthetic, social and spiritual powers of the human being according to their essential hierarchy, by and for the individual and social uses and directed towards the union of educand with his creator as the final end.

—**Redden and Ryan**

AIMS OF EDUCATION

Education is a purposeful and planned activity undertaken by the educator and the learner for achieving clearly defined objectives or ends in view. Without an end or objective no purposeful activity will have the real force which directs it and makes it meaningful. An aim is a predetermined goal which determines the individual to attain it through appropriate activities. Some suggested aims of education are discussed below (Fig. 5.1):

- **Individual aim:** Education should aim at the training and development of an individual. Only a well-trained individual can understand his rights and obligations towards the society. Biologists recognize every individual as different from another. Naturalists make nature supreme which would make an individual what he ought to be. Psychologists favour flexible curriculum development based on individual mental capacity and emotional disposition. Though qualities of individual aim, criticism says that it makes education selfish and self-centred and ignores society and culture. Some important individual aims of education are as follows:
  - Development as an individual of a human being
  - Moral and spiritual development
  - Cultural development

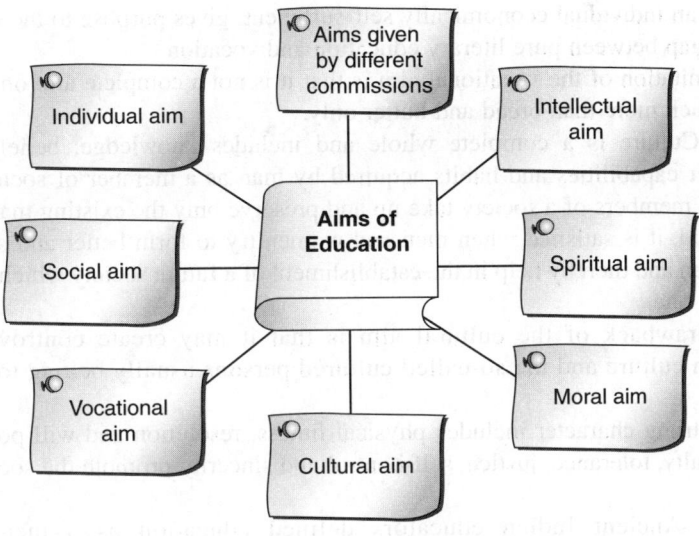

FIGURE 5.1

Aims of education.

- Harmonious development
- Promote positive physical development
- Provide a sense of complete living
- Development of a right personality
- Development of good citizenship
- Development of good leadership
- Vocational development of an individual
- Emotional and mental development
- Create national consciousness
- Promote good social development
- Character building

- **Social aim:** An individual is born with certain potential and natural endowments. It is the task of education to develop these into distinct individual personality. Personality development does not take place in a vacuum. It takes place in association with others, in cooperative living and in working together for the welfare of group or society. As per historical evidences, in ancient Sparta, it was believed that each individual was born not for himself but for his country. A socially efficient individual conforms to certain standards of conduct known as *moral conduct*. John Dewey once said that in the democratic and technological environment the aim of education should be to enable the individual to control his environment and fulfil his responsibilities. He further added that all education proceeds by the participation of an individual in the social consciousness of race. This process begins almost at birth and is continually shaping individual powers.

   The critics consider the social aim makes an individual only a tool of the government. The extreme notion of an all-powerful state or society ignores the legitimate needs, desires and interests of the individual and suppresses his creative power.

- **Vocational aim:** Education should have a utilitarian aim. This means that education should help an individual earn his livelihood himself which is an essential function of life that cannot be ignored.

This aim makes an individual economically self-sufficient, gives purpose to the educational activity and bridges the gap between pure literary education and vocation.

The major limitation of the vocational aim is that it is not a complete aim on its own as life and education are much more than bread and butter only.

- **Cultural aim:** Culture is a complete whole and includes knowledge, belief, art, morals, law, custom and other capabilities and habits acquired by man as a member of society. True education is not satisfied if members of a society take up and preserve only the existing manners and customs. On the other hand, it is satisfied when men and women try to form better and still better habits of thought and action and thereby help in the establishment of a future society which is an improvement over the existing one.

  The major drawback of the cultural aim is that it may create controversies as there is high diversity in culture and the so-called cultured persons usually belong to the high strata of society.

- **Moral aim:** A strong character includes physical fitness, resolution and will power. Moral virtues like honesty, loyalty, tolerance, justice, self-control and sincerity promote the social efficiency of an individual.

- **Spiritual aim:** Ancient Indian educators defined education as a means for salvation. Dr Radhakrishnan said that the aim of education is neither national efficiency nor world solidarity but making individual feel that he has within himself something deeper than intellect, call it spirit, if you like. But spiritual aim does not find any place in the western education system.

  The criticism follows the spiritual aim by mentioning that it might lead us to an attitude of escapism, renunciation of the world and complete inaction. Only the realization and preaching of this philosophy is not enough but practising it in daily life is also mandatory.

- **Intellectual aim:** Education in ancient times did not have much vocational aim but emphasized mostly on the development of intellectual powers and imbibing culture. Knowledge aim is the exact antithesis of vocational aim. The former glorifies material possessions while the latter emphasizes intellectual possessions.

- **Aims of education as stated by Secondary Education Commission, 1952–53:** The Secondary Education Commission formulated the following aims of education:
  - *Development of democratic citizenship:* It includes developing clear thinking, clear speech and writing, receptivity to new ideas, social justice, tolerance, patriotism and internationalism.
  - *Improvement of vocational efficiency:* It refers to the appreciation of dignity of work and promotion of technical skills.
  - Development of personality by inculcating creative energy, interest and the development of hobbies.
  - Development of qualities of leadership.

- **Aims of education as stated by Kothari Commission Report, 1966:** This report gave a four-fold aim of our national education system which are as follows:
  - Increasing productivity
  - Achieving social and national integration
  - Accelerating the process of modernization
  - Cultivating social, moral and spiritual values

- **Aims of education as stated by Education Commission, 1964–66:** It mentioned a five-fold programme on educational aims which are stated below:
  - Relating education to productivity
  - Strengthening social and national integration
  - Consolidation of democracy through education
  - Development of social, moral and spiritual values
  - Modernization of society through the awakening of society through curiosity, development of attitudes and values and building up certain essential skills.

I. AIMS OF NURSING EDUCATION

Nursing education has its aims in common with the aims of education in general as well as specific. The nursing education aims are determined by the health needs of the society, needs of students, philosophy of nursing, current trends in education and nursing and advancement in science and technology. The many nursing aims are listed below:

- *Intellectual aim:* Theoretical and practical knowledge is essential for rendering intelligent and efficient nursing services. Professional nursing practice is based on scientific principles and evidence-based practice.
- *Leadership aim:* Nurses plan, organize and manage health care activities and programmes. They have to evaluate the quality and structure of health care services. They have to coordinate and collaborate on the health care services. Thus, education aims at identifying potential nursing leaders.
- *Professional development aim:* Each individual nurse should be educated in a manner to enable her to develop the appropriate skills and attitude essential for professional practice.
- *Personality development aim:* Nursing education should aim at an all-round development of the individual in all aspects. The nurse should grow and develop as a person of self-awareness, self-direction and self-motivation.
- *Generating and utilizing research evidences:* Evidence-based practice and ongoing research is vital for the growth of the nursing profession. Therefore, nursing education must pay emphasis on the utilization and development of resource evidence.
- *Ensuring a safe, quality and cost-effective case:* It is the prime responsibility of the nursing education that it equip its professionals to provide safe, quality and cost-effective care to the common man.

II. FACTORS AFFECTING AIMS OF EDUCATION

Educational aims are affected by certain factors such as philosophy of life, elements of human nature, religious reasons, political ideology, socioeconomic reasons, cultural reasons and the intention of exploring new knowledge, which are described as follows (Fig. 5.2):

- *Philosophy of life:* Both educational aims and philosophy of life are very closely related just like two facets of the same coin. Education is the best means of propagation of the philosophy of life and philosophy gives the basis for aims of education.
- *Elements of human nature:* Human nature is always considered for determining educational aims. Idealism infolding divinity in man is considered as the main aim of education.

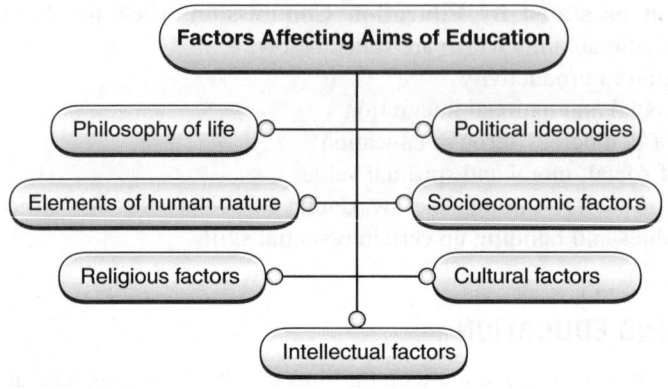

FIGURE 5.2

Factors affecting aims of education.

- *Religious factors:* Religion is an inseparable determinant of educational aims. In India, Buddhism focuses on adoption of *ahimsa* and truth in the education system and Sikhism focuses on patriotism as the aim of education.
- *Political ideologies:* Political ideologies certainly have a say in determining educational aims. The educational aims of a democratic political system can be quite different from that of an autocratic political set-up.
- *Socioeconomic factors:* These factors play an important role affecting the aims of education. The social system, social ideology and economy of a country are important factors to affect the aims of education.
- *Cultural factors:* Education plays an important role in transmitting cultural heritage and traditions from one generation to another. Culture also develops educational aims by itself.
- *Intellectual factors:* As education is fully scientific today, it has to aim at exploring new information and knowledge.

FUNCTIONS OF EDUCATION

Education is the process of living through a continuous reconstruction of experiences. It is the development of all those capacities in an individual which will enable him to control his environment and fulfil his possibilities. A child is born with certain endowments which are developed in accordance with the demands of the society through education. Education enables the child to manipulate his environment. Thus, education provides important functions towards the individual as well as the society. Functions of education can solely be for an individual or towards the society and nation at large. Some essential functions of education are discussed below (Fig. 5.3):

I. FUNCTION OF EDUCATION TOWARDS AN INDIVIDUAL

Education participates in the growth and direction of an individual as described below:

- *Growth and development of individual:* Johann Heinrich Pestalozzi said when we leave the earth carelessly to nature, it bears weeds and thistles. The same way when we leave child's education to

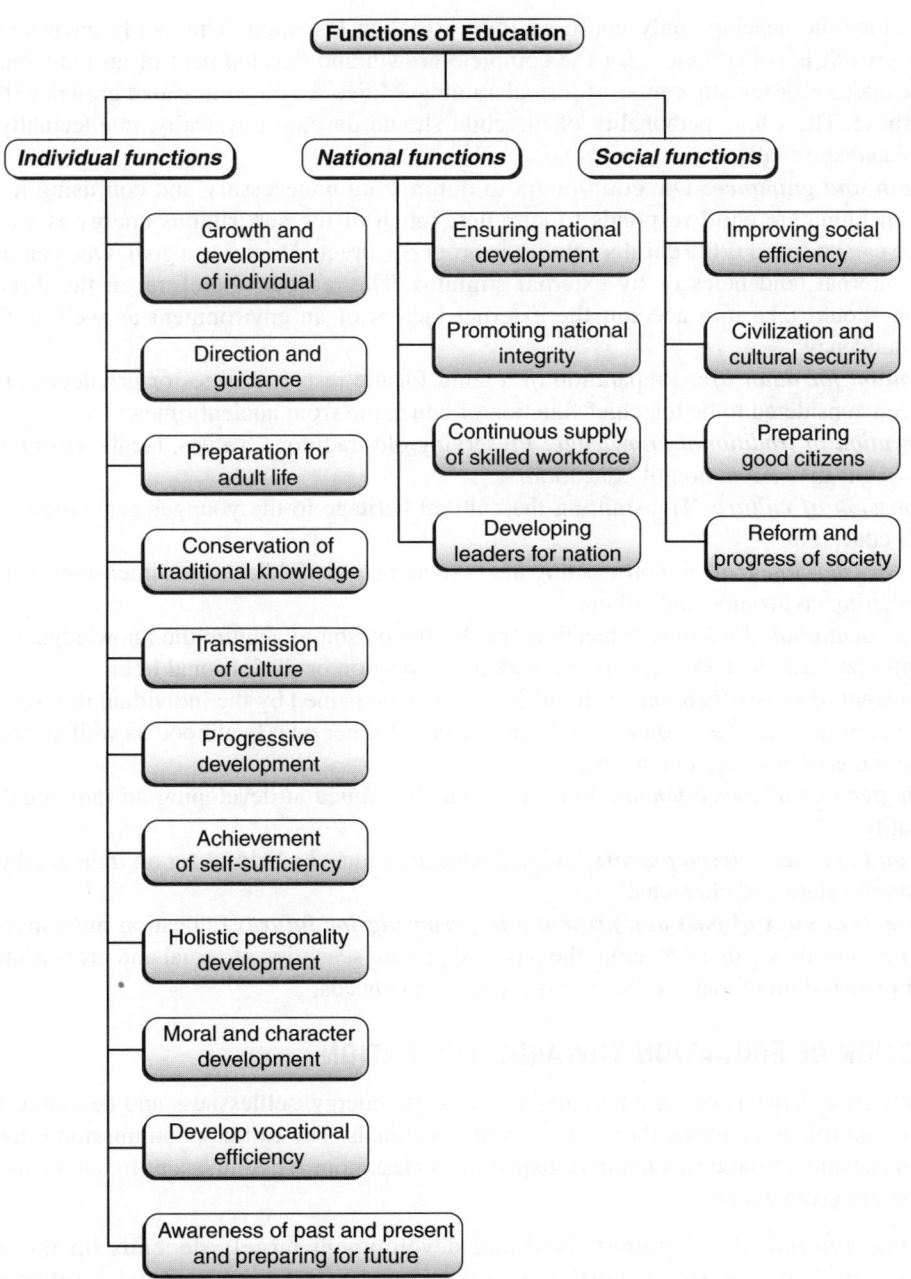

FIGURE 5.3

Functions of education.

nature alone, he develops only confused impressions in his mind. Thus, only environmental and natural growth is not sufficient for the complete growth and development of an individual. To this must be added a systematic course of formal training. Moreover, only one-sided growth will not serve the purpose. The whole personality of the child should develop physically, intellectually, morally, socially and spiritually.

- *Direction and guidance:* Direction refers to minimizing unnecessary and confusing movements. When an immature child responds to stimulus, much of the superfluous energy is wasted. This wastage can be saved if the child's activity is properly directed towards a goal. One can be directed by his internal tendencies or by external stimulus. The teacher, therefore, in the direction programme should take into account the external factors of an environment as well as the child's inborn tendency.
- *Preparation for adult life:* Preparation of a child for the responsibilities or privileges of adult life have been considered to be the chief function of education from ancient times.
- *Conservation of traditional knowledge:* Preserving old traditions, values, ideals, customs and way of thinking is also a function of education.
- *Transmission of culture:* Transmitting the cultural heritage to the younger generation is achieved through education.
- *Progressive development:* Reconstructing new experiences, unfolding new dimensions of knowledge and furthering civilization and culture.
- *Develop vocational efficiency:* Education enables the person to acquire the knowledge and skills to efficiently perform the tasks related to a particular vocation or professional field.
- *Achievement of self-sufficiency:* Self-sufficiency can be gained by the individual through education because after the due education person is able to earn for her own livelihood as well as become cognitively and economically independent.
- *Holistic personality development:* Education must be aimed at developing an individual's holistic personality.
- *Moral and character development:* An ideal education must be helpful for an individual to develop good moral values and character.
- *Creating awareness of past and present and preparing for future:* Education must make an individual become knowledgeable about the past and present scenarios of social and professional pursuit as well prepare him to manage future expectations and needs.

II. FUNCTION OF EDUCATION TOWARDS THE NATION

National progress depends on an individual's hard work, energy, selflessness and devotion. Education plays important role to inculcate these qualities in individuals. The Kothari Commission Report rightly said that the destiny of India was being reshaped in its classroom. The important functions of education for a nation are given below:

- *Ensuring national development:* National development largely depends on the education of a country. It is directly proportional to the literacy rate as well as availability of human resources.
- *Promoting national integrity:* India is a country of diversity having a strong sense of casteism, communalism, provincialism, regionism and linguistic antagonism that could serve as barriers to national integration. Education can be helpful in breaking these barriers and can promote national integration.

- *Continuous supply of skilled workforce to the nation:* Every country requires a skilled workforce for the smooth functioning of its service sector. It is the main national function of education to ensure the continuous supply of skilled workforce to the country.
- *Developing leaders for the nation:* Leaders are the main role players in the overall development of a country. Leaders are essentially required in social, economic, political and cultural sectors and education can realize this requirement by preparing leaders to meet a country's present and future needs.

III. FUNCTION OF EDUCATION TOWARDS THE SOCIETY

As biological life maintains and transmits by nutrition and reproduction, the same way social life is maintained by education. Education is necessary and an inevitable result of the society's needs to guide the growth and development of its younger members to produce an improved generation. History bears evidence that as education advances, civilization also advances. Some selected social functions of education are as follows:

- *Improving social efficiency:* Education ensures the overall holistic development of individuals, who could be good individuals in a society. It ultimately promotes social efficiency and the society flourishes in the right direction.
- *Civilization and cultural security:* Education teaches individual gain civic sense so that a positive civilization can be expected for its members. In addition, education must ensure cultural security so that important traditional culture can be preserved and utilized by the future generations.
- *Preparing good citizens:* The main function of education is to prepare good citizens in a country so that a civilized society can be expected and each individual has the privilege of enjoying full social freedom, human honour and rights.
- *Reform and progress of society:* The progress of a society primarily depends on education. Mahatma Gandhi once said that education acts as fertilizer for social growth and progress. Growth is the law of nature and human existence requires reforms to meet new demands and needs. Therefore, social reform and progress of a society is also one of the important functions of education.

PHILOSOPHIES OF EDUCATION

The term *philosophy* has a Greek origin, i.e. *philosophia*, which is made up of two words, viz. *phileo* and *sophia*. *Phileo* means 'love' and *sophia* means 'wisdom'. The literal meaning of *philosophy* is 'love of wisdom' or 'passion of learning'.

I. DEFINITIONS OF PHILOSOPHY

It is said that education without philosophy is blind and philosophy without education is invalid (Thomas, 1968). Philosophy is the earliest and the most original intellectual discipline. It is one of the oldest and most respected disciplines of knowledge. It is rather difficult to define philosophy in a way that is universally acceptable. Some of the most accepted and prevailing definitions of philosophy are given below.

Philosophy is the science of knowledge.

—Fitch

Philosophy is the science of sciences.

—Coleridge

Philosophy is a search for comprehensive view of nature, an attempt at a universal explanation of the nature of things.

—Alfred Weber

Philosophy is critical reviewing of just those familiar things.

—John Dewey

Philosophy is the critical science of universal values.

—Windlband

Philosophy is concerned with everything as a universal science.

—Herbert Spencer

Philosophy is a persistent effort of both ordinary and pertinent people to make life as intelligible and meaningful as possible.

—Bramold

Philosophy, like science, consistent of theories of insight arrived at as a result of systemic reflection.
—Joseph A. Leighton

II. PHILOSOPHY, EDUCATION AND THEIR INTERDEPENDENCE

Philosophy and education are interdependent in nature and that can be clearly understood from the following facts (Fig. 5.4):

- The philosophy of great philosophers reflects from their educational systems and they are great educators of their times.
- Education and philosophy have a common end, i.e. wisdom and common means directed towards the end, i.e. inquiry. Separation of philosophy and education would frustrate wisdom. Philosophy can provide the direction and guidance to behave intelligently in the educational process.
- For the educator, philosophy aims at improving the quality of life because it helps us gain a wider perspective on human existence and the world around us.
- The chief task of philosophy is to state the aspects of a good life whereas for education the chief task is how to make life worth living. So, philosophy and education are mutually reconstructive, i.e. they function with a mutual give and take.
- Philosophy handles goals while education provides the means to achieve those goals. In this sense, philosophy of education is a distinct but not a separate discipline. The process of philosophizing about education requires an understanding of education and its problems.

Ross stated that philosophy is the contemplative side while education is the active side. It can be concluded that philosophy is the theory while education is the practice. Practice unguided by theory is aimless and inconsistent just as theory which cannot be translated into practice is useless and confusing.

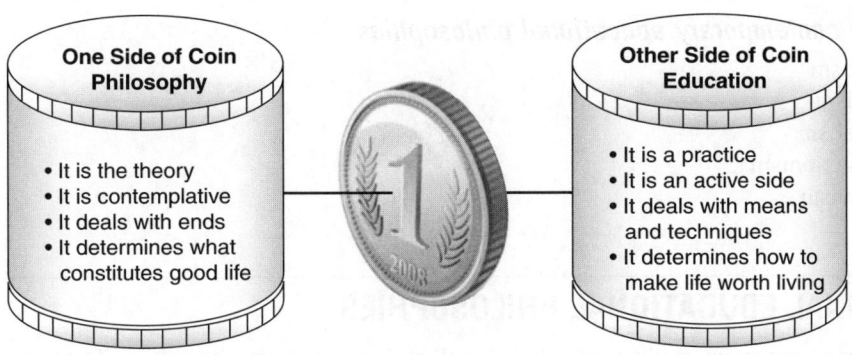

FIGURE 5.4

Interdependence of philosophy and education as two faces of a coin.

III. CLASSIFICATION OF EDUCATIONAL PHILOSOPHIES

There are various schools of educational philosophies. Some of the main traditional and modern contemporary educational philosophies are discussed below (Fig. 5.5):

A. Traditional educational philosophies

- Naturalism
- Idealism
- Pragmatism
- Realism

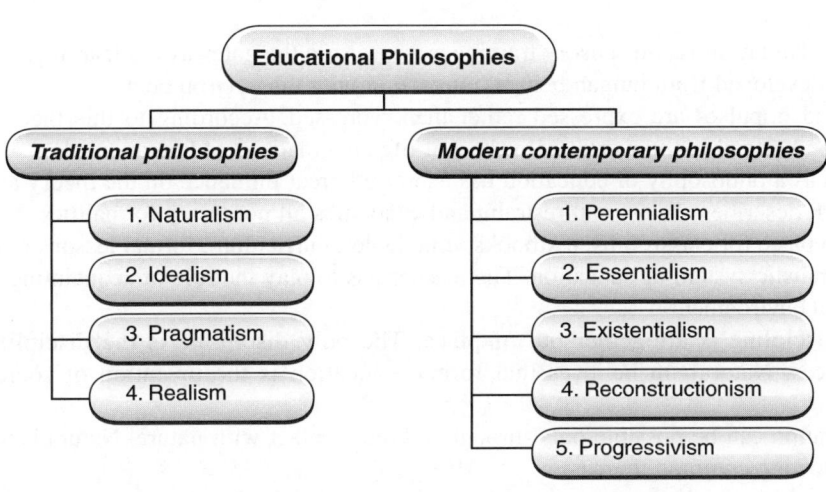

FIGURE 5.5

Classification of educational philosophies.

B. Modern contemporary educational philosophies

- Perennialism
- Essentialism
- Existentialism
- Reconstructionism
- Progressivism

TRADITIONAL EDUCATIONAL PHILOSOPHIES

In this chapter, the main traditional educational philosophies are discussed. These are naturalism, idealism, pragmatism and realism (a brief review may be seen in Table 5.1).

I. NATURALISM

The basic concepts of naturalism are as follows:

- The concept of *naturalism* as a philosophy of education occurred during the 18th century.
- Naturalism is based on the basic assumption that nature as a total system explains all existence including human beings and human nature.
- According to naturalists the material and the physical world is governed by certain laws, and man, who is the creator of the material world, must submit to it.
- It denies the existence of anything beyond nature, behind nature and other than nature such as supernaturalism.
- In terms of epistemology or theory of knowledge, naturalists highlight the value of scientific knowledge.
- Francis Bacon emphasizes the inductive method for acquiring scientific knowledge through specific observation, accumulation and generalization. He also lays emphasis on empirical and experimental knowledge.
- Naturalists also lay stress on sensory training as senses are the gateways to learning.
- Values are developed from human beings' interaction with the environment.
- Instincts and impulses are expressed rather than repressed. According to this theory, there is no absolute good or evil in the world. All values of life are creations of human needs.
- Naturalism as a philosophy of education has exercised great influence on the theory and practice of education. It describes all external restraint and condemns all necessary formalities.
- There is no place for classrooms, textbooks, time tables, curriculum, formal lessons or examinations in the naturalistic system of education. The teacher has to play the role of acquainting children with their natural environment.
- External discipline is altogether out of place. The only discipline is the discipline of natural consequences. Naturalism believes that formal education is the invention of society and so is artificial.
- Good education can be possible only through a direct contact with nature. Naturalism in education has the following common themes:
  - Look to nature and human nature as part of the natural order for the purposes of education.
  - The key to understanding nature is through the senses. Sensation is the basis of our knowledge of reality.
  - Because nature's processes are slow, gradual and evolutionary, our education should be steady too.

Table 5.1 Brief Description About Traditional Philosophies of Education

Concept of Philosophy	Organization and Aims of Education	Curriculum	Methods of Education	Role of Teacher	Discipline
1. Naturalism: Chief proponents were Rabindranath Tagore, Jean Jacques Rousseau, Johann Heinrich, Pestalozzi and Herbert Spencer					
Educating the human generations about and in the nature rather than artificial environment by keeping in mind the individuality of each child.	Nature is considered the classroom. Emphasis on open air schools to teach through direct experience with nature.	Basis of curriculum development was child's nature, interest and needs. Stressed on subjects dealing with nature such as physics, chemistry, biology, language and mathematics. Tagore also stressed on teaching spiritual values of nature.	As natural as possible considering individual differences. Noble efforts for planned living with nature. Direct experience of nature through observation, excursion, experimentation, play–way and Dalton plan methods.	Teacher is an observer and facilitator of the child to develop in nature; teacher facilitates best possible natural environment for prompt learning.	No emphasis on external rigid discipline; recommended free discipline to child in nature for optimum desired learning.
2. Idealism: Chief proponents were Dr Radhakrishnan, Sir Aurobindo, Plato, Ross and Socrates					
It believes that the act of knowing takes place within the mind for three values, i.e. intellectual, aesthetic and moral values and the purpose of education is the development of the student's mind and self.	Well-planned formal classrooms or formal place of teaching–learning activity is recommended.	The basis of curriculum is inculcating intellectual, aesthetic and moral values or discipline. The intellectual value is represented by subjects such as language, literature, science, mathematics, history and geography; aesthetic through arts and poetry and moral through religion, ethics and metaphysics. Dr Radhakrishnan also advocated for physical education.	Idealism recommended formal classroom teaching methods such as lecture, discussion, presentation and group interaction. Knowledge is transferred from the more mature person (teacher) to the less mature person (pupil) through formal and well-planned teaching–learning methods.	Teacher is considered as centre of education where pupil catches fire from teacher who is himself a flame. Teacher must be ideal and a role model for the child both intellectually and morally. The teacher should exercise great creative skills in providing opportunity for the pupil's mind to discover, analyse, unify, synthesize and creative application of knowledge to life.	Idealism believes in interconnection of discipline and interest. Advocates discipline for self-realization of individual. It does not favour rigid discipline but advocates spontaneous and self-discipline.

Continued

Table 5.1 Brief Description About Traditional Philosophies of Education—cont'd

Concept of Philosophy	Organization and Aims of Education	Curriculum	Methods of Education	Role of Teacher	Discipline
3. Pragmatism: Chief proponents were Williams James, John Dewey, Charles Sanders Pierce, S Kil Patrick and Margaret H					
It considers self-activity as the basis of all teaching–learning processes in context of cooperative activity; to create optimistic men, who are the architects of their own fate by the process of their efforts. Education should be according to the child's aptitudes and abilities, where he is respected and education is planned to cater to his inclinations and capacities; however he develops in social context.	Aim of education is to teach one how to think so that one can adjust to an ever-changing society. In order to produce creative, resourceful and adaptable children we should have conditions in the school which are conducive to the creation of these qualities of mind. Recommends formal schools to have activity-oriented learning based on the needs, interest, aptitude and capabilities of the individual student.	Pragmatists believe in a broad and diversified curriculum, which is composed of both content and process and subjects ranging from humanities to geography and sciences.	Teaching–learning process is a social process where the sharing of experiences between the teacher and the student takes place. Preferred methods are project method and activity-oriented learning.	Role of a teacher is not that of a dictator or a task master but as a leader of group activities. Teacher acts as catalyst where he suggests a problem to students and stimulates them to find a solution. Teacher is a mentor with resources to guide the students.	Pragmatism does not believe in traditional firm discipline, however it advocates for freedom of self-discipline in a free and conducive teaching–learning environment.
4. Realism: Chief proponents were Aristotle, Johann Friedrich Herbart, Herbert Spencer, John Locke and Franklin Bobbitt					
Realism makes the human being understand and enjoy society in the true sense by getting the multidimensional real joy of life in reality. It also aims for education to make the life of a man useful, where a man can enjoy his activities and comfort in reality. Education should equip individuals to a best possible meaningful life through	Realism emphasizes on scientific attitude based on realistic principles, where the child can extend his knowledge, which he learns through books. It has given due emphasis on formal schools, which provides adequate opportunity for learners to learn the vocational skills through observation, experimentations and examinations	Selection of the curriculum for the students must be based on their abilities, interest and capabilities so that education helps the student to adjust to changing circumstances of the society. It also emphasizes on subject matters of real-life use such as science, mathematics, hygiene and vocational subjects. Vocational content has given prominent stress on the curriculum.	Realism believes in objectivity, knowledge of scientific evidences and reality. Methods of teaching should be according to needs, interest and capabilities of students. Vocational education should equip the individual with capacities to earn livelihood such as experimentation, examination and observation.	Teachers must focus on the development of vocational skills in the learners, so that they can be equipped with qualities of race preservation and vocational behaviour activities. Teacher acts as a mentor, and must be a role model and skilled to demonstrate vocational skills to the learners.	Realism believes in an optimum level of discipline without imposing undue stress on the learners.

A. Chief proponents of naturalism

There are many great names associated with naturalism but the eminent ones are as follows:

- Jean Jacques Rousseau
- Johann Heinrich Pestalozzi
- Herbert Spencer
- Rabindranath Tagore

B. Naturalism and aims of education

The main aims of education according to naturalism are given below:

- Development of self-realization, self-expression and self-preservation in children.
- Cultivating self-restrain and a sense of moral values.
- Making a child adjust himself both physically and psychologically to his immediate environment and to the challenging surroundings in his life.
- Equipping the child to struggle for existence and ensuring his survival by making him the fittest.
- Promoting better humanity through the transmission of not only physical characteristics but also moral values.
- Promoting the perfect development of individuality in a child through the development of natural endowments, into a joyous, rational, balanced, useful and natural person.
- Customizing the teaching–learning process according to the child's nature, tenderness, capacities, likes and dislikes.

C. Naturalism and organization of education

- According to naturalists, the existence of school is a natural necessity. All of us know that man is the most dependent creature of God as compared to other animals because of the long period of infancy and a child's consequent dependence on adults. The offsprings of other animals have negligible periods of infancy, whereas the human offspring requires at least a few years to perform simple functions of day-to-day living. Because of this important dimension of the dependent nature of man, education becomes an urgent necessity and so do educational institutions like schools.
- Naturalism attaches less importance to the existence of a formal school and textbooks because it hinders the natural development of children. For Rousseau 'everything is good as it comes from the hands of author of nature, but everything degenerates in the hands of man.' According to him, nature is the only pure, clean and ennobling influence. Human society is thoroughly corrupt. Therefore, a man should be freed from the bondage of society, and he should be prepared to live in the state of nature. Human nature is essentially good, and it must be given full opportunities for free development in a free atmosphere.
- Gandhi's philosophy of education is also naturalistic in setting as he believes in the essential goodness of a child's nature. According to him, children should be educated in an atmosphere of freedom, freedom from superimposed restriction and interferences. His main emphasis is on activity or learning by doing and he shows an aversion to artificiality and pedantry. Being a naturalist, he attempts to liberate education from the four walls of the classroom and wishes it be given in a wider sphere of the natural surroundings of a child.

D. Naturalism and methods of education

- The school to the naturalist is in no way different from the home; Frobel called the school as *kindergarten* or *garden for children* whereas Montessori calls it *Case-de-Bambini* or *home for* the children.

- According to Pestalozzi, there should be no difference between school and home. Tagore also believes that education given in natural surroundings develops intimacy with the world. He puts more faith on the individual rather than institutions. Nature, to him, is the focus where the interests and aspirations of human beings meet. It is therefore essential not only to know nature, but to live in nature. *School*, according to him, is like a large home where the children and teachers live together with their families sharing a common life of high aspirations, planned living and noble efforts in contact with nature on one hand, and with the spirit of joy on the other.
- Naturalism also believes in the principle of individual differences which means that every child has a unique capacity to acquire knowledge. The pace of learning is also unique. The school should have respect for personal diversity and it should cater to the varied and different interests of the child.
- Naturalists advocate the methods of teaching that offer the child an opportunity for self-education, self-expression, creative activity and integrated growth in an atmosphere of unrestrained freedom.

E. Naturalism and curriculum

- Naturalists emphasize the study of sciences dealing with nature such as physics, chemistry, biology, zoology and botany.
- They also give importance to the study of language and mathematics.
- Naturalism gives a very insignificant place to spiritualism in the curriculum. However, naturalists like Rabindranath Tagore do emphasize spiritual values together with the study of literature and sciences, to facilitate the harmonious development of a child.
- At the same time, teaching of religion according to Tagore can never be imparted in the form of lessons, but should be imparted by actual practice. By religion he does not mean, the religion of man or any narrow sectarianism. According to him, truth is the basis of all religions.
- Spencer, an extreme naturalist, thinks that human nature is strictly individualistic and self-preservation is the first law of life. He wants all activities to be classified in order of their importance and priority should be given to activities that minister self-preservation. Thus, he assigns a special place to *laws of life and principles of physiology* in the curriculum. He gives a very high place to science, which he considers best both for intellectual and moral discipline. According to him, all studies should be correlated with science.
- T.H. Huxley does not agree with Spencer for giving undue importance to science. He wants aesthetic culture to be imparted to children as a subject of priority.
- Rousseau promotes negative education, a typical feature of the naturalistic philosophy: the subordination of the child to natural order and his freedom from the social order. He defines negative education as one which perfects the senses that are the instruments of knowledge before giving them this knowledge directly.
- For naturalists, genuine education is based on the laws of readiness and needs of human beings. According to them child's nature, interests, and needs provide the basis of curriculum.

F. Naturalism and teacher

- According to naturalists, the teacher is not only the provider of information, ideas, ideals and will power or a moulder of character but is the observer and facilitator of the child's development. Ross stated that teacher in a naturalistic set-up is only a setter of the stage, a supplier of materials and opportunities, a provider of an ideal environment, a creator of conditions under which natural development takes place. Teacher is only a noninterfering observer.

- Like Rousseau, Tagore is also an individualist and a naturalist. He says that everyone is unique and every individual is different from another. He believes that the natural teachers, i.e. the trees, dawn, evening, moonlight, etc., nourish the child's nature spontaneously. Nature inspires human beings differently at different stages of human development. He gives an important place to the teacher because according to him a real teacher humanises the learning process and activates the mind instead of stuffing it. It is the teacher who kindles independent thinking, imagination and judgement.
- Rousseau said that the teacher should not be in a hurry to make the child learn but should be patient, permissive and nonintrusive. Demonstrating great patience, the teacher cannot tell the student what the truth is but rather must stand back and encourage a student's self-discovery. Naturalists view that the teacher is not one who stresses on books, recitations and massing information in literary forms rather he should give emphasis on learning by doing.

G. Naturalism and discipline
- Naturalism has given no emphasis on external rigid discipline. However, he recommended free discipline to child for optimum desired learning to take place in nature.
- Naturalists believed that external discipline should be altogether out of place in education. The only discipline is the discipline of natural consequences. Naturalism also believes that formal education is the invention of society which is artificial. Therefore, rigid man-made discipline must be avoided in the teaching–learning process.

II. IDEALISM

The basic concepts of idealism are as follows:

- Idealism is the oldest system of philosophy known to man. Its origin goes back to ancient India in the East and to Plato in the West. Generally, idealists believe that ideas are the true reality. According to them, the human spirit is the most important element in life.
- All of reality is reducible to one fundamental substance: spirit. The universe is viewed as essentially nonmaterial in its ultimate nature. Matter is not real; rather it is a notion, an abstraction of the mind. It is only the mind that is real. Therefore, all material things that seem to be real are reducible to mind or spirit.
- For idealists, all knowledge is independent of an experience of sense. The act of knowing takes place within the mind. The mind is active and contains innate capabilities for organizing and synthesizing the data derived through sensations.
- Idealists advocate the use of intuition for knowing the ultimate. Man can immediately apprehend some truth without making use of any of his senses. Man can also know the truth through the acts of reason and examine the logical consistency of his ideas.
- Idealists like Plato believe that the spirit of man is eternal. Whatever he knows is already contained within his spirit.
- In idealist axiology, or value theory, values are more than mere human preferences; they really exist and are inherent intrinsically in the structure of the universe. Value experience is essentially an imitation of the Good, which is present in the absolute universal realm of ideas. According to them values are eternal. They believe in three spiritual values: *the truth, the* beauty and *the goodness.* The truth is an intellectual value, the beauty an aesthetic value and the good a moral value.

- The purpose of education is the development of the mind and self of the pupil according to idealism. Idealists like to educate the child for mainly two reasons. First, education is a spiritual necessity and second education is also a social necessity. The school should emphasize on intellectual activities, moral judgement, aesthetic judgement, self-realization, individual freedom, individual responsibility and self-control in order to achieve this development.
- In essence, idealists advocate that:
  - Education is a process of unfolding and developing that which is a potential in the human person. It is unfolding of what is already enfolded.
  - Learning is a process of discovery in which the learner is stimulated to recall the truth present within the mind.
  - The teacher should be a moral and cultural exemplar or model of values that represents the highest and best expression of personal and human development.

A. Chief proponents of idealism

There are a number of great names associated with idealism, a few important ones are as follows:

- Plato
- Guru Nanak Dev Ji
- Rabindranath Tagore
- Mahatma Gandhi
- Dayananda Saraswati
- Sri Aurobindo
- Dr Sarvepalli Radhakrishnan
- Socrates
- Ross

B. Idealism and aims of education

The main aims of education according to idealism are given below.

- Exaltation of the human personality which leads to perfection in the individual.
- Ensuring self-realization of the individual towards duties of self, cleanliness, satisfaction of all desires, self-control, self-sacrifice, punctuality and regularity, avoidance of obscenity, profanity and immoral language.
- Ensuring the individual realize unity within him and establish harmony between his nature and ultimate universe. Indian idealism advocates for liberation (*mukti* or *nirvana*) as the ultimate aim of life.
- Providing a means for students to acquire achievement in art, literature, mathematics and sciences, so that a man can invent, create and produce new ideas and objects of the community and society.
- Provide an opportunity for the acquisition and enrichment of cultural heritage. Promoting the development of moral sense and moral values, so that he can distinguish between right and wrong.
- Promoting the development of self-culture, which includes polite behaviour, good manners, self-control, respect for others opinion, cooperativeness, reliability, liberality, generosity, sincerity and perseverance.
- Promoting universal education without discrimination in gender, cast, creed, religion, region, culture, country and language.

C. Idealism and organization of education

- Idealism recommends well-planned formal classrooms or a formal place for teaching–learning activity where the teacher is considered as a mature person gets an opportunity to share or transfer his knowledge to students.

D. Idealism and methods of education

- Idealism recommends formal classroom teaching methods such as lectures, discussions, presentations and group interaction, self-activity, project methods, questioning and role play.
- Knowledge is transferred from a more mature person (teacher) to a less mature person (pupil) through formal and well-planned teaching–learning methods.

E. Idealism and curriculum

- Idealism emphasizes the spiritual side of a man. For idealists, curriculum is based upon the idea or assumption of the spiritual nature of man. They are of the view that the curriculum is a body of intellectual or learned disciplines that are basically ideational or conceptual. They arrange their curriculum in the form of a hierarchy in which the general discipline occupies the top most position and gradually comes down to the particular subjects in their relationship to general discipline.
- Plato, a great exponent of idealism, conceives of the curriculum from the point of ideas. He believes that the highest idea of life is the attainment of the highest good or God; hence curriculum ought to impart inherent values to enable the educand (student) to attain his highest good. The spiritual values, according to him are truth, beauty and goodness. These three values determine three types of activities: intellectual, aesthetic and moral. Each type of activity is represented by different subjects and should form a part of the curriculum. Intellectual activities are represented by subjects such as language, literature, science, mathematics, history and geography; aesthetic activities will be possible through the study of art and poetry and moral activities are possible through the study of religion, ethics and metaphysics.
- Ross talks of two types of activities, i.e. physical and spiritual, to be included in an idealistic curriculum. Physical activities include subjects such as health and hygiene that foster physical skills (such as gymnastics and athletics) that lead to good health and fitness and thus make the pursuit of spiritual values possible. Spiritual pursuits imply intellectual, aesthetic, moral and religious studies. Hence, subjects such as history, geography, language, fine arts, morality, ethics, religion, science, mathematics and others should be included in the curriculum.
- Sri Aurobindo in his *Integral Philosophy of Education* gives importance to moral, religious and physical education. By moral education, he means the training of moral faculty, i.e. the ability to distinguish between right and wrong. Another important thing in moral education is the value of suggestion. A suggestion by the teacher has to be exercised by personal example, daily talks and *svadhyaya* or reading good books. Narration of the deeds of great men in an interesting style always makes a large amount of impression on the young minds. In addition, Aurobindo advocates that religious education should be imparted not only through religious books or religious sermons but by the practice of religious life and spiritual self-training. Theoretical teaching of religion must be complemented with actual practice. Along with moral and religious education, he stresses on the importance of physical education. With regard to physical education he says, 'if our seeking is for a total perfection of the being, the physical part of it cannot be left aside; for the body is the material basis, the body is the instrument which we have to use.'

- Another Indian idealist Dr Radhakrishnan wants to make moral education a compulsory part of education at the primary and secondary level. Without moral education, he states, 'the educational institutions cannot fulfil their objectives of educating the youth of the country.' According to him the greatness of a country cannot be measured by its physical civilization but by its moral and spiritual advancement. He also supports religious education which for him is not the instruction of a particular religion but a means for developing spiritual intuition because the aim of religion is spiritual and not merely a change in metaphysical ideas. Further he suggested the inclusion of physical education in the curriculum. In his words, 'the body is the means of the expression of the human soul; physical education therefore must be properly given.'

F. Idealism and teacher

- Idealism believes in the maxim that pupils catch fire from a teacher who is himself a flame. Idealists have high expectations of the teacher. The teacher must be ideal both intellectually and morally to serve as an example for the student. They believe that the teacher is an important ingredient in a child's education. The teacher should not only understand the stages of learning but also maintain constant concern for the ultimate purpose of learning.
- Some idealists emphasize the importance of emulation in learning. They feel the teacher should be the kind of person we want our children to become. Socrates has been used by idealists not only as a prototype of learning but also as a model for emulation.
- In this connection, Dr Radhakrishnan opines, 'the type of education which we may give to our youth depends on the fact that what type of teachers we get.' According to him, teachers have a special place in the formation of the mind and heart of the youth. Besides knowledge and scholarships, the teacher should be devoted to teaching. It is the teacher who has to provide the right environment in the school. He must be himself an ideal person in order to exercise wholesome influences on the young ones. It is the teacher's forceful personality, his effective methods, his sense of dedication to the work which encourages the child to perceive him as exemplary. The teacher must also exercise great creative skill in providing opportunities for the students' mind to discover, analyse, unify, synthesize and create applications of knowledge to life and behaviour. The teacher should respect the learner and assist the learner to realize the fullness of his or her own personality. To the idealist 'the school is a garden, the educand (student) is a tender plant, and the educator the careful gardener.'
- In the words of Ross, 'the educator constitutes the special environmental factor whose function is to lead the child nearer to reality, to guide him towards his utmost possible perfection.' J. Donald Butler has identified the desired qualities of a good teacher. According to him, the teacher should:
  - Personify culture and reality for the student
  - Be a specialist in the knowledge of the pupils
  - Be the kind of person who commands the student's respect by virtue of what he is himself
  - Be a personal friend of the individual student
  - Awaken students' desires to learn
  - Be a master of art of living
  - Be one who capably communicates on his subject
  - Appreciate the subject he teaches
  - Aid in the cultural rebirth of generations

G. Idealism and discipline

- Interest and discipline are interconnected devices of education. The concept of interest and discipline can be better understood with the help of another concept called *effort*. By interest, we mean the totally positive attraction of a child for the work at hand without any conscious or voluntary exertion and also a minimum persistence on the part of the teacher.
- Effort is the conscious and voluntary exertion by the student for doing the work without any self-interest. By discipline, we mean some extraneous action by the teacher to stimulate the pupil to complete the task in hand.
- According to Home, interest and effort cannot be distinctly separated as interest evokes effort and effort may give rise to interest. Effort is not a substitute to interest, but it supplements interest. It acts as a faithful friend. He says, 'effort is the will to do one's duty.'
- Idealist educators like Fredrick Froebel, the founder of the kindergarten, emphasize the principle of the learner's own self-activity. The learners self-activity is related to the learner's interests and willingness towards an effort. Students have their own intuitive self-interest, which attracts them to certain acts, events and objects for which they readily put in effort.
- *Gentile* finds discipline that is separated from the constructive teaching process as undesirable. According to him, discipline should be considered as an end product instead of an input and it is a part of the teaching process and should be in the teacher's personality. Teacher should achieve discipline through freedom and not conversely. But today education has bypassed this concept by beginning with discipline and moving towards freedom. Idealists do not favour rigid discipline. In fact, their theory of discipline is based on their concept of freedom. Freedom does not mean waywardness, it implies responsibility. It should be regulated, guided and restrained freedom.
- Mahatma Gandhi also believed that real freedom comes through self-discipline; discipline that arises spontaneously from the inner spring of life rather than that which is imposed from without. His concept of discipline is a synthesis of both freedom and external control. Idealists believe that human behaviour should have internal rather than external control. Discipline begins externally but ends internally through self-control.

III. PRAGMATISM

The basic concepts of pragmatism are as follows:

- Pragmatism is popularly regarded as an indigenous American philosophy. But its roots can be traced to ancient Greek philosophy.
- The term *pragmatism* is derived from the Greek word *pragma* which means 'work'. Heraclitus and Sophist of ancient Greece are considered to be pragmatic in their approach to life.
- There were other contemporaries such as Protagoras and Gorgias. The background of pragmatism is associated with the works of Francies Bacon, John Locke, Jean Jacques Rousseau and Charles Darwin. But the philosophical elements that give pragmatism a consistency and system as a philosophy in its own right are primarily the contributions of Charles Sanders Pierce, William James and John Dewey though they differ considerably in their methods and conclusions. Pierce's view of pragmatism is oriented towards physics and mathematics and Dewey's towards social science and biology. James's philosophy, on the other hand, is personal and psychological, and is motivated by religious considerations.
- Pragmatists reject metaphysics as a legitimate area of philosophical inquiry. Reality, they opine, is determined by an individual's sense experience. Man can know nothing beyond his experience. Questions

relating to the ultimate nature of man and the universe simply cannot be answered because these problems transcend one's experience. For example, there is no way for any living being to determine whether there is life after death, because one cannot experience life after death while living. Any conclusion we make about life after death in merely conjecture or a guess.

- Pragmatists believe that reality is in constant flux. There is nothing in the world which is static, permanent or eternal. According to pragmatism, knowledge based on experience is me, genuine and worthy of acquisition. Since the phenomena are constantly changing, knowledge and truth must change accordingly.
- Knowledge which is helpful in solving present-day problems is most preferred. Pragmatists emphasize on functional knowledge and understanding.
- Pragmatism does not believe in standard, permanent and eternal values. According to this philosophy, values are derived from the human condition. Because man is a part of the society the consequences of his actions are either good or bad according to their results. If the consequences are worthwhile, the value of the action is proven to be good. Thus, values in ethics and aesthetics depend on the relative circumstances of situations as they arise. Definitive values cannot exist.
- Pragmatism, being a practical and utilitarian school of philosophy, has influenced education to the maximum extent. It considers activity as the basis of all teaching and prefers self-activity in the context of cooperative activity. It creates optimistic men who are the architects of their own fate by the process of their efforts. Pragmatists want that education should be according to one's aptitudes and abilities.
- Individuals must be respected and education should be planned to cater to their inclinations and capacities. Individual development, however, must take place in a social context.
- According to pragmatism, the aim of education is to teach individuals how to think so they can adjust to an ever-changing society. To produce creative, resourceful and adaptable children, we should have conditions in the school which are conducive to the creation of these qualities of mind.
- Children should not be asked to work according to predetermined goals. They should determine their goals according to their needs and interests and in conformity with the demands of the activities that they have undertaken. For them the teaching–learning process is a social process where the sharing of experiences between the teacher and the student takes place.

A. Chief proponents of pragmatism

Many great names are associated with pragmatism but the important ones are as follows:

- Williams James
- John Dewey
- Charles Sanders Pierce
- S. Kil Patrick
- Margaret H.

B. Pragmatism and aims of education

- *All-round development of the individual:* Pragmatism believes in the holistic development of physical, psychological, social, moral and esthetical domains of an individual so that an individual's full potential can be utilized to live a fruitful life.
- *Personal and social adjustment of an individual:* Human beings are social animals; however, they have to fulfil their personal as well social needs to attain ultimate satisfaction in life. Pragmatism

believes that education must equip the individual to have a harmonious adjustment in the achievement of personal and social needs.

- *Learning through activity and experience:* Pragmatism believes that education must be based on the activity and experiences of an individual so that it can help the individual in the creation of new values, activities and experiences that are essential for a man to be a social being.
- *Reconstruction of experiences:* Pragmatism emphasizes on the adaptation of an individual on contraction and reconstruction of experiences to develop specific capabilities in an individual to control the new or existing environment.
- *Creation of new moral and aesthetic values:* The main aim of education is to develop the individual's moral and aesthetic values so that these new values can serve as a guiding path to handle and manage the new complex life environment.

C. Pragmatism and organization of education

- The aim of education in pragmatism is to teach one how to think so that one can adjust to an ever-changing society. To produce creative, resourceful and adaptable children, we should have conditions that are conducive to the creation of these qualities of mind in schools. They recommend formal schools to have activity-oriented learning based on the needs, interests, aptitude and capabilities of individual students.

D. Pragmatism and methods of education

- Pragmatism primarily believes in the principle of learning by doing, where the learner is encouraged to learn in real-life situations by self-activity, self-effort and creative activity like project methods and practice-oriented learning.
- Pragmatism also advocates for programmed learning in either real-life situations or artificial situations such as real-life laboratories or simulated laboratories for practical learning of the individuals.

E. Pragmatism and curriculum

- According to pragmatists, the focus of education is a good life in the present and future. The standard of social good is dynamic so it should be tested and verified through changing experience. John Dewey, however, is of the view that acquaintance with past experience is very important for handling the present and the future effectively.
- School curriculum should reflect the society. Pragmatism refused to the traditional approach to subject matter curriculum which is associated with formal schooling, where knowledge is fragmented or compartmentalized.
- Dewey viewed that all learning should be contextual to the given time, place and events. For example, history is taught to students without considering its relevance to everyday life.
- Dewey recommended three levels of curricular organization: (a) making and doing, (b) history and geography and (c) organized sciences.
  - The first curricular level, making and doing, engages students in activities and projects based on their experiences. This idea is similar to that of Mahatma Gandhi, who is considered as an idealist, a naturalist as well as a pragmatist. He believes in the principle of learning by doing. There is a lot of similarity between the craft-centred activities advocated by him and the project method of Dewey. Though Rabindranath Tagore is a naturalist, his views regarding curriculum are pragmatic in nature. To him, curriculum is not a number of subjects to be learnt but relevant activities to be undertaken.

- The second level curriculum, history and geography, helps in enlarging the scope and significance of the child's temporal and spatial experience to the larger community and the world.
- The third stage of curriculum is that of the organized subjects, the various sciences, i.e. bodies of tested knowledge. Pragmatists endorse a more general education than narrow specialization.

F. Pragmatism and teacher

- Pragmatism neither treats the teacher merely as a spectator like naturalism nor regards him as a pragmatist, the teacher is not a dictator or task master but a leader of group activities.
- The chief function of a pragmatic teacher is to suggest problems to his pupils and to stimulate them to find solutions. Teachers should not try and pour information and knowledge into the puppet, because what students learn depends on their own personal needs, interests and problems.
- Dewey views the teacher as a resource person who guides rather than directs learning. The teacher's role is to guide learners who need advice or assistance and the direction comes from solving particular problems. Educational aims always belong to the learner majorly rather than the teacher. Since pragmatists are concerned with teaching children how to solve problems, they should select real-life situations that encourage the problem-solving ability in children. For a problem to be solved correctly, the learner needs to establish a correct procedural sequence with the help of teacher guidance to solve a particular problem.
- A pragmatist teacher needs to be patient, friendly, enthusiastic and cooperative. Although coercion might force students to achieve immediate results, it is likely to limit the flexibility needed for future problem solving.
- The teacher's control of the learning situation is ideally indirect rather than direct. Direct control, coercion or external discipline generally fails to enlarge the learner's internal disposition and does not in any way contribute to the learner in becoming a self-corrected person.
- As a resource person, the pragmatic teacher needs to be noninterfering or what Dewey refers to as *permissive* and allow students to make errors and to experience the consequences of their actions. In this way, the teacher helps students become self-directed individuals. For Dewey, permissiveness does not mean that children's whims should dictate the curriculum. Rather, the teacher as a mature person should exercise professional judgement and expertise so that the consequences of action do not become dangerous to the students or their classmates.
- The pragmatic teacher should constantly be aware of the motivation factor. Dewey opined that children are naturally motivated and the teacher should capture and use the motivation that is already present.
- Dewey also pointed out that the teacher should respect the principle of individual differences and treats students accordingly. A pragmatic teacher wants his students to think and act for themselves, to do rather than to know and to originate rather than to repeat. The pragmatic teacher is a pragmatist first and a teacher afterwards.

G. Pragmatism and discipline

- Pragmatism advocates a discipline that can be maintained through play as work. It is the mental attitude that converts work into play and vice versa. For example, a football game becomes work if it is played due to some external pressure and difficult algebraic sums become a play if solved out of zeal.
- Pragmatism does not believe in external discipline exercised by the authority of the teacher.
- Discipline is based on the principles of child's activities and needs, and the interest of the child should be aroused and satisfied.

- Control is achieved from the cooperative aspect of shared activity, which involves working with the fellow mates.
- There is no place for rewards and punishments. In pragmatism as every activity is to be pursued in a social setting where the teacher should come down to the children's level, mix with them, share their interests and participate in their activities.

IV. REALISM

The basic concepts of realism are as follows:

- Realism is also known as *objectivism* and basically opposes idealism and has the opposite viewpoints of spiritualism. However, realism propagates for the true and real in daily life.
- Scientific development ultimately gave birth to realism, through experimentation, examination and observation, what is found true and evident and considered real and is the basis of realism. Therefore, realism is directly associated with man and society.
- Realism makes human beings understand and enjoy the society in the true sense by getting multidimensional real joy of life in reality.
- Realism aims at education in making the man's life useful, where a man can enjoy his activities and comfort in reality.
- The main types of the realism are naïve realism, representationism, neorealism and critical realism.

A. Chief proponents of realism

Many great names are associated with realism, the important ones are as follows:

- Aristotle
- Johann Friedrich Herbart
- Herbert Spencer
- John Locke
- Franklin Bobbitt

B. Realism and aims of education

Realism propagates for the following aims of education:

- Education can facilitate the individual enjoy a happy, comfortable, integrated and meaningful life.
- Franklin Bobbitt mentioned that the basic aim of education is bringing happiness in life of an individual that can be achieved by fulfilment of human responsibilities and obligations such as activities concerned with language, hygiene, citizenship activities, ordinary social activities, leisure activities, activities of mental health, religious activities, activities concerning race preservation, vocational behaviour activities and vocational activities.
- Realism emphasizes on developing a man's capabilities of earning by vocational means.
- It also emphasizes on developing and strengthening the wisdom and power of decision making.
- Education must develop the capacity to patiently fight and struggle against adverse situations arising in everyday life.
- Education must enable individuals to develop the capacities to handle the reality of life and making the child successful in fighting with routine and adverse difficult situations.

C. Realism and organization of education

- Realism emphasizes on scientific attitude based on realistic principles, where the child extends the knowledge he learns through books. Spiritual needs are not given due consideration as a real need of education.
- It gives due emphasis on formal schools that provide adequate opportunity for learners to learn vocational skills through observation, experimentations and examinations.

D. Realism and methods of education

- Proponents of realism believe objectivity and knowledge of scientific evidences and reality are key in deciding what methods should be used for the teaching–learning process. Teaching methods should be according to the needs, interest and capabilities of student.
- Vocational education equips the individual with capacities to earn livelihood and enjoy leisure time utilization through experimentation, examination and observation.

E. Realism and curriculum

- Selection of curriculum for students must be based on their abilities, interest and capabilities so that education helps the student to adjust to changing circumstances of the society. The curriculum must have practical utility and must equip the child to adjust to the needs of the day-to-day life.
- Realism emphasizes on subject matters of real life use such as science, mathematics, hygiene and vocational subjects. Vocational content has given prominent stress on curriculum.

F. Realism and teacher

- Teachers must focus on the development of vocational skills in learners so that they can be equipped with qualities of race preservation and vocational behavioural activities.
- According to realism, teachers are the mentors who must be role models and skilled to demonstrate the vocational skills to their learners.

MODERN CONTEMPORARY EDUCATIONAL PHILOSOPHIES

Modern contemporary educational philosophies are also known as *normative philosophies*. These are actually the theories of education that are based on the results of philosophical thought and of factual inquiries about human beings and the psychology of learning. However, they guide about what education should be, what dispositions it should cultivate in learners, why it ought to cultivate them, how and in whom it should do so and what forms it should take. Some of the major modern contemporary education philosophies are discussed below (a brief review may be seen in Table 5.2).

I. PERENNIALISM

The basic concepts of perennialism are as follows:

- It is oldest and most conservative educational philosophy that has roots in realism and relies in the past views about changes in the nature of universe, human beings, knowledge, truth, virtue, etc.
- The major aim of education is to ensure that students acquire understanding about the great ideas of western civilization that focuses on enduring truths which are constant, not changing, as the natural and human worlds at their most essential level, do not change.

Table 5.2 Brief Description About Modern Contemporary Educational Philosophies of Education

Concept of Philosophy	Organization and Aims of Education	Curriculum	Methods of Education	Role of Teacher	Discipline
1. Perennialism: Chief proponents were Thomas Aquinas, Robert Hutchins and Mortimer Adler					
Education ensures that students acquire an understanding about the great ideas of civilization. These ideas have the potential for solving problems in any era. The focus is to teach ideas that are everlasting, to seek enduring truths which are constant, as the natural and human worlds at their most essential level.	The aim of education is to develop the rational person, who has intellectual abilities to uncover universal truth. Character training is also important for moral and spiritual development of an individual.	Accepts little flexibility in the curriculum that emphasizes on language, literature, mathematics, arts and sciences. Common curriculum for all the students with minimal opportunities for elective subjects. Teaching-learning process must create liberalism, tolerance and discretion among learners.	Perennialism portages for the educational methods, which promotes constant teacher-taught interaction such as oral exposition, lecture and explication. Emphasis is placed on teacher-guided seminars, where students and teachers engage in mutual inquiry sessions. Students may also learn directly from reading and analysing the great books.	Teacher must be competent and master of his subject so that he can help their students to develop the power to think deeply, analytically, flexibly and imaginatively. Teacher is also authoritative and a guide of the students.	Education should be organized and conducted in a manner that problem of indiscipline does not arise at all.
2. Essentialism: Chief proponents were William Bagley, Arthur Bestor, Admiral Hyman Rickover, James D. Koerner, Paul Copperman and Theodore Sizer					
Essentialists believe that there is a common core of knowledge that needs to be transmitted to students in a systematic, disciplined way. The emphasis is placed on intellectual and moral standards that schools should teach and preparing students to become valuable members of society.	Essentialism has recommended for the formal schools or teaching-learning places. The aims of education is to promote intellectual growth and academic competitiveness of the individual to become a model citizen.	This philosophy recommended intellectual content with quality and capacity of the learner. The recommended subjects are English, mathematics, natural science, history and foreign languages.	Essentialism recommended formal and well-planned classroom teaching methods such as lectures, discussions, presentations and group interaction.	Teacher must be a master of subject matter and role model for learners with high level of authority and control over teaching–learning process and learner.	Essentialism believes in rigid discipline and devoted hard work of learners in his studies.

Continued

Table 5.2 Brief Description About Modern Contemporary Educational Philosophies of Education—cont'd

Concept of Philosophy	Organization and Aims of Education	Curriculum	Methods of Education	Role of Teacher	Discipline
3. Existentialism: Chief proponents were Soren Kierkegaard, Friedrich Nietzsche, Maxine Greene, George Keller and Van Cleve Morris					
This philosophy believes that education must develop the consciousness about the freedom of choices among learners because a man becomes what he chooses for his self. Education must equip the individual for better choices.	The ultimate aim of education is to develop child's knowledge about human conditions and the choices that person has to make for self. Therefore organization of education must be formal with sufficient opportunities of choices.	Curriculum must be that which provides the free opportunities for children to select from many available learning situations and choosing the subjects that learner wish to learn. Humanities are commonly given tremendous emphasis, which helps the student to unleash their own creativity and self-expression.	Existentialism promotes the methods of education which emphasizes on self-activity of the learner such as self-expressive activities, experimentation, methods and media that illustrate emotions, feelings and insight.	Teacher must promote freedom for a learner to make personal choices and individual self-definition.	Existentialism believes in self-discipline but not in the strict discipline. Teacher creates an environment in which students may freely choose their own preferred way.
4. Reconstructionism: Chief proponents were Theodore Brameld, George Counts and Paulo Freire					
This philosophy of education believes on reorganizing and restructuring the process of education to being about social and cultural contrastive changes in community, society and country, where emphasis is placed on cultural pluralism, equality, futurism, national interest-oriented education.	Reconstructionism recommends for formal as well as informal ways of organizing the education so that desired aim of education can be achieved to bring the reconstruction of the society.	Curriculum should be conceived with a new socioeconomic and political interest. Therefore, the subject content must be oriented towards aspects of new changes expected social, economic and political discipline such as sociology, economics and science and technology.	This philosophy of education believes that teaching methods must be organized in manner that student become self-reliant, education must be activity oriented to develop necessary activities and abilities.	The role of a teacher is to take the social responsibilities and along with students must become the agent to improve society.	This philosophy of education propagates about optimum level of discipline but not a rigid discipline.
5. Progressivism: Chief proponents were Horace Mann, Henry Barnard and Johan Dewey					
Progressivism believe that learning must be through problem solving and scientific inquiry in a cooperative and self-discipline way, which promote the democratic living and transmits the culture of society while preparing students to adapt in changing world.	Progressivism recommended democratic school procedures, which promote the community and social reforms. The aim of education is to promote the democratic social living.	Progressivism recommended curriculum, which is interdisciplinary in nature, which promotes written textbooks and subject content that are the part and process of learning rather than ultimate source of knowledge. Further, curriculum is based on child's interest, problems	Child is considered as learner rather than subject, who primarily learned through cooperative group activities and experiences.	Teacher must act as guide for problem solving, leader for group activities and partner in planning the learning activities.	Has not recommended any sort of specific formal discipline.

- The curriculum focuses on attaining cultural knowledge and stressing on students' growth in enduring disciplines.
- *Perennial* means 'everlasting', like a perennial flower which grows year after year. Some ideas have lasted over a long time and are as relevant today as when they were first conceived. Perennialism urges these ideas should be the focus of education. When students are immersed in the study of those profound and enduring ideas, they will appreciate learning for themselves and become true intellectuals.

A. Chief proponents of perennialism

Many great names are associated with perennialism but the important ones are as follows:

- Roots lie in the philosophy of Plato and Aristotle
- Thomas Aquinas
- Robert Hutchins
- Mortimer Adler

B. Perennialism and organization of education

- Aims to rigorously develop students' intellectual powers, in a classroom-centred environment by the teachers.
- It further aims to develop a rational person who has intellectual abilities to uncover the universal truth.
- Character training is also important for moral and spiritual development of an individual. It further develops the power of an individual to think deeply, analytically, flexibly and imaginatively.
- Perennialists criticize the vast amount of discrete factual information students are required to absorb. Perennialists urge schools to spend more time teaching how these concepts are meaningful to students.

C. Perennialism and curriculum

- Accepts little flexibility in the curriculum that emphasizes on language, literature, mathematics, arts and sciences.
- This philosophy allows no curricular electives except in the choice of a second language.
- Common curriculum for all students with minimal opportunities for elective subjects. The teaching–learning process must create liberalism, tolerance and discretion in the learners.
- Perennialists oppose vocational curriculum or life-adjustment courses because they believe that this type of curriculum blocks the opportunity to fully develop students' rational powers.

D. Perennialism and methods of education

- Greater emphasis is placed on students and teachers engaging in Socratic dialogues or mutual inquiry sessions to develop an enhanced understanding of concepts.
- They recommend that students learn directly from reading and analysing great books.
- Perennialism portages for the educational methods that promote constant teacher–student interaction such as oral exposition, lecture and explication.
- Students must spend considerable time in classroom for mastering the three 'Rs', *Reading*, *Riling* and *Rithmetic*.

E. Perennialism and teacher

- The teacher must be competent and a master of his subject so that he can help his students develop the power to think deeply, analytically, flexibly and imaginatively.
- They must also be authoritative and a guide to manage a classroom as well as the teaching–learning activities.

F. Perennialism and discipline

- Education should be organized and conducted in a manner such that problems of indiscipline do not arise at all. Perennialism believes on laying a significant amount of external discipline on the learner along with a good amount of freedom to think rationally and logically.

II. ESSENTIALISM

The basic concepts of essentialism are as follows:

- This philosophy has its roots in both idealism and realism that has a primary focus on the development of academic standards and improving the mind and workability of a child.
- *Essentialism* means a 'traditional' or 'back to the basics' approach towards education. It strives to instill in students the essentials of academic knowledge and character development.
- The term *essentialism* was popularized in the 1930s by the American educator William Bagley.
- It is a dominant approach to education in America from the beginnings of American history. Early in the twentieth century, essentialism was criticized for being too rigid to prepare students adequately for life.
- But with the launching of Sputnik in 1957, interest in essentialism revitalized. Among the modern supporters are members of the President's Commission on Excellence in Education.
- Essentialists believe this conservative perspective is on intellectual and moral standards that schools should teach in a systematic and disciplined way.
- The schooling should be practical which may prepare students to become valuable members of the society. It should also focus on facts, the objective reality and train students to read, write, speak and compute logically.

A. Chief proponents of essentialism

Many great names are associated with essentialism but the important ones are as follows:

- William Bagley
- Arthur Bestor
- Admiral Hyman Rickover
- James D. Koerner
- Paul Copperman
- Theodore Sizer

B. Essentialism and organization of education

- Essentialism recommends that formal schools or teaching–learning places and classrooms should be oriented around the teacher.
- It emphasizes that American schools should transmit the traditional and moral values and intellectual knowledge that students need to become ideal citizens.
- The aims of education are to promote intellectual growth and academic competitiveness of the individual.

C. Essentialism and curriculum

- This philosophy recommends intellectual content with quality and capacity of the learner. Essentialists emphasize on instruction in natural science.
- Essentialists urge that the most essential or basic academic skills and knowledge such as mathematics, natural science, history, foreign language and literature form the foundation of curriculum.

D. Essentialism and methods of education

- Essentialism recommends formal and well-planned classroom teaching methods such as lecture, discussion, presentation and group interaction.
- It believes that elementary students should receive instructions for writing, reading, measurement and computers.
- Even while learning art and music, the subjects associated with the creativity development, the students are required to master information and basic techniques, moving from less to more complex skills and knowledge.

E. Essentialism and teacher

- The teacher must be a master of subject matter and a role model for learners with a high level of authority and control over the teaching–learning process and the learner.
- Teachers decide what students should learn and place little emphasis on student interests, especially when students divert their time and attention away from academic curriculum.
- Teachers focus on achievement test scores as a means of evaluating the student's progress.

F. Essentialism and discipline

- Essentialism believes in a significant amount of external discipline and complete devoted hard work of learners in their studies.
- Students should be taught hard work, discipline and respect authoritatively. Teachers are to help students keep their nonproductive instincts such as aggression or mindlessness in control.

III. EXISTENTIALISM

The basic concepts of existentialism are as follows:

- Existentialism refers to a set of ideas about human existence beyond the terms used in ancient philosophy and objective science. Jean Paul Sartre mentioned that 'man is nothing else but what he makes of himself', which is the essential principle of existentialism.
- This philosophy believes that education must develop a consciousness of the freedom of choice in learners because a man becomes what he chooses for his self.
- Education must provide the individuals with opportunities so they can make wise choices and live a meaningful and productive life.
- Individuals are responsible for determining for themselves what is 'true' or 'false', 'right' or 'wrong' and 'beautiful' or 'ugly.' There is no existence of any source of objective and authoritative truth about metaphysics, epistemology and ethics.
- Existentialists believe that there exists no universal form of human nature and each of us have the free will to develop as we see fit.

A. Chief proponents of existentialism

Many great names are associated with existentialism but the important ones are as follows:

- Soren Kierkegaard
- Friedrich Nietzsche
- Maxine Greene
- George Keller
- Van Cleve Morris

B. Existentialism and organization of education

- The subject matter is secondary in helping the students appreciate themselves as unique individuals with responsibility for their thoughts, feelings and actions.
- The ultimate aim of education is to develop a child's knowledge of human conditions and the choices that a person has to make for himself. The organization of education must be formal with sufficient opportunities for choices.

C. Existentialism and curriculum

- Existentialist advocates education of the whole person and not just the mind. Although many existentialists provide some curriculum, existentialism affords students great freedom in their choice of subject matter. Students are given a wide variety of options to choose from.
- Curriculum must provide free opportunities for children to select from the many available learning situations and choose the subjects that the learner wishes to learn.
- The humanities are explored as a means of providing students with vicarious experiences that will help unleash their own self-expression.

D. Existentialism and methods of education

- Existentialist methods focus on the individual. Learning is self-paced, self-directed and includes a great deal of individual contact with the teacher, who relates to each student openly and honestly.
- Existentialism promotes the methods of education which emphasize on self-activity of the learner such as self-expressive activities, experimentation and methods and media that illustrate emotions, feelings and insight.

E. Existentialism and teacher

- The teacher must promote the freedom for a learner to make personal choices and individual self-definition.
- The teacher's role is to expose students to various paths they may take in life and create an environment where they can freely select their own way.

F. Existentialism and discipline

- Existentialism believes in self-discipline but not in a rigid and strict discipline.

IV. RECONSTRUCTIONISM

The basic concepts of reconstructionism are as follows:

- Reconstructionism is a philosophical theory with the belief that societies should continually reform themselves in order to establish more perfect governments or social networks. Thus social questions will emerge as there are quests to create a better society and worldwide democracy.

- Reconstructionism is an ideology that emphasizes on the importance of changing for the better. In other words, reconstructionism is a philosophy that centres on the idea of constant change.
- This philosophy of education believes on reorganizing and restructuring the process of education to bring about social and cultural contrastive changes in community, society and country, where emphasis is placed on cultural pluralism, equality, futurism and national interest-oriented education.
- Reconstructionists encourage others to make necessary changes that will be beneficial to their future. These are positive changes that will help make life better and solve social problems. These changes are completed through a systematic outlook called the *reconstructionist philosophy*.

A. Chief proponents of reconstructionism

Many great names are associated with reconstructionism but the important ones are as follows:

- Theodore Brameld
- George Counts
- Paulo Freire

B. Reconstructionism and organization of education

- Reconstructionism recommends for formal as well as informal ways of organizing education so that the desired aim of education can be achieved to bring about reconstruction of the society.

C. Reconstructionism and curriculum

- Reconstructionism is more concerned with the broad social and cultural fabric in which humans exist. Reconstructionist educators focus on a curriculum that highlights social reform as the aim of education.
- Curriculum should be conceived with the new socioeconomic and political interest. Therefore, the subject content must be oriented towards aspects of new changes and expected social, economic and political disciplines such as sociology, economics, science and technology.
- Curriculum focuses on student experience and taking social action on real problems (violence, hunger, international terrorism, inflation and inequality). Strategies for dealing with controversial issues, inquiry, dialogue and multiple aspects are also the focus of the curriculum.

D. Reconstructionism and methods of education

- This philosophy believes that the educator does not deposit information into students' heads and teaching and learning is a process of inquiry in which the child must reinvent the world.
- This philosophy of education believes that the teaching methods must be organized in a manner such that the student becomes self-reliant. Education must be activity oriented to develop necessary activities and abilities.
- Community-based learning and bringing the world into the classroom are also considered as effective methods and strategies of education in reconstructionism.

E. Reconstructionism and teacher

- The role of a teacher is to take social responsibilities and become an agent to improve society along with students.

F. Reconstructionism and discipline

- This philosophy of education propagates about the optimum level of discipline but does not stress on rigid discipline.

V. PROGRESSIVISM

The basic concepts of progressivism are as follows:

- Progressive philosophy believes that the school must play a leading role in preparing citizens for active civic participation in a democratic society.
- Progressivism believes that learning must be done through problem solving and scientific inquiry in a cooperative and self-discipline way, which promotes democratic living and transmits the culture while preparing students to adapt in changing world.
- Progressivists believe that education should focus on the whole child rather than on content or the teacher.

A. Chief proponents of progressivism

Many great names are associated with progressivism but the important ones are as follows:

- Horace Mann
- Henry Barnard
- Johan Dewey

B. Progressivism and organization of education

- This educational philosophy stresses on active experimentation by students.
- Learning is embedded in the queries of learners that arise through experiencing the world. The learner is a problem solver and thinker who learns through her individual experiences in the physical and cultural context.
- Progressivism recommends democratic school procedures that promote community and social reforms. The ultimate aim of education must be to promote democratic social living.

C. Progressivism and curriculum

- Curriculum is drawn from student interests and questions. The scientific method is used so that students can study matter and events systematically.
- Progressivism recommends curriculum that is interdisciplinary in nature, which promotes written textbooks and subject content as part and process of learning rather than the ultimate source of knowledge. Further, curriculum is based on child's interests, problems and life affairs.

D. Progressivism and methods of education

- A child is considered as a learner rather than a subject who primarily learns through cooperative group activities and experiences.
- Lessons that are planned provoke curiosity to make school interesting and useful.
- Students are active learners. The students interact with one another and develop cooperation and tolerance for different points of view.

E. Progressivism and teacher

- Effective teachers provide experiences so that students can learn by doing.
- The teacher must act as a guide for problem solving, as a leader in group activities and as a partner in planning learning activities.

F. Progressivism and discipline

- Progressivists believe that education should be a process of ongoing growth, not just a preparation of becoming an adult. Therefore, they do not recommend any sort of specific formal discipline. However, they believe in an individual's self-discipline and self-governance.

CURRICULUM

The term curriculum has been derived from a Latin word *'Currere'* means 'to run', 'to run a course' or 'the path' that one takes up to achieve the goal. Thus, one can say that the curriculum is a pathway to achieve the educational goals. Originally, it meant the process and ways of passing the knowledge from one generation to the next. A common understanding of the curriculum is a programme of studies with specified course, leading to an academic certification, diploma or degree. However, in broader context curriculum is anything and everything that teaches a lesson, planned or otherwise.

Pedagogically, curriculum is the description of course content, learning experiences and the course of studies to be taken up by the particular group of students to obtain a particular degree, diploma or certification. Curriculum is one of the most important components of education system, where traditionally it was subject or content centred, while in modern era it is learner or life centred. Therefore, it is essential that curriculum must be revised from time to time based on the needs of the learner, the society and the nation.

I. DEFINITION

The curriculum is defined differently by different authors and there is a lack of consensus on meaning of curriculum. Some of the important definitions of the curriculum are as given below:

Curriculum is a tool in the hands of the artist (teacher) to mould his material (the pupil) in accordance with his idea in his studio (school).
—**Cunningham**

A systematic arrangement of the sum total of selected learning experiences planned by the school or a defined group of students to attain the aims of a particular educational programme.
—**Florence Nightingale International Foundation**

All the educational activities which are planned and guided by the school, whether they are carried out in groups or individually, inside and outside the school.
—**Kerry**

A curriculum is the offering of socially and scientifically valued knowledge, skills and attitudes made available to students through a variety of arrangements during the time they are at school, college or university.
—**Bell**

The curriculum includes all the learners' experience in or outside school that are included in a program which has been devised to help him developmentally, emotionally, socially, spiritually and morally.
—**Crow and Crow**

A curriculum is a plan or program of all experiences which the learner encounters under the directions of a school.

—**Tanner and Tanner**

Thus, a Curriculum is

- a programme of studies.
- a course of study.
- that which is taught in educational institute.
- a set of subjects and the course content.
- a set of performance objectives and learning experiences.
- everything that in planned by an educational institute.
- a series of experiences undergone by a learner in an educational institute.
- is everything that goes within the educational institute including extra-curricular activities, guidance and interpersonal relationships.

II. TYPES OF CURRICULUM

It is evident from the ancient Indian literature that human being even learns in womb and thereafter through the life experiences in family, society and the formal and informal means of teaching in an educational institute. In broader perspective, curriculum is everything through which the learner learns in this universe; thus, the types of curriculum may be the written curriculum, societal curriculum, hidden curriculum, the null curriculum, phantom curriculum, and concomitant curriculum and electronic curriculum, etc. The details of each type of curriculum are given below:

- *Written curriculum:* It is written format of curriculum draft, which is prepared by the specially constituted curriculum committee, which is used as guidelines for providing the learning experiences for the particular group of students. It is also known as formal syllabus for a particular programme. For example, a written curriculum guidelines are prepared by the curriculum committee of Indian Nursing Council of the B.Sc. Nursing programme, which is used the nursing colleges across India.
- *Societal curriculum:* The societal curriculum is unwritten form of curriculum, which informally teaches the learner. For example, a person learns from family, friends, community, media, religious organizations, etc.
- *Hidden curriculum:* Each institute has varying structure, organizational design and routines in the teaching–learning process and attitude and behaviour of teachers and administrators. Therefore, learner learns spontaneously many things differently through above-mentioned factors when even they are taught with the same written content/subjects in different schools/colleges or universities. For example, same written curriculum is followed for B.Sc. Nursing in each institute in India but one can observe the difference in graduate nurses prepared in different nursing institute because of existing hidden curriculum in the institutes.
- *The null curriculum:* There are certain areas/topics that are least important to be included in the written curriculum because of the changing needs and the trends, but teachers somehow convey the message to the learners that this is not an important topic in present context that may indirectly stimulate the learner to learn about this omitted topic in written curriculum. For example, inclusion

of smallpox in current curriculum of Indian medical or nursing courses may not be relevant but a message received from the teacher that it was a deadly disease of past era that does not exist in present time may stimulate the learner to learn about it.

- *Phantom curriculum:* The people learn many things through the messages prevalent in and through exposure of any type of media; especially the culture, subculture are learned through the media. For example, a budding Indian nurse watches a western nurse communicating with her clients in a documentary film; she may learn many things from her through the exposure of this form of media.
- *Concomitant curriculum:* The concomitant curriculum is an unwritten form of curriculum where learner learns what is taught or emphasized in the family milieu. The moral and ethical values and moulded behaviours are learned through family milieu.
- *Electronic curriculum:* The present era is the era of electronics, where in day-to-day life every one of us communicate as well as learn through electronic means either in formal or informal ways. Many of us use internet on regular basis for recreational purposes or for research or personal information gathering purposes, where we get opportunity to learn many things. For example, a budding nurse learns about a new emergency drug through a post made by her friend on Facebook account and so on.

III. TYPES OF CURRICULUM ORGANIZATION

The broad categories of types or pattern of curriculum organization are subject-centred curriculum, integrated curriculum, fusion curriculum, core curriculum and experience curriculum, which are discussed below:

- *Subject-centred curriculum:* It is a type of curriculum in which the content is organized based on the subjects to be cover in particular course. For example, the General Nursing & Midwifery (GNM) diploma, B.Sc. Nursing and M.Sc. Nursing degree curriculum prescribed by the Indian Nursing Council are the subject-centred curriculum.
- *Student-centred curriculum:* It is a type of curriculum in which the content is organized based on the nature, capabilities, interest, attitude and abilities of the students.
- *Correlated curriculum:* It is a type of curriculum, in which the content is organized in such a sequence that the content taught in one of the subject subsequently also helps to understand the problems in the other subject. For example, the content of microbiology is organized in such a manner that it is taught in the first semester of B.Sc. Nursing, so that students can easily understand the related topics of concurrently taught fundamentals of nursing subject, such as infections prevention, barrier nursing, medical and surgical hand washing.
- *Fusion curriculum:* In fusion curriculum, the two subjects are fused and are generally taught by the same instructor, such as in GNM diploma course the psychology and sociology are fused as behavioural sciences and anatomy and physiology are fused as biological sciences.
- *Integrated curriculum:* It is unification of all the subjects and experiences to cover in a particular course or programme. For example, the content of anatomy-physiology, pathophysiology, pharmacology and medical-surgical nursing is organized in manner that it had horizontal and vertical integration of subjects.
- *Core curriculum:* The term core curriculum, self-explanatory from the term itself, refers that the curriculum includes the core content or common to all the students and rest specialized content

are differently learned by the different students. For example, advance nursing practices, nursing education, nursing research and biostatistics subjects are core or common to all the M.Sc. nursing speciality students.

- *Experience curriculum:* In the experience curriculum, the content is organized in the form of real-life experience to teach the content through direct real-life experiences in the natural environment rather than the theoretical deliberation through classroom. For example, in the Florence Nightingale Model of curriculum of nursing, the nurses were predominantly taught through the real-life experience while working in hospital under supervision of experienced nurses; the same was followed in India before the university level nursing education era.

IV. CURRICULUM DEVELOPMENT PROCESS

The curriculum development is an ongoing process in each field of education including nursing education, which is a scholarly and creative process to develop and design an evidence-based, context-relevant and unified curriculum. Curriculum development in nursing education is generally developed by the regulatory bodies such as Indian Nursing Council and/or State Nursing Council to ensure the uniformity in minimum standards of nursing and midwifery education nationally. The curriculum developed at national level also facilitates the inclusion of national health issues in curriculum and a smooth movement of nurses from one state to other or even other countries. The curriculum process includes the following steps (Fig. 5.6):

A. Planning

This is the first phase of curriculum development process where issues/needs are identified for a new curriculum or in the existing curriculum; a curriculum development committee is identified and data are gathered, analysed and interpreted for need assessment and analysis for the development of particular curriculum. Through situation analysis, it is assessed that who will be the students? What will be their preentry level of education? What they have already learned before admission in particular programme? What will be expected from the passing out graduates? And ideally what should be taught and which learning experiences are to be given during the particular course, so that these students develop adequate knowledge base and skills. In addition, curriculum models are also reviewed by the curriculum committee so as to decide that based on mission, vision and philosophies of particular course/programme and national interests, which curriculum model will be most suitable for developing the curriculum for the particular programme.

The identification and formulation of curriculum committee is also a crucial decision to be made during this phase of curriculum development, where it must be ensured that members chosen for the curriculum committee should be national-level specialists, leaders, experts and researchers in the particular discipline, who have deep understanding of traditional as well as modern developments in the particular fields and are aware about the latest curriculum research findings, which are relevant for particular discipline.

B. Design the content and methods

In this phase of curriculum development, the intended outcomes are stated, the relevant content is selected and experiential methods are designed. The content of the curriculum is designed based on present and expected future trends in healthcare system, morbidity trends, education system, societal system, available teaching–learning resources, clinical facilities and prospective students. Traditionally nursing curriculum had been the subject and

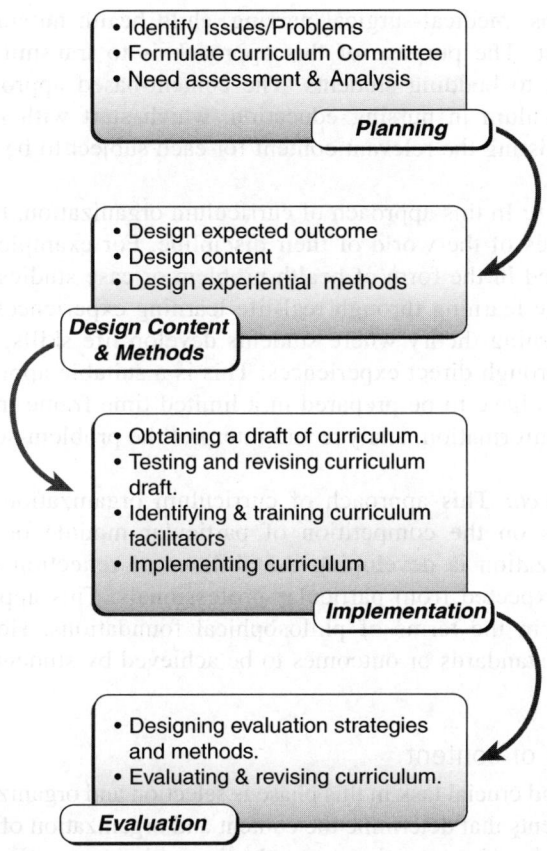

FIGURE 5.6

Curriculum development process

semester-oriented curriculum, but recently many countries have emphasized on the module curriculum, which involves the division of curriculum in units/modules and where students are assessed at the end of each unit/module through which students earn specific credits to obtain a particular professional qualification. There are three important things to be developed in macrocurriculum, i.e. programme outcomes, content guidelines and teaching approaches and schedules of teaching–learning during the particular programme period. The outcomes or objectives could be the programme objectives, level objectives, course objectives and unit objectives. There are three basic approaches of curriculum organization, i.e. organizing the curriculum by content, process and outcome. The curriculum could be pure form of one approach or mix and match of more than any one approach of curriculum organization.

- *Content-based approach:* In this approach of curriculum organization, the focus remains on inclusion of fundamental as well as core subjects relevant for a particular discipline. For example, including anatomy, physiology, biochemistry, psychology and sociology as fundamental subject and nursing foundations, medical-surgical nursing, child health nursing, mental health nursing as core nursing subject. The purpose of this approach is to transmit the worthwhile body of acuminated knowledge to budding students. The content-based approach is most widely used in designing the curriculum in nursing education, which start with listing the subjects to be included, followed by listing the relevant content for each subject to be included in the particular programme.

- *Process-based approach:* In this approach of curriculum organization, the focus remains towards the learner's experiences of the world of their discipline. For example, experiences of nursing, health, disease presented in the form of health problem or case studies. The purpose of this approach is to provide the learning through real-life learning experiences. This approach is based on the experiential learning theory where students develop life skills, such as problem-solving and critical thinking through direct experiences. This is a suitable approach for the programmes where the professionals have to be prepared in a limited time frame in which teachers help the students to search the information, analyze and interpret the problem-solving during the real-life experiences.

- *Outcome-based approach:* This approach of curriculum organization focuses on inclusion of expected competencies on the competition of particular module or course. The purpose of this curriculum organization is developing the abilities of reflection on problem and abilities to perform the tasks expected from particular professionals. This approach is very difficult to pin down the content in the terms of philosophical foundations. However, it proceeds from defining the minimum standards or outcomes to be achieved by students at the end of particular course or degree.

a. Criteria for selection of content

The next most important and crucial task in this phase is selection and organization of content and learning experiences. The elements that determine the content and organization of curriculum are the educational philosophy, content, learning experiences, evaluation and outcome (Fig. 5.7).

The following criteria may be kept in mind while selecting the content and learning experiences for the particular curriculum:

- *Validity and meaningfulness:* The selected content must be meaningful for the particular programme and it must be duly validated by the experts of the particular discipline. The content also must reflect the scientific thinking and evidence-based practices. The content must focus towards fundamental knowledge rather than the superficial information; it mean learning the principles rather than only the facts.

- *Relevance to the social, economic, occupational, judicial, political, technical and geographic context:* The curriculum content must be the socially, economically, occupationally, judicially, politically, technically and geographically relevant. In 1980s, World Health Organization (WHO) has recommended community-based curriculum, where healthcare professionals must be initially placed for community field experience followed

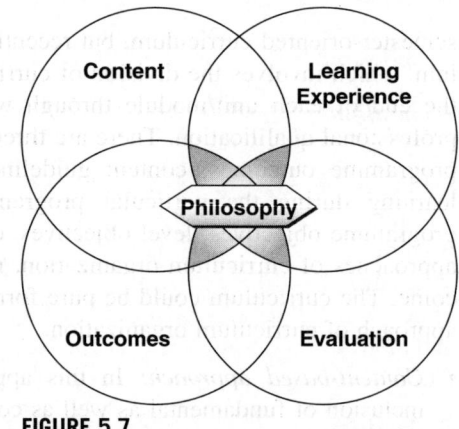

FIGURE 5.7

Elements determining content and organization of curriculum

by the long-term hospital experience, so that they understand community and family dynamics before understanding the diseases and their management.

- *A balance between breadth and depth:* It is a serious dilemma in each of the course and discipline that what to teach and how much to teach and what to be left. One school of thought says that it is better to know everything but other school of thought supports that it is better to master one area rather than knowing only little about everything. The content-based approach of curriculum organization supports the ideas of covering everything though it could be only superficial but the process-based and outcome-based approaches of curriculum organization support the idea of mastering the one area rather than covering everything superficially. Therefore, it is essential for the curriculum development experts to maintain balance between breadth and depth of curriculum content, so that most of the essential areas are covered and mastery in essential areas is also achieved.

b. Principles for organization of content

It is essential that curriculum is a 'coherent set of course' where there is optimum level of horizontal as well as vertical relationship of subjects/content, so that a smooth transition may be ensured from one unit/module to another and one course to another. The following criteria may be kept in mind while organizing the content and learning experiences for the particular course:

- *Principle of continuity:* The content presented in the curriculum must be in continuity, so that students can experience smoothness in learning the topics. The continuity must be in terms of complexities, breadth, depth and sophistication required. To maintain the continuity in the content, the vertical and horizontal strands are used.
- *Principle of order:* Principle of learning experience referred to the sequencing of the learning experiences and presentations of concepts. To ensure the principle of order in content organization, following teaching–learning maximums may be used:
  - *Simple to complex:* For example, teaching tables before teaching multiplications.
  - *Chronological:* First including concept and definition followed by the causes, pathophysiology, clinical manifestation, diagnostics test, treatment and nursing management.
  - *Whole to part:* Teaching complete healthcare system than teaching each part of system in detail.
  - *Part to whole:* Teaching cell, followed by tissue, organs and systems of the body.
  - *Health to illness:* Teaching physiology before the pathology.
- *Principle of integration:* It is essential to organize the content of curriculum, which is horizontally and vertically integrated to avoid the compartmentalized learning.

C. Implementation

After preparing the final draft of the curriculum, the curriculum is tested and revised. In this phase, the facilitators are identified and trained, who are going to facilitate the implementation of the curriculum and finally implement the curriculum in the real field. It is not easy to implement a new curriculum because of teacher's resistance to accept the change, lack of acceptance of new responsibilities due to change in curriculum and lack of knowledge and skill in implementation of new curriculum. The effective implementation of new curriculum may be ensured through facilitative leadership, training and motivation of people involved in the change process, creating conducive environment for implementation of change in curriculum, effective monitoring and support in curriculum implementation.

D. Evaluation

This is the final phase of the curriculum development in which the evaluation strategies and methods are identified and they are utilized for evaluation of implemented curriculum. The curriculum evaluation is designed to assess logic and coherence of curriculum concepts, design, implementation and utility; in addition to the fairness, objectivity, comprehensiveness, credibility, usefulness and effective communication may also be assessed. The major purpose of curriculum evaluation is to ensure the continuous improvement in the curriculum draft. The curriculum evaluation could be internal versus external, formative versus summative, holistic versus specific and high stakes versus low stakes. The evaluation process includes the following main steps:

1. Defining standards against which evaluation will be done.
2. Collecting the information after implementation of curriculum from different stakeholders.
3. Analyzing and synthezing the results.
4. Preparing the recommendations for improvement of curriculum.

V. DETERMINANTS OF CURRICULUM/FACTORS INFLUENCING CURRICULUM DEVELOPMENT

The curriculum development is influenced by many factors, such as educational psychology, educational philosophies, society, economic status, political will, scientific and technical development, available resources and capabilities, interest, attitude and abilities of students. The detail about determinants of curriculum development is given below (Fig. 5.8):

- *Student:* The interest, attitude, abilities and capabilities of the learners are the most important factors which determine the development of the content in the curriculum. For example, the curriculum for the anatomy subject will not be similar for the Auxiliary Nurse Midwifery programme and Bachelor of Science in nursing programme.
- *Educational philosophy:* The type of educational philosophy followed for the development of the curriculum is also the important determining factor for the curriculum development. For example,

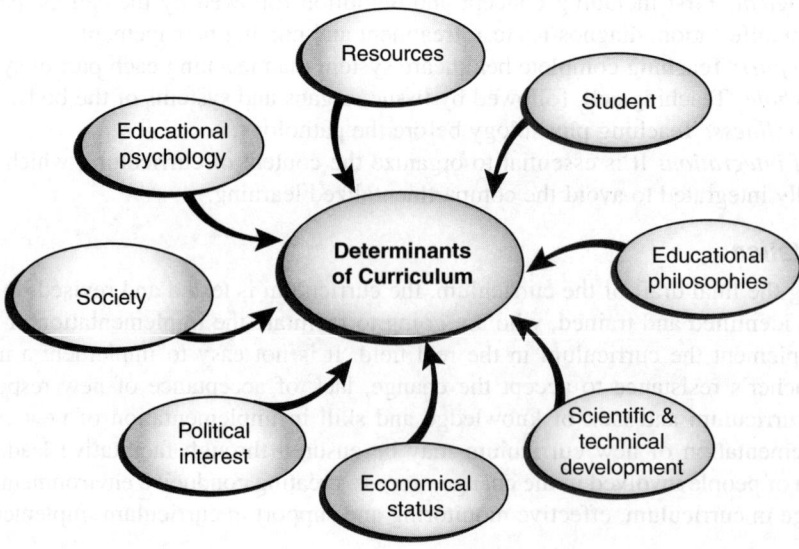

FIGURE 5.8

Determinants of curriculum development

the essentialism educational philosophy supports the outcome-based approach of curriculum development, whereas the realism and idealism support the content-based approach in curriculum development.

- *Society:* The person getting education in any of the discipline ultimately has to go back and work in the society. So it is essential for the curriculum development committee to consider the social factor while developing the curriculum. It is essential to know that what particular society will be expecting from the particular group, so that content may be designed accordingly.
- *Political interest:* In any country including India, political will is very important factor for the success of any of the programme. Therefore, political interest is also very important determinant of the curriculum development.
- *Economic status:* Nothing can be possible without the availability of the finance. Therefore, curriculum development committee should consider the economic factor as one of the crucial determinant factors for the curriculum development.
- *Scientific and technical development:* Scientific and technical development is the main driving force behind the development of the any of the field. Thus, scientific and technical development is also a significant determinant factor for the curriculum development for the particular discipline.
- *Resources:* The needs of resources are the paramount important factor in planning, implantation and evaluation of any programme. Thus, the curriculum development is also largely depends on the available resources with particular organization, institute or country for the success of it. The important resource factors that may affect the curriculum development are the available teaching–learning infrastructure, faculty, teaching–learning aids and finance.

VI. MODELS FOR CURRICULUM DEVELOPMENT

The curriculum development model is a format for curriculum design or pattern of configuration and arrangement of one or more key curriculum components to meet the unique needs, contexts and/or purposes. The use of curriculum development models may offer the greater efficiency and productivity in curriculum development process. Many models of curriculum development have been proposed by different educationists to increase academic rigor, sharpen student's critical thinking and analytical reasoning and provide them exposure to a richer subject matter. The four popular models of curriculum development are discussed in this chapter, i.e. The Tyler Model, The Taba Model, The Oliva Model and The Saylor, Alexander and Lewis Model of curriculum development.

A. The Tyler model

- It is the most popular model of curriculum development, which was introduced by Relph W. Tyler in 1949. It is also known as 'classic model' or 'prescriptive model' of curriculum development.
- It is a linear model, means it proposes an order/sequence of how to progress the different steps of curriculum development.
- It is a prescriptive model, means it suggests what 'ought' to be done.
- It is a deductive model, which proceeds from the general to specific. For example, it proceeds from examining from the needs of society to specifying the educational objectives.
- The main features of Tyler model are as follows:
  - It was recommended in Tyler's model that the curriculum developers initially may collect the information/data from three main sources (student, society and subject matter) to identify general objectives.

- Then numerous identified general objectives are screened through two screens, i.e. (a) philosophical screen and (b) psychological screen, to obtain significant and feasible objectives. The objectives that are unaligned with philosophical and psychological screen are omitted at this stage.
- Finally, the most significant and feasible objectives are obtained, which are popularly known as instructional objectives.
- These identified instructional objectives are used as base to plan learning experiences and evaluation methods.

B. The Taba model

- Hilda Taba proposed this model in her book *Curriculum Development: Theory and Practice* published in 1962, which is also known as 'interactive model' or "instructional strategies model'.
- It is also a linear and prescriptive model of curriculum development.
- It is an inductive model, which starts with the actual development of curriculum material leading to generalization of curriculum.
- She proposed that curriculum should be designed by the teacher rather than the higher authorities; thus this model is also known as grass-roots approach of curriculum development.
- The Taba's model is built on five steps, i.e. (a) produce pilot units, (b) testing experimental units, (c) revise and consolidate, (d) develop framework and (e) install and disseminate new unit. The following seven steps were proposed by Taba in her grass-roots model to produce a new unit in which teachers would have major contribution:
   i. *Diagnosis of need:* It was proposed that curriculum development must start with the identification of students' needs by the teachers because majority of students are immature to think critically and identify their needs.
   ii. *Formulation of objectives:* The student's need identification should be followed by the formulation of objectives, which is to be accomplished in a particular educational programme.
   iii. *Selection of content:* After formulation of objectives, the content is selected, which must be in concurrence with formulated objectives. The validity, relevance and significance of the content also must be ensured during this step.
   iv. *Organization of content:* Then the content must be organized in a sequence considering the learner's maturity, interest and capabilities. The sequence of content organization also must be logical and in coherence.
   v. *Selection of learning experiences:* In this step of model, teacher selects the instructional methods, which involve the students with the content.
   vi. *Organization of learning activities:* The learning activities also must be organized in sequence considering the content as well as the learner's interest, abilities and capabilities.
   vii. *Evaluation and means of evaluation:* Finally, the teachers who are the curriculum designers must determine the procedures to evaluate the learning outcomes and also determine what has been accomplished.

C. The Oliva model

- This deductive model of curriculum development was given in 1976. It is also a liner and prescriptive model of curriculum development.
- The main features of this model are as follows:
  - This is a 12-step model offering development of a school curriculum, which has two phases (a) curriculum development and (b) instructions.

- It is proposed that the aims of education are developed based on societal and student's needs, i.e. needs of particular student, needs of particular community and needs of particular subject taught.
- It was also recommended that the evaluation process should be through selection of tools to evaluate instructions and learner's performance and evaluation of entire curriculum programme.
- The 12-steps of the model are as follows:
    - **i.** To state the aims and beliefs of education.
    - **ii.** To analyze needs from general to specific.
    - **iii.** To specify curriculum goals.
    - **iv.** To specify curriculum objectives.
    - **v.** To organize and implement the curriculum.
    - **vi.** Increased specification of goals.
    - **vii.** Increased specification of objectives.
    - **viii.** Selection of instructional strategies.
    - **ix.** Selection of evaluation techniques.
    - **x.** To implement instructional strategies.
    - **xi.** To evaluate instructions.
    - **xii.** To evaluate entire curriculum.
- This model accomplishes two main purposes, i.e. (a) suggest a system that curriculum planner might wish to follow and (b) serve as the framework for explanations of phases or components of the process for curriculum improvements.

D. The Saylor, Alexander and Lewis model

- This deductive model was given by Galen Saylor, William Alexander and Lewis in 1974. It is also a linear and prescriptive model of curriculum development.
- It was believed in this model that the curriculum plan is not a single document but many smaller plans for each domain of the curriculum.
- In this model, it was viewed that the curriculum development consists of the following four steps:
    - **i.** *Specifying major educational goals, objectives and domains:* This model believes that curriculum planning starts with specifying the major educational goals, objectives, which are to be achieved. These main goals, objectives and domains are specified considering several external factors, such as educational research evidences, inputs of particular society/community and accreditation standards. Furthermore, it was believed that each major goal represents a curriculum domain and four major goals or domains are proposed in this model, which are (a) personal development, (b) social competence/human relations, (c) continued learning skills and (d) specialization.
    - **ii.** *Curriculum designing:* After specifying the main goals, objectives and domains, the next step is to design the curriculum, which involves the selection of appropriate learning opportunities for each goal or domain. It is also decided at this stage that how and when these learning opportunities will be provided and what will be main bases and sources for development of curriculum content.
    - **iii.** *Curriculum implementation:* In this step, the designed curriculum is implemented by the teachers, where they identify the instructional objectives, relevant teaching methods and strategies to achieve the expected learning outcomes.

iv. *Evaluation:* Finally, it is examined that whether the expected learning outcomes are achieved or not, which is proposed to be done using variety of evaluation techniques and tools. It was recommended that the evaluation process should be comprehensive in natures involving the entire educational process including curriculum plan, instructional methods/strategies and achievement of planned learning outcomes.

REVIEW QUESTIONS

Long-Answer Questions

1. Describe the philosophy of education.
2. Discuss the aims of education.
3. Discuss about social aim of education.
4. Describe the aims of nursing education.
5. Briefly explain the philosophies and aims of education.
6. Discuss the relationship between education and philosophies.
7. Define education and discuss the various aims of education.
8. Explain the various philosophies of education and formulate a philosophy for a B.Sc. Nursing programme.
9. Describe idealism.
10. Define education and discuss the functions of education.
11. Describe pragmatism.
12. Discuss the traditional philosophies of education.
13. Discuss the differences between philosophy and education.
14. Define curriculum and discuss the curriculum development process.

Short-Answer Questions

1. Define education, as given by Mahatma Gandhi.
2. List down the methods of teaching under Naturalism.
3. Mention four educational philosophies.
4. Discuss briefly the four aims of education.
5. Mention four aims of nursing education.
6. List down the types of education.
7. Discuss any four principles of pragmatism.
8. Define philosophy.

Multiple-Choice Questions (MCQs)

1. The term *education* is derived from a
   (a) Latin word
   (b) Sanskrit word
   (c) Chinese word
   (d) Greek word

2. The word *education* means
   (a) An act of teaching
   (b) An act of training
   (c) An act of teaching and training
   (d) An act of learning
3. Which aim of education allows the student to develop themselves into distinct individual personality?
   (a) Individual aim
   (b) Social aim
   (c) Vocational aim
   (d) Moral aim
4. The aim of education 'achieving social and national integration' was stated by
   (a) Secondary education commission
   (b) Kothari commission
   (c) Education commission
   (d) Planning commission
5. Which of the following factors plays an important role in transmitting the cultural heritage and traditions from one generation to another?
   (a) Religious factors
   (b) Cultural factors
   (c) Intellectual factors
   (d) Philosophy of life
6. Which of the following is not a function of education towards nation?
   (a) Ensuring national development
   (b) Promote national integrity
   (c) Preparing good citizen
   (d) Developing leader for nation
7. _____ is the social function of education.
   (a) Civilization and cultural security
   (b) Preparation for adult life
   (c) Transmission of cultural
   (d) Moral and character development
8. Philosophy is defined as
   (a) Science of knowledge
   (b) Science of facts
   (c) Review of universal things
   (d) Critical review of critical science
9. Which of the following is not a traditional philosophy of education?
   (a) Naturalism
   (b) Idealism
   (c) Pragmatism
   (d) Essentialism

10. The concept of philosophy 'educating the human generation about and in the nature rather than artificial environment by keeping in mind the individuality of each child' is based on
    (a) Naturalism
    (b) Idealism
    (c) Pragmatism
    (d) Essentialism
11. Which of the following philosophy recommended well-planned classroom for teaching–learning activity?
    (a) Naturalism
    (b) Pragmatism
    (c) Idealism
    (d) Realism
12. Naturalism philosophy emphasizes
    (a) Rigid discipline to child
    (b) Free discipline to child in nature
    (c) Spontaneous and self-discipline to child in nature
    (d) No discipline to child in nature
13. Existentialist method focuses on
    (a) Individual
    (b) Group
    (c) Society
    (d) Nation
14. Reconstructionist educators should emphasize on curriculum that highlights
    (a) Social reforms
    (b) Traditional facts
    (c) Scientific knowledge
    (d) Logical studies
15. _____ believe that education should focus on whole child rather than content or teacher:
    (a) Reconstructionists
    (b) Existentialists
    (c) Progressivists
    (d) Naturalists

Answers of the Multiple-Choice Questions

1. (a), 2. (c), 3. (a), 4. (b), 5. (b), 6. (c), 7. (a), 8. (a), 9. (d), 10. (a), 11. (c), 12. (b), 13. (a), 14. (a), 15. (c)

FURTHER READING

Acemoglu, D., Johnson, S., & Robinson, J. A. (2001). The colonial origins of comparative development: An empirical investigation. *American Economic Review*, 91(5), 1369–1401.

Armstrong, J. S. (1979). The natural learning project (pp. 5–12). North-Holland: Elsevier.

Armstrong, J. S. (1983). *"Learner responsibility in management education, or ventures into forbidden research (with comments)"*. How the world's best-performing school systems come out on top. Mckinsey.com. September 2007.

Asimov, M. S., & Bosworth, C. E. (1999). *The Age of Achievement* (vol. 4, pp. 33–35). Motilal Banarsidass.

Barbe, W. B., Swassing, R. H., & Milone M. N. (1979). *Teaching through modality strengths: Concepts and practices*. Columbus, OH: Zaner-Bloser.

Blurton, C. (1999). *New directions of ICT-use in education (PDF)*. Retrieved 2007–02–06.

Bowles, S., & Herbert, G. (2011). *Schooling in capitalist America: Educational reform and the contradictions of economic life*. Chicago, IL: Haymarket Books. Retrieved 21 October 2011.

Cahn, Steven M. (1997). Classic and contemporary readings in the philosophy of education (p. 197). New York McGraw Hill.

Card, D. (1999). Causal effect of education on earnings. In O. Ashenfelter & D. Card (Eds). Handbook of labor economics (pp. 1801–1863). Amsterdam: North-Holland.

De Grauwe, A. (2009). *Without capacity, there is no development*. Paris: UNESCO-IIPE.

Dewey, J. (1916/1944). *Democracy and Education* (pp. 1–4). New York: The Free Press.

Dubois, H. F. W., Padovano, G., & Stew, G. (2006). Improving international nurse training: an American–Italian case study. *International Nursing Review*, 53(2), 110–116.

Finn, J. D., Gerber, S. B., & Boyd-Zaharias, J. (2005). Small classes in the early grades, academic achievement, and graduating from high school. *Journal of Educational Psychology*, 97(2), 214–233.

Frankena, W. K., Raybeck, N., & Burbules, N. (2002). Philosophy of Education. In J. W. Guthrie (Ed). *Encyclopedia of education* (2nd ed.). New York Macmillan Reference.

Gutek, G. L. (2009). *New perspectives on philosophy and education* (p. 346). New Jersey: Pearson Education, Inc.

Hanushek, E. A. (2005). *Economic outcomes and school quality*. International Institute for Educational Planning. Retrieved 21 October 2011.

Hanushek, E. A., & Woessmann, L. (2008). The role of cognitive skills in economic development. *Journal of Economic Literature*, 46(3), 607–608.

Harriman, P. (1935). Antecedents of the Liberal Arts College. *The Journal of Higher Education*, 6(2), 63–71.

Heckman, J. J., Lochner, L. J., & Todd, P. E. (2006). Earnings functions, rates of return and treatment effects: The Mincer equation and beyond. In E. A. Hanushek, & F. Welch (Eds). *Handbook of the economics of education* (pp. 307–458). Amsterdam: North Holland.

Kneller, G. (1964). *Introduction to the Philosophy of Education* (p. 93). New York: John Wiley & Sons.

Locke, J. (1996). *Some thoughts concerning education and of the conduct of the understanding* (p. 10). R. W. Grant, & N. Tarcov (Eds). Indianapolis: Hackett Publishing Co., Inc.

May, S., & Aikman, S. (2003). Indigenous education: Addressing current issues and developments. *Comparative Education*, 39(2), 139–145.

Mincer, J. (1970). The distribution of labor incomes: a survey with special reference to the human capital approach. *Journal of Economic Literature*, 8(1), 1–26.

Munari, A. (1994). Jean Piaget (1896–1980). *Prospects: the quarterly review of comparative education*, XXIV(1/2), 311–327.

Noddings, N. (1995). *Philosophy of education* (p. 1). Boulder, CO: Westview Press.

Pashler, H., McDonald, M., Rohrer, D., & Bjork, R. (2009). Learning styles: Concepts and evidence. *Psychological Science in the Public Interest*, 9(3), 105–119.

Phenix, P. H. (1963). Educational theory and inspiration. *Educational Theory*, 13(1), 1–64.

Potashnik, M., & Capper, J. (2005). *Distance education: Growth and diversity (PDF)*. Retrieved 2007-02-06.

Rizvi, S. H. (2006). Avicenna/Ibn Sina (c. 980–1037), *Internet Encyclopedia of Philosophy*.

Robinson, K. (2006). *Schools kill creativity*. Monterrey, CA: TED Talks.

Russell, G. A. (1994). *The 'Arabick' interest of the natural philosophers in seventeenth-century England* (pp. 224–262). Leiden, The Netherlands Brill Publishers.

Schofield, K. (1999). *The purposes of education*. Brisbane, Australia: Queensland State Education board.

Steer, L., & Baudienville, G. (2010). *What drives donor financing of basic education?* London: Overseas Development Institute. news room/latest news/press_releases/2010/2010_02_23_AEW_launch_en. Transparency.org (2010-02-23). Retrieved on 2011-10-21.

Swassing, R. H., Barbe, W. B., & Milone, M. N. (1979). *The Swassing-Barbe modality index: Zaner-Bloser modality kit*. Columbus, OH: Zaner-Bloser.

Thomas, G. W. P. (1968). *Introduction to philosophy*. London: Novello and Company.

Thomson, I. (2002). Heidegger on ontological education. In M. A. Peters (Ed). *Heidegger, education, and modernity* (pp. 141–142). New York: Rowman and Littlefield.

Tremblay, E. (2010). Educating the mobile generation: Using personal cell phones as audience response systems in post-secondary science teaching. *Journal of Computers in Mathematics and Science Teaching*, 29(2), 217–227.

UNESCO (2008). *Education For All Monitoring Report 2008, Net Enrollment Rate in primary education*.

Webb, D. L, Metha, A., & Jordan, K. F. (2010). *Foundations of American education* (6th ed.) (pp. 55–91, 77–80, 192–193). Upper Saddle River, NJ: Merill.

Whyte, C. B. (1989). Student affairs: The future. *Journal of College Student Development*, 30(1), 86–89.

Teaching–learning process

6

The tragedy in life doesn't lie in not reaching your goal. The tragedy lies in having no goal to reach.
—Benjamin Mays

LEARNING OBJECTIVES

This chapter is designed to enable the reader to

- Understand the concept and nature of teaching and learning
- Describe the characteristics, principles and domains of learning
- Recognize the factors influencing learning
- Discuss the characteristics, principles and maxims of teaching
- Identify the meaning, characteristics, importance, domains and types of educational objectives
- Demonstrate skills in framing the educational objectives
- Explain meaning, functions, importance, characteristics, prerequisites, types and format of lesson planning
- Design the format of lesson plan to use for teaching the assigned group
- Explain the meaning, dimensions, principles, problems and strategies of classroom management and role of teacher in it

KEY TERMS

INTRODUCTION

Teaching and learning activities are twin activities involved in the total educational process. Teaching and learning are closely related and they are reciprocal to each other. Teaching cannot be thought without an idea of learning and learning is not possible without teaching activities. The main focus of teaching is to facilitate learning, where the teaching–learning process occurs smoothly and continuously. The teaching–learning process has four pillars: teacher, student, learning process and learning activities. Interaction between the teacher and learners is the core of the teaching–learning process.

MEANING OF LEARNING

Learning is said to be equivalent to change, modification, development, improvement and adjustment. It is a comprehensive term which leaves permanent impressions on individuals. Learning is central to our behaviour as we learn to speak, write, think and perceive. Our attitudes and emotional expressions are also learned behaviours.

Meaning of efficient learning: Efficiency in learning can be measured by three factors, namely accuracy, speed and retention. The meanings of accuracy, speed and retention are given below:

- *Accuracy:* How accurately do learners remember?
- *Speed:* How soon do learners remember?
- *Retention:* How long do learners remember?

DEFINITIONS OF LEARNING

Learning is acquisition of habits, knowledge and attitudes. It involves new ways of doing things and it operates in an individual's attempt to overcome obstacles or to readjust to new situations. It represents progressive change in behavior. It enables him to satisfy interests to attain goals.

—Crow and Crow

Any activity can be called learning so far as it develops the individual and makes his/her behavior and experiences different from what that would otherwise have been.

—Woodworth R.S.

Learning is a process that results in the modification of behavior.

—J.F. Travers

Learning may be considered as a change in insights, behavior, perception, motivation or a combination of these.

—M.L. Bigge

Learning is the process by which behavior is originated or changes through practice and training.

—Kingsley H.L. and Garry R.

Learning is the process by which an activity originates or is changed through reacting to an encountered situation, provided that the characteristics of the change in activity cannot be explained on the basis of native responses tendencies maturation or temporary states of the organism.

—B.L. Hilgard

Learning is the acquisition of new behavior or strengthening or weakening of old behavior as the result of experience.

—H.P. Smith

Learning is the process by which an organism is satisfying its motivation, adopts and adjusts its behavior in order to overcome obstacles or barriers.

—Hunter and Hilgard

Learning is an episode in which a motivated individual attempts to adapt his behavior to succeed in a situation, which he perceives as requiring action to attain a goal.
—Pressey, Robinson and Horrocks

Learning can be defined as changing one's potential for seeing, feeling and doing through experiences partly perceptual, partly intellectual, partly emotional and partly motor.
—W.C. Morse and G.M. Wingo

There are three important factors in the definition of learning:

- Learning brings change in behaviour (usually for betterment).
- Change takes place through practice or experience and not due to maturation.
- The change in behaviour should be relatively permanent lasting for years, months or weeks.

CONCEPT OF LEARNING

People learn, but they also forget. Learning may or may not be useful in few situations. According to Crow and Crow, learning is the acquisition of knowledge, habits and attitude in an individual for the betterment of self and society.

According to Woodworth, the process of acquiring new knowledge and new responses is the process of learning. Learning is not only getting knowledge of the subject matter or skills in art by study, by experience or by being taught, it is also an acquisition of habits, attitudes, perceptions, preferences, interests, social adjustments, values and ideals. Learning is a modification of observation, overt activity, thinking and associated motivational and emotional reactions.

A change in behaviour may occur through maturation which implies progressive advancement towards maturity. Learning is a change in performance through conditions of activity, practice and experience. In classroom situations, the activity or experience which leads to change in performance may be listening or judging, reading or reciting or observing a demonstration of a procedure. Through these activities or experiences an effective teacher can bring out changes in behaviour. Desirable changes are those changes that serve educational purposes, aims, objectives and goals.

A learning pyramid is depicted in Fig. 6.1, which illustrates the average retention rate among students through the different learning methods.

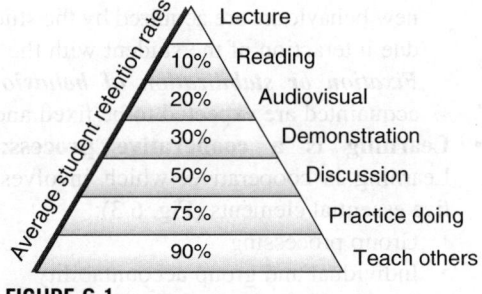

FIGURE 6.1
Learning pyramid.

NATURE OF LEARNING

Following are some of the significant views about the nature of learning:

- **Behaviourist view:** Learning is a change in behaviour as a result of experience. Men and other living beings react to the environment.

- **Gestalt view:** According to this view, learning depends on gestalt or configuration (wholeness of the situation). Learning is a total reaction to the total situation.
- **Hormic view:** This view was developed by McDougall. It stresses on the purposeful nature of learning, i.e. learning is a goal-directed activity.
- **Trial and error view:** This view was put forward by Thorndike. He conducted many experiments on dogs, cats and fish and concluded that most learning takes place by trial and error.
- **Learning is a process which involves a series of steps (Fig. 6.2):**
  - *Motive of the learner:* Motive or need arises first. Motive is the force that impinges or compels the individual to behave or react or do a particular task.

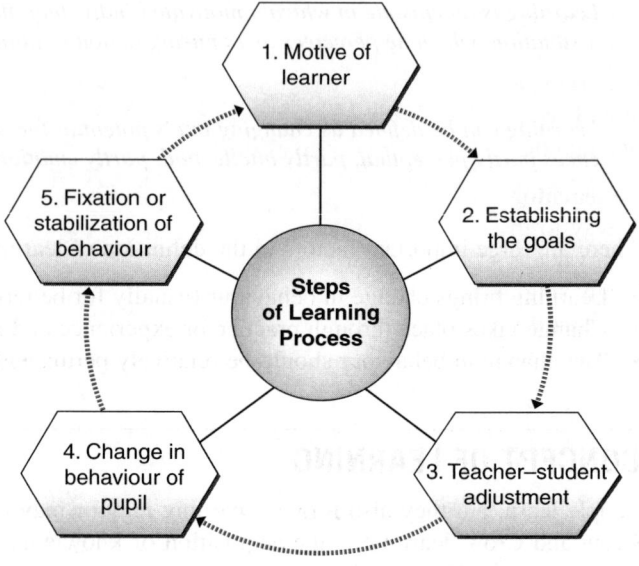

FIGURE 6.2

Learning process.

- *Establishing goals:* If a motive or need is present, the goal is set up by the teacher and learner.
- *Teacher–student adjustment:* Adjustment on the part of the students and teacher to each other and the environment.
- *Change in the student's behaviour:* During this phase, inappropriate behaviours are dropped and new behaviours are acquired by the student. Changes in behaviour in an individual take place after due interaction of the student with the educational environment and/or teacher.
- *Fixation or stabilization of behaviour:* Later the changes in the behaviour of the learner acquainted are expected to be fixed and stabilized for permanence.
- **Learning is a cooperative process:** Learning is cooperative, which involves five essential elements (Fig. 6.3):
  - Group processing
  - Individual and group accountability
  - Promote face-to-face interaction
  - Positive interdependence
  - Learning social skills

CHARACTERISTICS OF LEARNING

Learning is the acquisition of knowledge and/or skill through education and experience. Our ability to learn and our intellectual

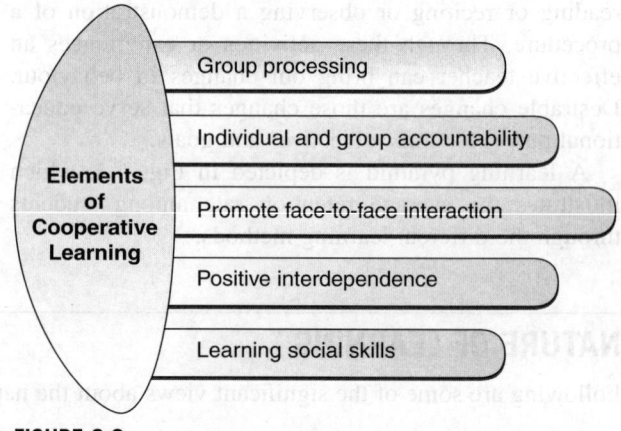

FIGURE 6.3

Elements of cooperative learning.

capacity are intangibles. These intangibles are our greatest assets because everything we do to reinvent and update our knowledge allows us to grow from where we are today to where we want to go. Learning is a prerequisite to growth, some may think that learning is a luxury for a few individuals or learning should be concerned with our early years. It should be looked at as something beyond formal schooling. Detailed discussion about the characteristics of learning is given below (Fig. 6.4):

- **Learning is unitary:** The process of learning helps the learner respond as a whole person in a unified way to the whole situation or total pattern. He responds intellectually, emotionally, spiritually and physically and these occur simultaneously. He reacts to the whole learning situation rather than to any single stimulus.
- **Learning is individual and social:** Learning is in a sense an entirely individual matter. Each individual must learn his or her own activity. In a larger sense, all learning is social, as it takes place in response to the environment in which there are other individuals as well as physical things. Learning is social because it takes place as a type of response to an individual's social environment. It is

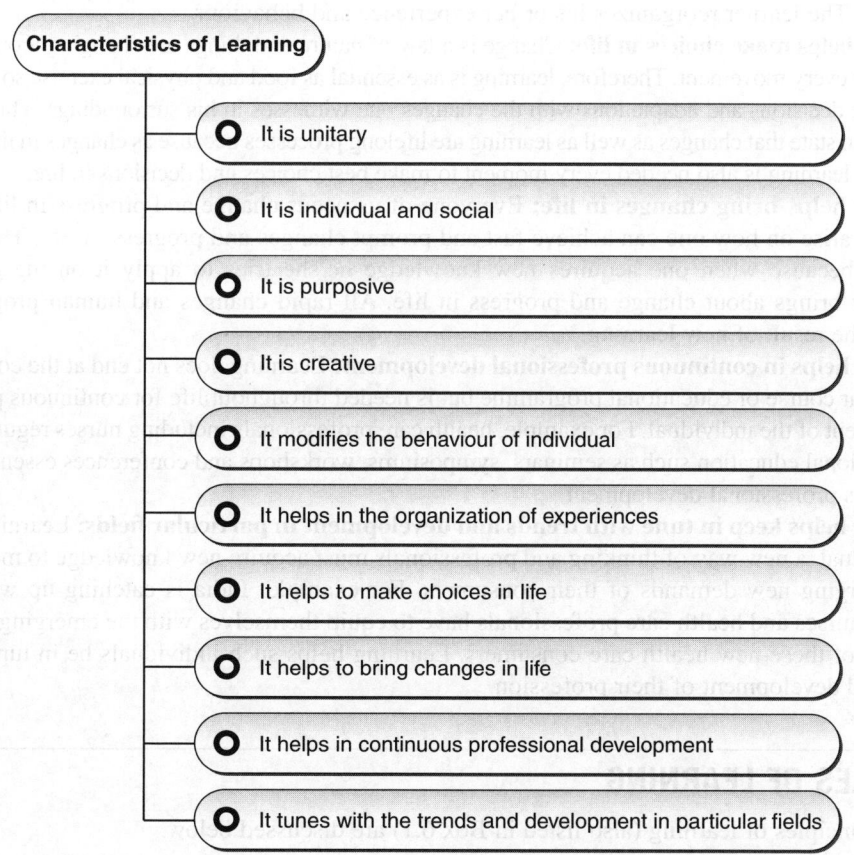

FIGURE 6.4
Characteristics of learning.

important that each person do his or her own learning irrespective of their individual differences, their capacities and level of intelligence.

- **Learning is purposive:** Learning is not only active but active in a specific direction. It helps the individuals achieve goals or purposes in their life. Learning cannot be meaningful and efficacious without persistent selective and purposeful effort. Learning not only contributes to an individual's purposes at times but enables him/her to make more intelligent adjustments in future.
- **Learning is creative:** Human learning is both selective and creative. Man is the only creature on earth who is not merely a creature but a creator as well. Learning helps a man to be more creative in life. It is the process of personal choice making. Learning helps him be creative for the betterment of the society.
- **Learning modifies the behaviour of the individual:** Learning affects the conduct of the individual. True learning takes place only when the individual acquires a type of knowledge or a skill that changes his or her attitudes and appreciations in response to a real need and modifies his or her conduct in accordance with new learning and therefore is changed.
- **Learning helps in the organization of experiences:** The process of learning is not mere acquisition of facts and skills through drill and repetition. It involves organization and evaluation of learning materials. The learner reorganizes his or her experience and behaviour.
- **Learning helps make choices in life:** Change is a law of nature and things are changing around us in the universe at every movement. Therefore, learning is as essential as food and physical exercise so that one can make wise decisions and adaptations with the changes one witnesses in his surroundings. Thus it will not be wrong to state that changes as well as learning are lifelong processes because as changes in life take place every day, learning is also needed every moment to make best choices and decisions in life.
- **Learning helps bring changes in life:** Everyone of us needs change and progress in life; however questions arise on how one can achieve fast and prompt changes and progress in life. The answer is learning, because when one acquires new knowledge he/she tries to apply it on the ground that ultimately brings about change and progress in life. All rapid changes and human progress in the world is the result of new learning.
- **Learning helps in continuous professional development:** Learning does not end at the completion of a particular course or educational programme but is needed throughout life for continuous professional development of the individual. For example, health care professionals including nurses regularly engage in professional education such as seminars, symposiums, workshops and conferences essential for their continuous professional development.
- **Learning helps keep in tune with trends and development in particular fields:** Learning provides an individual, a new way of thinking and professionals must acquire new knowledge to meet the pace with emerging new demands of their consumers. For example, India is catching up with medical tourism; nurses and health care professionals have to equip themselves with the emerging health care demands of these new health care consumers. Learning helps such individuals be in tune with new trends and development of their profession.

PRINCIPLES OF LEARNING

The main principles of learning (also listed in Box 6.1) are discussed below.

- **Brings progressive change in behaviour:** Learning brings progressive change in behaviour as the individual reacts to situations and this is how learning leads to improvement in an individual.

BOX 6.1 PRINCIPLES OF LEARNING

I. *Basic fundamental principles of learning*
   Learning is
   - motivated by adjustment with new things
   - universal in nature
   - never-ending growth
   - a continuous process
   - goal directed or purposive
   - active and creative
   - aroused by individual and social needs
   - response of the whole individual to the total situation
   - transferable
   - possible on cognitive, affective and conative side
   - a process not a product
   - Learning brings progressive change in behaviour of learner

II. *Ten principles of learning given by JTFSL**
   Learning is
   - a constant interaction between learner and environment
   - an outcome of stimulation and motivation of learner
   - an active process
   - ongoing, developmental and cumulative process
   - an outcome of cooperation and support
   - an essential influence of environment
   - through practice, feedback and evaluation
   - a formal as well as an informal act
   - an individual phenomenon
   - an act of self-awareness

*The Joint Task Force on Student Learning.

- **Learning is motivated by adjustment:** The individual has to adjust to the new environment.
- **Learning is universal in nature:** Man is a rational animal and learns more than other animals from nature; however learning does occur in other animals, since it is an omnipresent phenomenon.
- **Learning is never-ending growth:** Every individual has an inspiration to learn more. One achievement leads to further incentive, pursuit and effort. Therefore, learning is the never-ending growing phenomenon of an individual.
- **Learning is a continuous process:** Learning is continuous and not restricted to the childhood but grows with life. Death is the end of learning.
- **Learning is goal directed or purposive:** When the purpose or goal of learning is clear, vivid and explicit, learning becomes meaningful and effective to the learner.
- **Learning is active and creative:** Learning largely depends on the activities of a learner. It is said no learning can take place where there is no self activity. Learning results from the activity and experience.
- **Learning is aroused by individual and social needs:** Learning depends on individuals: their needs, problems, interests, attitudes, ambitions and needs of the society. Learning may be quick and fast for some individuals and in others it may be slow or steady. No learning can take place in the absence of social environment.

- **Learning is the response of the whole individual to the total situation:** Learning does not take place in one dimension at a single time; it usually happens in a holistic manner and takes place in several dimensions together (such as cognitive, affective and psychomotor). Generally, individuals respond to the total situation in a wholesome manner rather than in an impendent and isolated manner.
- **Learning is transferable:** Learning is a transferable phenomenon, which may transfer from one learning generation to the next generation learners. A transfer of learning content may take place but the amount of transfer may vary from situation to situation and from individual to individual. Transfer occurs when there is similarity of content, techniques, ideals, procedures, interest and attitudes.
- **Learning is possible on cognitive, affective and conative side:** Acquisition of knowledge is cognitive, modification of emotions is affective and acquisition of skills and habits is conative learning. Generally, learning takes place in these three dimensions.
- **Learning is a process not a product:** Learning is an ongoing process as it goes on and on and is a never-ending process; death of an individual is considered as the end point of learning. Therefore, it is considered a lifelong process rather than an end product of a particular point of life.

I. JTFSL's PRINCIPLES OF LEARNING

The Joint Task Force on Student Learning (JTFSL) created by the American Association of Higher Education gave ten principles of learning, as discussed below:

1. *Learning is a constant interaction between the learner and environment:* Learning is fundamentally about making and maintaining connections; biologically through the neural network; mentally between concepts, ideas and meanings and experimentally through interaction between the mind and the environment, self and others, generality and context, deliberation and action.
2. *Learning is an outcome of stimulation and motivation of the learner:* Learning is enhanced when taking place in the context of a compelling situation that balances challenges and opportunities, stimulates and uses the brain's ability to conceptualize quickly and its capacity and need for contemplation and reflection upon experiences.
3. *Learning is an active process:* Learning is considered as an active process rather than passive. It is commonly said that one can take a horse to the water but cannot make it drink water until and unless the horse itself does it. The same way, learning is also an active process and cannot be achieved passively.
4. *Learning is a continuous ongoing, developmental and cumulative process:* Learning is considered as a continuous ongoing, developmental and cumulative process. It is a regular process of the storing of new knowledge over the past knowledge that leads to ultimate development of an individual.
5. *Learning is an outcome of cooperation and support:* Learning cannot be imagined without the help, cooperation and support of other individuals in the society. For example, learning occurs with the help of a teacher who teaches; a headmaster who coordinates in the educational activity and a writer who writes the textbook and so on.
6. *Learning has an essential influence of environment:* It is generally believed as well as empirically provided that learning is largely influenced by the environment and even some educationists believe that environment is the most important and crucial factor leading to learning. They believe that a man cannot force other men but it is the conducive educational environment created by one mature man that ultimately leads to learning in other individuals.

7. ***Learning takes place through practice, feedback and evaluation:*** Learning requires consistent practice as practice makes a man perfect. In addition, frequent evaluation and feedback to the learners also helps them in improvement during the ongoing learning process.

8. ***Learning is a formal as well informal act:*** Learning takes place formally as well as informally. Formal learning occurs during a planned teacher–taught interaction such as classroom teaching, interaction during a formal couching session and so on. Informal learning takes place during informal interaction of learning in the educational environment such as campus social interactions, active community activity participations and so on.

9. ***Learning is an individual phenomenon:*** Every individual is a unique creature of nature; therefore, he/she also learns in a unique pattern.

10. ***Learning is an act of self-awareness:*** In the true sense, learning is more of knowing about the self and then learning about others. Learning leads to great strength of introspection and ultimately improved self-awareness.

DOMAINS OF LEARNING

Learning does not take place in an aspect. It is identified that learning mainly occurs in three areas: intellectual, emotional and motor aspects, also called cognitive, affective and psychomotor domains of learning (Fig. 6.5). These domains are discussed below.

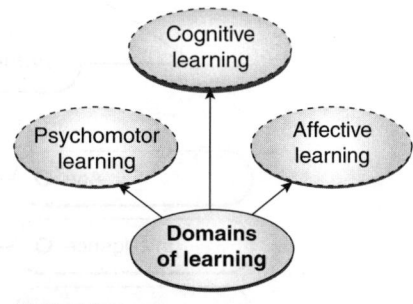

FIGURE 6.5

Domains of learning.

- **Cognitive domain:** This domain includes intellectual skills such as thinking, knowing and understanding. Cognitive learning is generally provided starting from a simple to a complex manner, which requires various teaching–learning and evaluation methods. The teaching–learning methods or strategies used to achieve this domain of learning are lectures, discussions, lectures enforced with discussion, seminars, panel discussions, conferences, etc. This domain of learning has further sublevels that are expected to be achieved by a learner, i.e. knowledge, comprehension, application, analysis, synthesis and evaluation. This domain of learning is generally evaluated by formal written examinations such as essay-type or objective written examinations.

- **Affective domain:** This domain includes feelings, emotions, interests, attitudes and appreciations. This domain of learning has further sublevels that are expected to be achieved by a learner, i.e. receiving, responding, valuing, conceptualizing, organizing and characterizing. The teaching strategies needed for the successful achievement of this domain of learning are simulations, role-plays, discussions, etc.

- **Psychomotor domain:** This domain of learning is also known as the *conative* or *skill learning domain*. This domain involves learning motor skills that require the acquisition of combined psychological and masculine ability to perform a task. Examples are taking blood pressure, performing head-to-toe assessment. This domain of learning has further sublevels that are expected to be achieved by a learner, i.e. impulsion, imitation, manipulation, coordination and habit formation. Teaching–learning strategies involve demonstrations, laboratory practice, skill practice on simulators, clinical practice, case studies, clinical conferences, etc.

FACTORS INFLUENCING LEARNING

Factors influencing learning are classified under two main headings: intrinsic and extrinsic factors (Fig. 6.6). Details of the intrinsic and extrinsic factors influencing learning are given below.

I. INTRINSIC FACTORS

Intrinsic factors are from within the individual learner such as age, intelligence, attention, interest, holistic health, maturation, fatigue, insight, ability, capacity and motivation.

- *Age:* Age can impact the capability to learn. A child can learn faster and an aged person will have difficulty learning the modern ways of knowledge.
- *Intelligence:* Mental ability of an individual can affect learning. Individuals with subaverage intelligence will learn later than individuals with normal intelligence level.

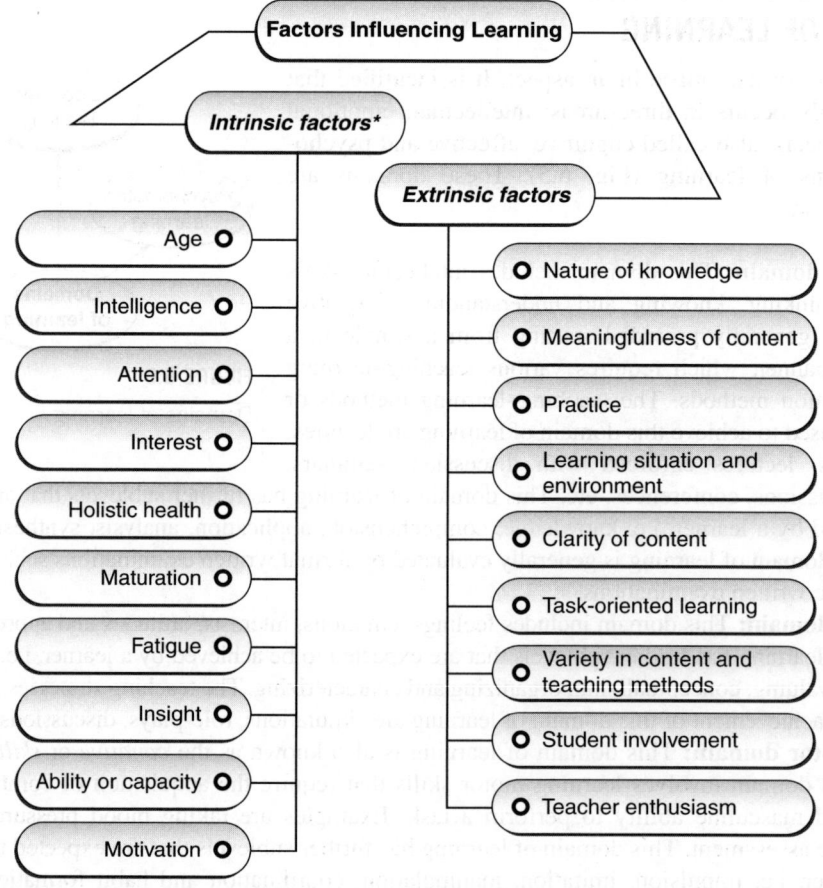

FIGURE 6.6

Factors influencing learning.

Indicates that the factors belong to the learner.

- *Attention:* Attention plays an important role in the education and training process. Attention is not static. It fluctuates from one object to another. Inattention by trainees is responsible for poor learning.
- *Interest:* Interest is an inner disposition or a tendency of readiness to perceive. Effective learning requires assimilation and interest. Interest should be aroused before learning begins and for satisfactory results it should be maintained throughout the learning period.
- *Holistic health:* Physical and intellectual health promotes effective learning. Without sound intellectual or physical health, an individual is unable to fulfil the demands of the learning process.
- *Maturation:* Learning depends on intellectual age. Maturation means intellectual, social maturity and psychological readiness. The changes associated with normal growth are called *maturation*.
- *Fatigue:* Every physical activity involves the consumption of energy. Human efficiency is the ratio between achievement and energy spent. Mental fatigue is caused by a loss of interest and the monotonous nature of work. When an individual is tired he/she cannot pay attention or concentrate towards learning activities.
- *Insight:* Insight also plays an important part in learning. Without clear insight it is impossible to achieve predetermined goals of learning. Insight is based on the ability of synthesizing the perceived facts and factors. It involves creative and imaginative thinking.
- *Ability or capacity:* Different species of animals have a different capacity to learn. Man is known to have a greater capacity to learn than other living beings. Even men vary in their ability to learn.
- *Motivation:* Motivation is a general term that encompasses the states of the individual under which he attends to certain aspects of his environment. As a result, his behaviour is both initiated and directed.

II. EXTRINSIC FACTORS

Extrinsic factors are from outside the individual learner and interfere directly or indirectly with an individual's learning process such as nature of knowledge, meaningfulness of content, practice, learning situation and environment, clarity of content, task-oriented learning, verity in content and teaching methods, student involvement and teacher enthusiasm.

- *Nature of knowledge:* If knowledge is interesting in nature, an individual can learn it more efficiently.
- *Meaningfulness of content:* Meaningless material can neither be learnt easily nor kept in memory for the long term. If the material is meaningful, the individual will learn it more effectively and easily.
- *Practice:* Practice, exercise, repetition or drill are interchangeable terms that are presumed to have something to do with learning. Simple acts are learnt in single trials, but complex acts are learnt through exercises or repeated trials.
- *Learning situation and environment:* A learner should have a conducive environment to learn that will promote the learning process. For example, adequate ventilation, lighting, temperature, odour free environment, absence of nose disturbance, rodent and insect free environment and availability of good library resources.
- *Clarity of content:* Clarity is the ability of the learner to clearly see, hear and understand what is being said. Threats to clarity include small fonts, slurred speech, obstructions to sight and ambiguous language.
- *Task-orientated learning:* People tend to learn better when they are engaged in tasks.

- *Variety in content and teaching methods:* A variety of ways used by the teacher can enhance the students' learning. Some people learn by listening, some by seeing and some by doing.
- *Student involvement:* Student involvement in the whole teaching–learning process is very crucial for his or her learning. Active involvement of students not only motivates them but also arouses interest in particular activities.
- *Teacher enthusiasm:* Enthusiasm of the teachers or presenters is contagious. If the teacher shows interest in a topic, the learners are more likely to be interested.

MEANING OF TEACHING

Teaching is a form of interpersonal influence aimed at changing the behavior potential of another person.

—American Educational Research Association Commission

Teaching is stimulation, guidance, direction and encouragement of learning.

—Burton

Teaching refers to activities that are designed and performed to produce change in student behavior.

—Clarke

Teaching is the means whereby the society trains the young in specific or selective environment as quickly as possible to adjust themselves to the world in which they live.

—Yoakm and Simpson

Teaching is concerned with growth and development of whole personality of the student—her mind, character and effective behavior.

—Thomas P. Green

Teaching is an arrangement and manipulation of situation in which there are gap and obstruction which an individual will seek to overcome and from which he/she will learn in the course of doing so.

—Johan Brubacher

CONCEPTS OF TEACHING

I. TRADITIONAL CONCEPT

Teaching used to be the act of imparting instructions and feeding the learner's mind with information in classroom situations. It emphasized on imparting instructions to learners in a classroom setting. In traditional classroom teaching, the teacher gives information to students or students can read from a textbooks. This method of teaching is not accepted by modern educators.

II. MODERN CONCEPT

Modern education has brought the child to the focus of the educative process. Teaching motivates the student to learn and acquire desired knowledge, skills and also desirable ways of living in the society. It is the process where the learner, teacher, curriculum and other variables are organized in a systematic and psychological way to attain some predetermined goals.

Following are some of the key views about the concept and meaning of education:

Gage's view
Teaching is a form of inter-personal influence aimed at changing the behavior potential of another person.

Ryburn's view
Teaching is a relationship which keeps the child to develop at his powers.

Brubacher's view
Teaching is an arrangement and manipulation of a situation in which there are gaps and obstructions which an individual will seek to overcome and from which he will learn in the course of doing so.

Green's view
Teaching is the task of teacher which is performed for the development of a child.

Morrison's view
Teaching is an intimate contact between a more mature personality and less mature one which is designed to further the education of the learner.

Smith's view
Teaching is a system of actions intended to produce learning.

Burton's view
Teaching is the stimulation, guidance, direction and encouragement of learning.

Hug and Duncan's view
Teaching is an activity—a unique, professional, rational human activity in which one creatively and imaginatively uses himself and his knowledge to promote the learning and welfare of others.

Sir Johan Adam's view
The teacher is maker of man.

H.G. Wells' view
Teacher is real maker of history.

NATURE OF TEACHING

Teaching has been viewed differently in different eras by different philosophers/educationists in different regions of the universe. The basic nature of teaching is discussed below.

- **Teaching is a tripolar process:** Teaching is tripolar process (Fig. 6.7). The three interconnected poles are teacher, pupil and subject matter.
- **Teaching is an interactive process:** Teaching is an interactive process. Interaction means participation of the teacher and student for mutual benefit to achieve objectives.
- **Teaching takes place at multiple levels:** There are multiple levels of teaching such as memory level, understanding level and reflective level.

- **Teaching must be planned:** Teaching is a planned activity. It is a systematic and organized process.
- **Teaching needs effective reciprocal communication:** Teaching can be made effective through the process of communication. Various communication skills dominate the process of teaching as it is between two or more persons influencing each other by their ideas.
- **Teaching is the motivation to learn:** Burton considers teaching as the stimulation, guidance, direction and encouragement for learning.
- **Teaching is guidance:** Students are guided to learn the right things in the right manner and at the right time through teaching.
- **Teaching is a professional activity:** Teaching is a professional activity involving the teacher and the student resulting in student development.

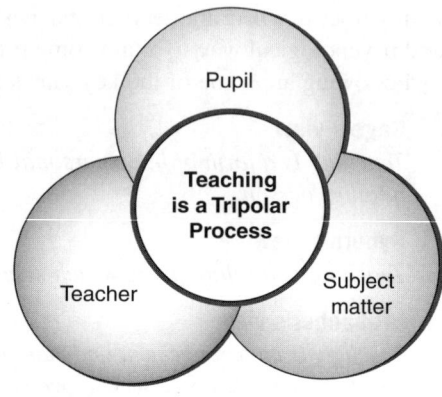

FIGURE 6.7

Teaching is a tripolar process.

- **Teaching is an art as well as science:** Teaching is a science as well as an art. The teacher has to adapt to various situations by using different techniques. Children are the raw materials the teacher has to deal with. A teacher's work is nothing less than that of an artist. Teaching has architectural functions to perform. It also involves art in the selection of proper techniques. The art of teaching is the ability to choose correct techniques at the right time.
- **Teaching helps attain information, knowledge and skills:** Teaching helps the learner attain information, knowledge of facts and skills for future use.

CHARACTERISTICS OF GOOD TEACHING

Teaching is a form of interpersonal influence aimed at changing the behaviour potential of another person and has the following main characteristics (Fig. 6.8):

- **Planned and systematic:** Good teaching is always planned and systematic. Planning involves careful selection, division and systematic revision of the subject matter.
- **Professional activity:** Teaching is a professional activity involving the teacher and students and results in student development'.
- **Preparation for life activities:** Good teaching helps the child develop physically, emotionally and spiritually to enable him to participate in life activities. According to Ryburn, 'teaching is a means of preparation and helping the pupil to live his life fully at a particular stage, it is also helping him to prepare for the future.
- **Training the emotions:** According to Ryburn, teaching should include training the child's emotions. Good teaching helps the students channelize and sublimate their emotions through activities like drama, singing, painting and games.
- **Matter of drawing out:** Good teaching is matter of drawing out rather than putting in anything. It provides suitable environment and activities for the development of a child's natural capacities.
- **Liberates the learner:** Successful teaching liberates and widens the intellectual horizon of the students. The ideal of good teaching is to liberate the student's mind from any fear he may incidentally feel

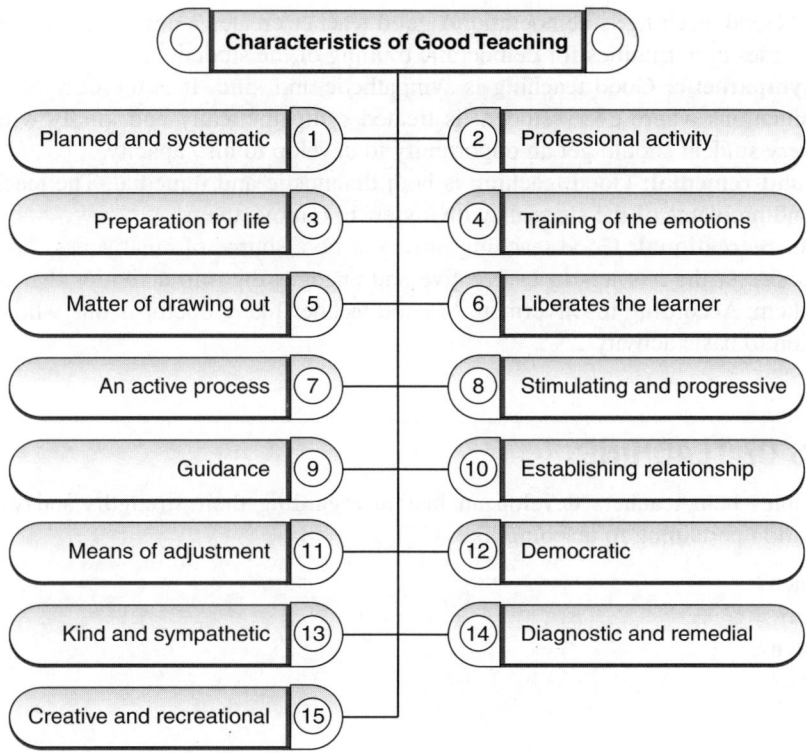

FIGURE 6.8

Characteristics of good teaching.

and develop independence in thought and method of procedure so that he may able to solve his problems independently and work out solutions.

- **An active process:** Good teaching emphasizes the importance of active participation in learning.
- **Stimulating and progressive:** Good teaching inspires and stimulates students for independent study, self-development and self-advancement.
- **Giving guidance:** Guidance is the core of teaching. The teacher guides the students to the right path. As Burton rightly remarked, 'teaching is the stimulation, guidance, direction and encouragement of learning'.
- **Establishing relationship:** Teaching is a tripolar process comprising the teacher, students and the subject. Hence the teacher has to know:
  - The nature of students, their individual differences in terms of abilities, aptitudes, interests, achievements and emotional development.
  - Himself through his feelings for students, knowledge and method of the teaching–learning process.
  - The subject and its orderly presentation to enable the students quickly grasp it.
- **Means of adjustment:** Good teaching helps students adjust themselves to their environment in an effective manner. The teacher helps the students adjust to the environment where they live in.

- **Democratic:** Good teaching is democratic. A good teacher creates a democratic environment in the class and provides opportunities for democratic training of the students.
- **Kind and sympathetic:** Good teaching is sympathetic and kind. It is the duty of a good teacher to provide situations where every student is treated sympathetically and kindly without room for scolding. Every student should get an opportunity to develop to his capacity.
- **Diagnostic and remedial:** Good teaching is both diagnostic and remedial. The teacher knows the difficulties and problems of the students with a view to remove them.
- **Creative and recreational:** Good teaching proves to be a source of creativeness and recreation. It awakens a desire in the learners to be creative and engages them in activities that are a source of pleasure to them. According to Silverman, 'a good teacher like a doctor is one who adds creativity and inspiration to basic activity'.

PRINCIPLES OF TEACHING

Teaching principles help teachers develop an insight regarding their strengths and weaknesses and provide information pertaining to teaching like:

- Whom to teach?
- Why to teach?
- Where to teach?
- What to teach?
- How to teach?
- When to teach?

The principles of teaching are discussed under two subheadings: general and psychological principles (Fig. 6.9).

I. GENERAL PRINCIPLES OF TEACHING

- *Definite aim:* Teaching should start with a definite aim that is of great help to both the teacher and the student. It makes the teaching and learning interesting, effective, precise and definite. Without definite aim the teacher might go astray and his teaching might lack coherence and definiteness. The students do not gain much if the lesson plan is haphazardly and aimlessly planned. Without definite aim, even the best lesson would fail to achieve its objectives.
- *Activity (learning by doing):* Teaching is effective when students actively participate in the lesson. Learning becomes active and quicker if the student is physically as well as mentally active. Students learn through self activity but the activity must be psychologically sound. Learning by doing removes the dullness of the lesson and puts children in life situations. The child engages himself fully and learns qualitatively as well as quantitatively. Teaching should be organized to provide the child with the maximum opportunity to learn by doing.
- *Principle of correlation (linking with actual life and other subjects):* Life and learning should become two poles of the same magnet; they are interdependent and cannot exist without one another. The teacher should not teach in water-tight compartments. Good teaching implies that learning must be vitally linked with the life of the learners and other subjects of their syllabus. For example, before teaching a topic in medical–surgical nursing, one must correlate it with the basic anatomy and physiology of a particular system.

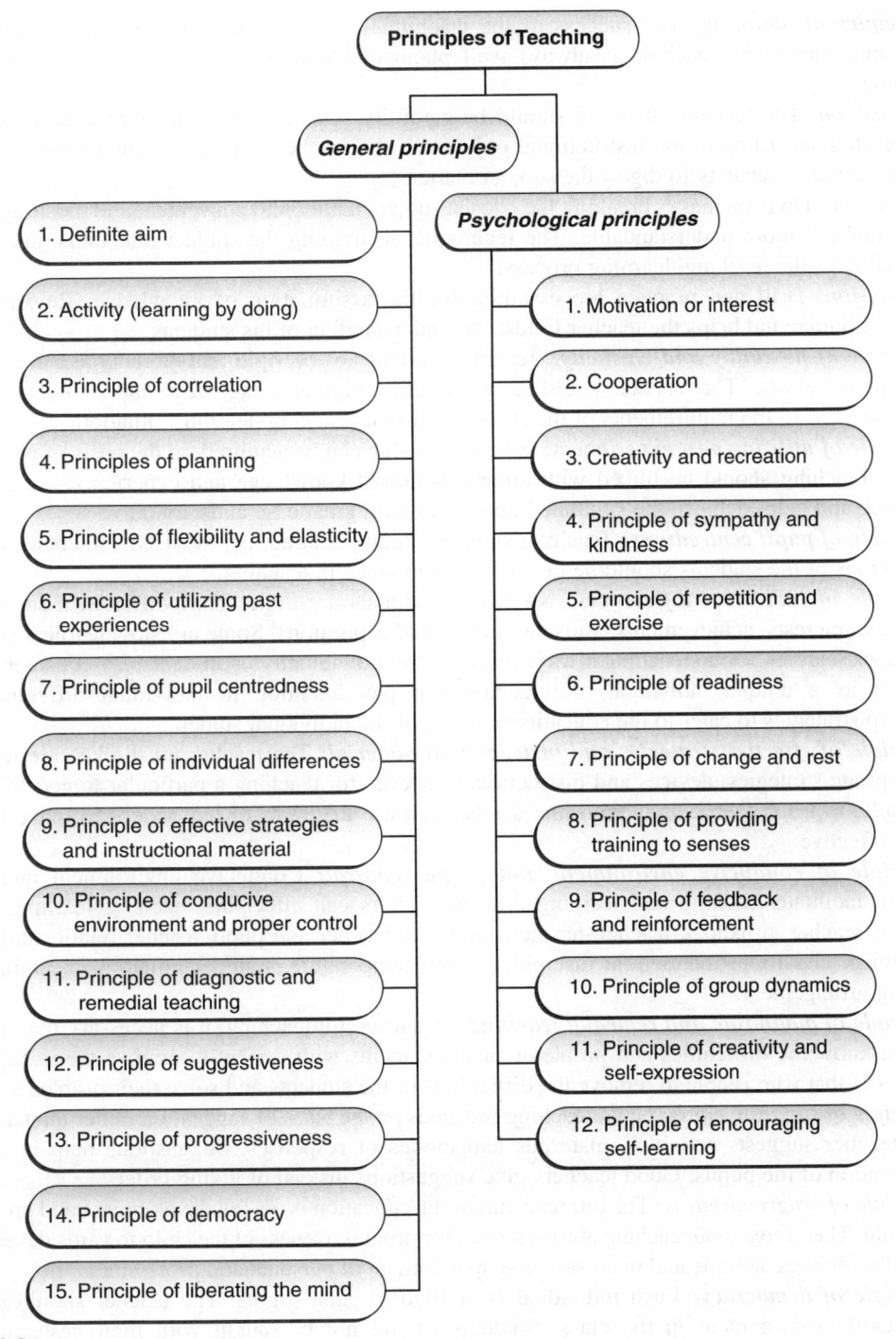

FIGURE 6.9

Principles of teaching.

- *Principles of planning:* The success of the teaching–learning process is directly proportional to planning. Successful teaching is always well planned. Planning involves selection, division and revision.
  - *Selection:* The teaching material should be carefully selected. The teaching material should be selected according to the instructional objectives, the teacher's ability to impart knowledge and the learner's capacity to digest the subject matter.
  - *Division:* Division makes breaking the chosen subject matter into convenient and meaningful units to make it more understandable. The technique of dividing the subject into units and subunits facilitates the teaching–learning process.
  - *Revision:* Drill and practice are essential for the assimilation of knowledge. Revision helps assimilation and helps the teacher to test the understanding of his students.
- *Principle of flexibility and elasticity:* Teaching should not be rigid and stereotyped. It should be flexible and elastic. The teacher should be resourceful, original, imaginative and creative enough to adapt himself to the requirements of the students and the teaching–learning situation.
- *Principle of utilizing past experiences:* New knowledge can be acquired on the basis of past experiences. Teaching should be linked with already acquired knowledge and experiences. It facilitates teaching and helps achieve the stipulated objectives with great ease and economy.
- *Principle of pupil centredness:* Teaching should be pupil centred, i.e. the needs, interests, abilities, aspirations of the students should be given due importance in teaching.
- *Principle of individual differences:* No two individuals are alike. They differ in their attitudes, abilities, interests, achievements, aims, ambitions and aspirations. Some are slow learners and some are quick learners. Good teaching always respects the individuality of students. By considering each student as a unique individual, the teacher can pay attention to individual differences and develop strategies to cater to the educational needs of the individual student.
- *Principle of effective strategies and instructional material:* The teacher must take care to choose appropriate strategies, devices and instructional material for teaching a particular topic/subject. For example, to teach foetal circulation, the teacher can use diagrams or live videos to make teaching more effective.
- *Principle of conducive environment and proper control:* Conducive environment and proper control facilitate teaching and learning. Various factors can affect the teaching–learning process such as teacher, principal, teacher–teacher, principal–teacher and pupil–teacher relationship, group dynamics, classroom interaction, discipline, room temperature, light, ventilation, cleanliness and seating arrangement.
- *Principle of diagnostic and remedial teaching:* In successful teaching, it is necessary that a teacher should know the difficulties and problems of the students with a view to remove them. Successful teacher is that who is able to remove the difficulties of the students and solve their problems.
- *Principle of suggestiveness:* Good teaching proceeds on the basis of suggestion rather than direction. The teacher suggests activities, materials and modes of responses. Suggestions help in securing cooperation of the pupils. Good teachers give suggestions instead of giving orders.
- *Principle of progressiveness:* The ultimate aim of the education is overall development and progress of the child. Therefore, good teaching always strives for progressiveness of the child towards development of skills, abilities, attitude and interest in essential domain of personal and professional life.
- *Principle of democracy:* Each individual is entitled to equal rights. The teacher should create a democratic environment in the class. Students should not be taught with their caste, creed or religion in mind.

- **Principle of liberating the mind:** The ideal of good teaching is to liberate the mind of students from any fear, which he may incidentally feel and to develop independence in thought and method of procedure so that he may be able to solve his problems independently and work out solutions.

II. PSYCHOLOGICAL PRINCIPLES OF TEACHING

- **Motivation or interest:** Teaching is directed towards promoting learning through motivating the learner or creating an interest in learning. Motivation is the key to the success of learning. Furthermore, motivation is like a petrol engine that drives the psychological engine. The teacher should properly motivate the students by creating interesting learning situations.
- **Cooperation:** Teaching is a cooperative affair between the teacher and the students. Poor cooperation leads to a poor teaching–learning process.
- **Creativity and recreation:** Teaching is not to be continued as a routine affair, but should arouse creativeness in the child. A sense of creativeness brings interest and pleasure in learning among learners, which ultimately leads to effective learning. Good teaching must strive to bring creativeness and a sense of recreation in the learners.
- **Principle of sympathy and kindness:** Successful teaching cannot take place in a situation that lacks sympathy and kindness with the interests and needs of the students. Students learn more when they are taught in a kind and polite manner.
- **Principle of repetition and exercise:** 'Practice makes a man perfect' is a well-known proverb. It applies well to the field of teaching and learning. If students are asked to repeat learning tasks, they will understand, retain and recall the subject matter more effectively.
- **Principle of readiness:** If students are not ready to learn, it is the teacher's duty to make them ready for learning. Teachers can choose the teaching tasks according to the student's psychology, i.e. their abilities, interests, attitudes, aspirations, maturation and development level.
- **Principle of change and rest:** Monotony fatigue and lack of attention decreases the speed of learning. Teaching–learning process followed by rest and change refreshes the mind and prepares the learners for more and effective learning.
- **Principle of providing training to senses:** Senses are gateways of knowledge. The power of observation, identification, discrimination, experimentation, application and generalization can be developed through proper training and functioning of the senses. The teacher should make proper arrangements for training the senses especially the senses of sight and hearing.
- **Principle of feedback and reinforcement:** Feedback about the progress of the student and further reinforcement are the most essential components of the teaching–learning process. Students are motivated for effective learning through timely and effective feedback and reinforcement.
- **Principle of group dynamics:** Group dynamics plays an important role in achievement of teaching objectives. Students tend to learn better in a group and also develop qualities of cooperation, mutual respect, sacrifice, etc. Therefore, the teacher should encourage group learning.
- **Principle of creativity and self-expression:** The development of the society and nation depends on creative ideas. It becomes imperative that the teacher should create situations in a classroom that inculcate creativity and self-expression in students. Usually, teachers feel happy if the students reproduce the same material in exactly the same manner. This practice can hinder a student's development and needs to be discouraged.
- **Principle of encouraging self-learning:** The teacher should inculcate habits of self-study, independent work and self-learning in the students by providing students with opportunities and training for this purpose.

MAXIMS OF TEACHING

The maxims of teaching may be defined as rules for presenting difficult terms and concepts to make them easy to comprehend in classroom teaching. A teacher employs some specific ways to organize teaching to make the terms and concepts communicable up to the cognition or rational process and level of learners. They are the guidelines for teaching. The maxims of teaching are very helpful in obtaining the active involvement and participation of learners in the teaching–learning process. They quicken the interest of the learners and motivate them to learn. They make students attentive to the teaching–learning process.

I. FEATURES OF MAXIMS OF TEACHING

- Maxim helps in organizing teaching–learning activities.
- It makes presentation of terms and concepts easily understandable.
- It enables teacher to make his communication for the mental level of the students.
- It is an important component of instructional procedure which is used in designing and presenting content in effective way.

II. ESSENTIAL MAXIMS OF TEACHING

Following are some of the essential maxims of teaching (Fig. 6.10):

- *From simple to complex or easy to difficult:* The nature of this maxim is more psychological that a child learns easy things and then proceeds towards complex things. For example, initially nursing students are taught about basic care procedures and then about complex procedures such as electro-cardiogram (ECG) and central venous pressure (CVP) monitoring.
- *From known to unknown:* This maxim is based on the appreciative mass theory of learning. It assumes that student-acquired knowledge is given by linking with actuarial knowledge so the student can learn better and retain for a longer time. Students have some knowledge and teachers should enlarge this knowledge. If we link new knowledge with the old knowledge we can make teaching clearer and effective. This maxim makes a link between the old and the new. If the teacher does not follow this maxim, then it is possible that students may be confused and may be interested in learning.
- *From part to whole:* B.F. Skinner gives emphasis on the part to whole maxim of teaching. He assumes that a student learns well if content is presented in small parts.
- *From whole to part:* According to the Gestalt school of psychology, whole is more important than parts. The whole is more motivating, understandable and effective than the study of various parts. A teacher should organize his activities in such a way that students can perceive the whole and then its parts because the whole attracts first. For example, while teaching *chambers of heart*, the teacher should show the entire heart first and then proceed with teaching the structure and functions of each part of the heart.
- *Proceed from concrete to abstract:* This is also a psychological rule of learning. Herbert said 'our lessons should start from the concrete and end in abstract'. A child's imagination is greatly aided by concrete material. 'Things first and words after' is a common saying. Rousseau said, 'things, things and things'. Children cannot think in abstractions in the beginning. Young children learn first from the things they can see and handle. Students learn from perception and experience about objects. After perception, concepts which are partially concrete and partially abstract in nature are formed.

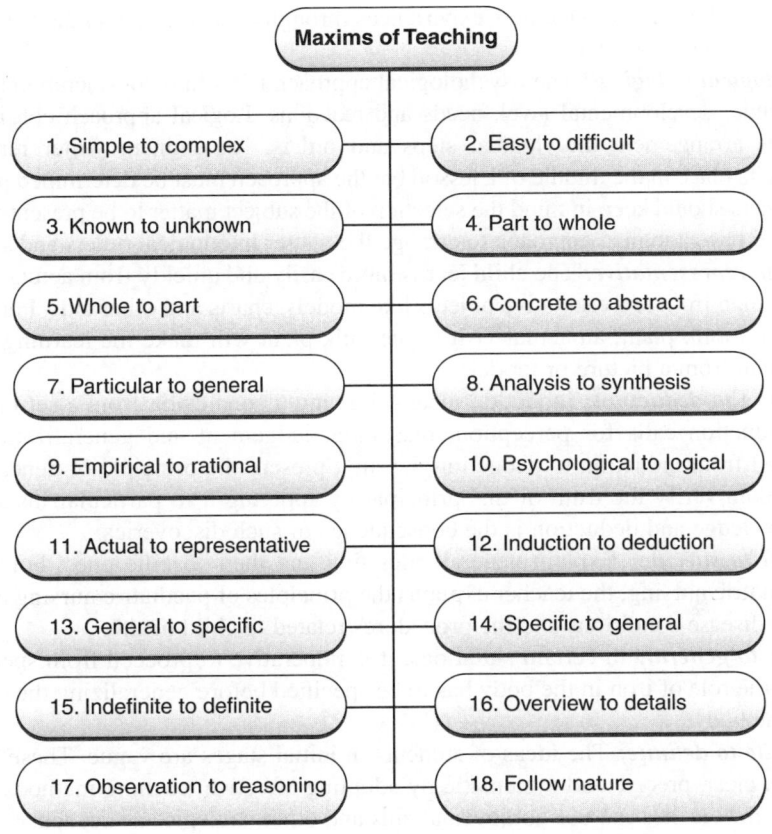

FIGURE 6.10

Maxims of teaching.

- *From particular to general:* Particular facts are easy to understand as compared to general facts. Particular facts and examples should be presented to the children before giving them general rules and principles. Particular is an inductive method and general is a deductive method. The process of induction is easier to comprehend than the so-called deductive one.
- *From analysis to synthesis:* Analysis and synthesis both are intellectual processes. This maxim is most frequently used in creative teaching. Analysis is an intellectual process. When a student comes to school, his knowledge is incomplete, indefinite and imperfect. Analysis makes the student's incomplete, indefinite and incoherent knowledge complete, definite and coherent. A teacher should begin teaching with analysis, so that complex problems are divided into systematic and comprehensible units. Synthesis must be performed in the end to make the knowledge definite and fixed. Analysis is useful for understanding and synthesis is useful for fixing this knowledge in students' minds.
- *From empirical to rational:* Empirical knowledge is based on the observations of students and has a significant role in a student's learning process. A student acquires most of his learning through observations. Learning by imitation is also based on observation. The activities of the teacher should be

so organized that they can provide new experiences through observation and the teacher should then proceed with the logical aspect.

- *From psychological to logical:* The psychological approach takes into consideration student interests, abilities, aptitude, developmental level, needs and reactions. Logical approach considers the subject matter and its arrangement into logical steps and orders. An eminent writer remarked, 'logical procedure has its place in the middle of a lesson but the approach must be determined psychologically'. First, the teachers should keep in mind the selection of the subject matter to be presented. After this, the teachers should have a logical approach to arrange the matter into logical orders and steps.

- *From actual to representative:* The child learns more easily and quickly from actual, natural and real objects rather than from representative objects like models, charts and other aids. For example, while learning about a milk plant, an actual visit to the milk plant will make the learning more vivid and rapid rather than from a picture or model.

- *From induction to deduction:* Induction means drawing a conclusion from a set of examples. The process of induction calls for perception, reasoning, judgement and generalization. The teacher should proceed from induction to deduction, i.e. first present the principle or generalization before students and then verify the truth of this principle by applying it to particular instances. Induction discovers knowledge and deduction is the consequence of such discoveries.

- *From general to specific:* Explain general rules first and then specific ones. For example, while teaching paediatric nursing, the teacher explains the principles of paediatric nursing and then teaches about various disease conditions and the procedures related to child health.

- *From specific to general:* In certain situations, it is imperative to proceed from specific to general. For example, the role of iron in the body has to be specified before generalizing the consequences of anaemia on the body.

- *From indefinite to definite:* The ideas of students in initial stages are vague. These ideas should be made definite, clear, precise and systematic by adopting effective teaching methods. To make these ideas definite, the teacher can use audiovisual aids and other strategies as needed.

- *Proceed from overview to details:* Students can easily comprehend if the teacher proceeds from an overview to details. For example, while teaching about the instruments used for performing an endoscopy, the teacher should introduce all instruments by listing down their names before explaining their uses and the ways to handle each instrument in detail.

- *From observation to reasoning:* The teacher has to provide an opportunity for the students to see and notice the factors involved in a particular topic or context before explaining the reasons associated with it or eliciting reasons from the students.

- *To follow nature:* This maxim of teaching is based on the philosophy of naturalism. Rousseau has given the concept to follow nature. The child is the centre of educational processes. A child should be given full freedom to learn according to his own ways. The teacher's role is to observe his behaviour and learning activities. There should be one teacher and one student in an ideal situation.

FORMULATION OF EDUCATIONAL OBJECTIVES

Objectives serve as a guiding path for people who move ahead; if someone is not certain of where he is going, he may end up at an unexpected place. Similarly, teaching–learning activities must begin with well-planned objectives so that the expected purposes of the planned teaching–learning activities can be efficiently achieved.

For an educational programme to be effective, the purposes and objectives are to be clearly stated so that it is easy to select the right subject content, learning experiences, clinical experiences and the right methods to evaluate student performance and the teaching–learning process. The objectives can either be teacher centred, student centred or subject content centred and must be planned keeping in mind the needs of the society, educational philosophy, values and circumstances under which students are expected to perform tasks in their life.

I. MEANING OF EDUCATIONAL OBJECTIVES

The words *aims*, *goals*, *objectives* and *targets* are often interchangeably used in relation to educational purposes. However, they are distinct and primarily the most commonly used terms for educational purposes to be achieved by students after undergoing the teaching–learning process.

> *Educational objectives are the results sought by the learner at the end of the educational program that is what the student should be able to do at the end of a learning period that they could not be beforehand.*
>
> **—J.J. Guilbert**

> *Educational objectives are the behaviors to be displayed by a learner, aims are for the teacher and the objectives are for the learners to achieve through the support and guidance of the teacher.*

> *Educational objectives are the statement of those changes in behavior that are desired as a result of specific learner and teacher activity which is a two-way process.*

II. FUNCTIONS AND IMPORTANCE OF EDUCATIONAL OBJECTIVES

The aim of education is to transfer knowledge to students and ensure their overall expected development. Crystal clear objectives are essential for the ultimate success of the teaching–learning process. Further, evaluation or assessment in the educational system will be aimless in the absence of clearly stated objectives. Therefore, before planning an educational activity one must have clearly stated educational objectives so that the teacher and learner are clear about what needs to be done to reach at these prespecified goals. Thus, educational objectives have a significant importance in the teaching–learning process as discussed below.

- Educational objectives are essentially important in the teaching–learning process, where the teacher and the learner get clear direction about where they are expected to reach at the end of a particular teaching–learning process.
- Educational objectives also help teachers plan appropriate evaluation methods and procedures for the students so that the students can be appropriately judged (whether the students have achieved the preset goals of a particular teaching activity or not).
- They are also important to inform the teacher and students of the gap between the expected and actual number of changes that have occurred in a particular student at the end of a particular teaching–learning activity.
- Educational objectives are responsible for providing direction to the teaching–learning as well as the evaluation process in a particular educational system.
- Educational objectives also help the teacher and the learner focus on a particular teaching–learning activity to achieve the specific predetermined educational goals.

- Educational objectives also help determine the educational recourse material, infrastructure, course content and curricular and cocurricular activities to achieve specific predetermined educational goals.
- Educational objectives provide an opportunity for the teacher to effectively monitor the teaching–learning process under the light of predetermined objectives.

iii. CHARACTERISTICS OF EDUCATIONAL OBJECTIVES

The well-stated objectives should be **SMART** (**S**pecific, **M**easurable, **A**ttainable, **R**ealistic and **T**ime bound) and **FOCUSED** (**F**easible, **O**bservable, **C**entred on students **U**nequivocally, **S**equentially appropriate, **E**ver relevant and **D**evelopmentally appropriate). The characteristics of the educational objectives are discussed below (Box 6.2).

- *Specific:* Educational objectives must be specific for a particular educational programme or learning instructions so that learners can achieve the specific goals of the educational programme or instructions.
- *Measurable:* Objectives must be stated in measurable terms rather than in an ambiguous nonmeasurable manner so that the teacher can evaluate the learners without any undue inconvenience. The teacher and the learner should be clear about what and how the evaluation is to be done towards the end of the programme or learning instructions.
- *Attainable:* Good educational objectives must be attainable within a stipulated time frame without undue wastage of time. Objectives that are too broad and require multiple cluster components to be achieved at one time may make educational objectives unattainable. Therefore, educational objectives must be planned with a single learning outcome and a narrow focus so they are attainable within a predetermined time frame.
- *Realistic:* Objectives must be planned keeping in mind the availability of basic resources and abilities and capabilities of the individual group of students so that they can be considered as realistic with reference to resources and individuality.
- *Time bound:* Well-written objectives must be time bound so that the teacher and the learner are clear about when learning has to be achieved and should motivate them do so accordingly.
- *Feasible:* Objectives must be feasible in terms availability of time, resources, attitude and intellectual abilities of the students.

BOX 6.2 CHARACTERISTICS OF EDUCATIONAL OBJECTIVES

Smart	Focused
S: Specific	F: Feasible
M: Measurable	O: Observable
A: Attainable	C: Centred on student
R: Realistic	U: Unequivocal
T: Time bound	S: Sequentially appropriate
	E: Ever relevant
	D: Developmentally appropriate

- *Observable:* The educational objective must be observable so that it can be observed and evaluated effectively. If an objective is not observable, it imposes a difficulty on the observation and measurement of learning in students. Verbs such as *to list*, *to compute* and *to define* make the stated educational objectives observable. On the contrary, verbs such as *to know*, *to understand* and *to enjoy* make the educational objectives unobservable.
- *Centred on student:* Good educational objectives are generally student centric and focus on what the student is expected to do rather than what the teacher is expected to do.
- *Unequivocal:* Ambiguous language or words should not be used while writing the objectives. Simple, precise and concise statements should be used while stating the educational objectives.
- *Sequentially appropriate:* Educational objectives must be sequentially appropriate that is preliminarily things that are expected to be achieved should be listed first followed by the complex things that should be achieved. For example, begin with define and then proceed towards enlisting and describing the complex parts of the topic or course content.
- *Ever relevant:* Objectives must always be relevant to a particular subject content and individual group of students. Further, objectives must be relevant to the level of expected learning as well as other teaching–learning factors.
- *Developmentally appropriate:* The educational objectives must be developmentally appropriate to a particular learner. They must be customized according to the intellectual, linguistic, social and moral developmental level of the learner.

IV. TYPES OF EDUCATIONAL OBJECTIVES

A. According to level of educational objectives

- *General/institutional objectives:* These objectives are known as *professional functions*, which are the statements identifying the major knowledge or skills that all students of a programme are expected to possess at the completion of their programme. They are short and relatively vague but they clearly define what students are expected to achieve at the end of their course or programme.
- *Intermediate objectives:* These objectives are also known as *departmental objectives* or *professional activities*. Intermediate objectives are a set of statements identifying the skills expected to be acquired by a group of students while studying in a particular department/division of their course or programme. However, these intermediate or departmental objectives must be consistent with institutional or general objectives of a particular programme.
- *Instructional objectives or specific objectives:* Instructional objectives are also known as *behavioural objectives* or *learning objectives* and are basically statements which clearly describe an anticipated learning outcome. They are brief and precise statements which clearly identify the basic skill or competence expected to be demonstrated by a group of students on the completion of a specific teaching–learning instructions.

B. According to taxonomy of educational objectives

- *Cognitive domain objectives:* The cognitive domain objectives (Bloom, 1956) involve knowledge and development of intellectual skills. This includes the recall or recognition of specific facts, procedural patterns and concepts that serve in the development of intellectual abilities and skills. There are six major categories: knowledge, comprehension, application, analysis, synthesis and evaluation, starting from the simplest behaviour to the most complex. The categories can be thought of as degrees of difficulty. The first ones must normally be mastered before the next one can take place.

- *Affective domain objectives:* The affective domain objectives (Krathwohl, Bloom and Masia, 1973) include the manner in which we deal with things emotionally such as feelings, values, appreciation, enthusiasms, motivations and attitudes. The five major categories are receiving phenomenon, responding to phenomenon, valuing, organizing and internalizing values (characterizing), from the simplest behaviour to the most complex.
- *Psychomotor domain objectives:* The psychomotor domain objectives (Simpson, 1972) include physical movement, coordination and the use of the motor-skill areas. The development of these skills requires practice and is measured in terms of speed, precision, distance, procedures or techniques in execution. The seven major categories are perception, set, guide response, mechanism, complex overt response, adaptation and organization, from the simplest behaviour to the most complex.

V. TAXONOMY OF EDUCATIONAL OBJECTIVES

The taxonomy for the educational objectives points out that they are concerned with intended behaviour or the behaviour to be learned by students rather than the actual behaviour learned from an educational objective (Bloom, 1956). In other words, taxonomy means 'a set of classification principles or structure and domains simply means category'.

Bloom's taxonomy divides educational objectives into three domains: cognitive, affective and psychomotor. Within these domains, learning at higher levels is dependent on having attained the prerequisite knowledge and skills at lower levels. The goal of Bloom's taxonomy is to motivate educators to focus on all three domains creating a more holistic form of education.

Bloom initially focused on the cognitive domain and later his colleagues published on affective domain. However, the details of the psychomotor domain were published by other authors later. The major categories in each domain are discussed below (Fig. 6.11).

I. Cognitive domain of educational objectives

The aspects of the cognitive domain revolve around knowledge, comprehension and critical thinking on a particular topic. This domain focuses on thinking skills. Traditional education tends to emphasize on skills in this domain, particularly the lower-order objectives. There are six levels in the cognitive domain, moving from the lowest order processes to the highest as discussed in Fig. 6.12 and Table 6.1.

II. Affective domain of educational objectives

The aspects in the affective domain describe the way people react emotionally and their ability to feel another living thing's pain or joy. Affective objectives typically target the awareness and growth in attitudes, emotion, motivation and feelings. There are five levels in the affective domain, moving from the lowest order processes to the highest as discussed in Fig. 6.13 and Table 6.2.

III. Psychomotor domain of educational objectives

The psychomotor domain describes about obtaining the skills or abilities to carry out physical tasks such as the skill of a nurse in catheterizing a patient or operating a mechanical ventilator. Psychomotor educational objectives usually focus on the expected changes in skills of an individual. Bloom and his colleagues did not offer subcategories of the psychomotor objectives but other authors (Dave, 1967; Simpson,

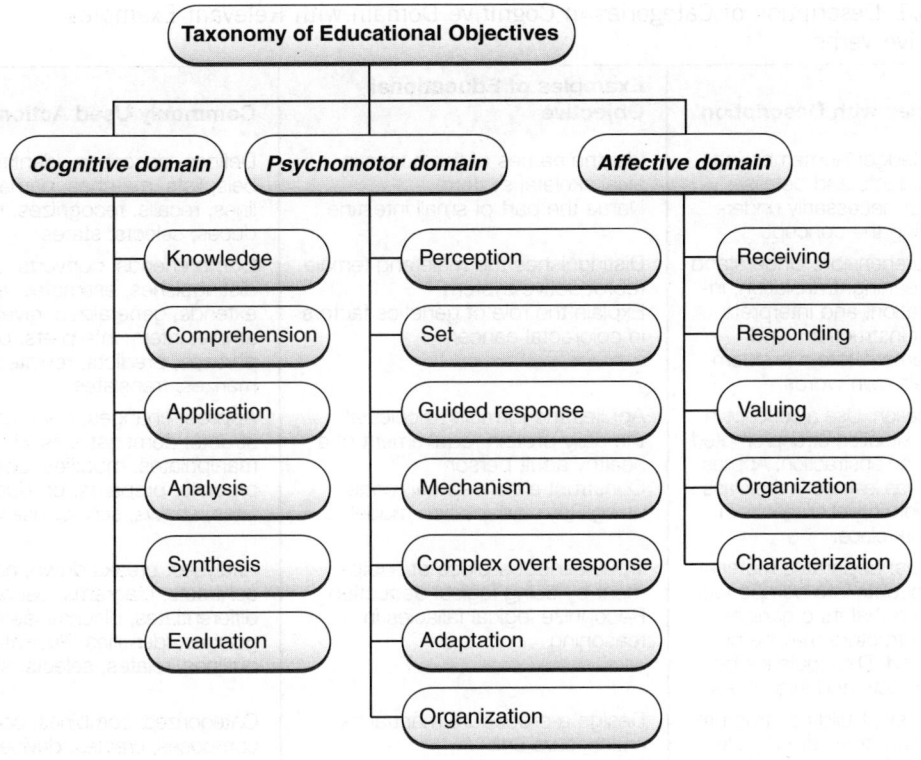

FIGURE 6.11

Bloom's taxonomy of educational objectives.

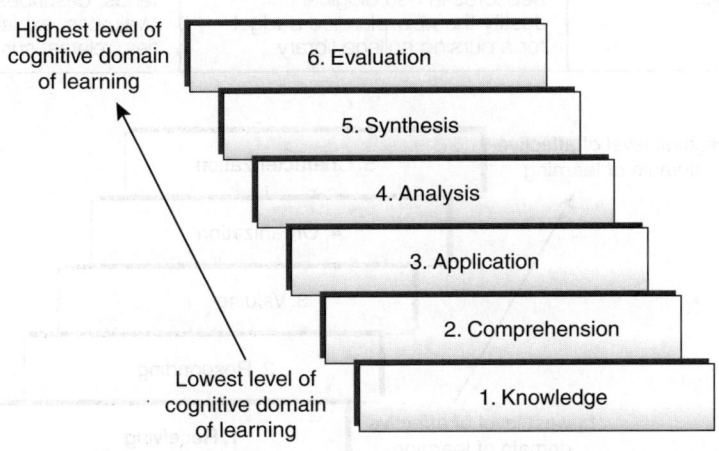

FIGURE 6.12

Categories of cognitive domain of the educational objectives.

Table 6.1 Description of Categories in Cognitive Domain with Relevant Examples and Active Verbs

Categories with Description	Examples of Educational Objective	Commonly Used Action Verbs
1. Knowledge: Remembering terms, facts and details without necessarily understanding the concept.	List the names of the bones in axial skeletal system Name the part of small intestine	Defines, describes, identifies, labels, lists, matches, names, outlines, recalls, recognizes, reproduces, selects, states
2. Comprehension: Understand the meaning, translation, interpolation, and interpretation of instructions and problems. State a problem in one's own words.	Distinguishes the male and female reproductive system Explain the role of genetics factors in colorectal cancer	Comprehends, converts, defends, distinguishes, estimates, explains, extends, generalizes, gives an example, infers, interprets, paraphrases, predicts, rewrites, summarizes, translates
3. Application: Use a concept in a new situation or unprompted use of an abstraction. Applies what was learned in the classroom into novel situations in the work place.	Applies the formula to calculate the daily protein requirement of a healthy adult person Construct a conceptual model using Roy's adaptation model	Applies, changes, computes, constructs, demonstrates, discovers, manipulates, modifies, operates, predicts, prepares, produces, relates, shows, solves, uses
4. Analysis: Separates material or concepts into component parts so that its organizational structure may be understood. Distinguishes between facts and inferences.	Troubleshoot a piece of equipment by using logical deduction Recognize logical fallacies in reasoning	Analyses, breaks down, compares, contrasts, diagrams, deconstructs, differentiates, discriminates, distinguishes, identifies, illustrates, infers, outlines, relates, selects, separates
5. Synthesis: Builds a structure or pattern from diverse elements. Put parts together to form a whole, with emphasis on creating a new meaning or structure.	Design a procedure manual for critical care unit Plan a staff requirement for a newly opened 20 bedded surgical unit	Categorizes, combines, compiles, composes, creates, devises, designs, explains, generates, modifies, organizes, plans, rearranges, reconstructs, relates, reorganizes, revises, rewrites, summarizes, tells, writes
6. Evaluation: Make judgements about the value of ideas or materials.	Select a most practical solution for reduction in prevalence of bedsores in neurological unit Justify the new planned budget for a nursing college library	Appraises, compares, concludes, contrasts, criticizes, critiques, defends, describes, discriminates, evaluates, explains, interprets, justifies, relates, summarizes, supports

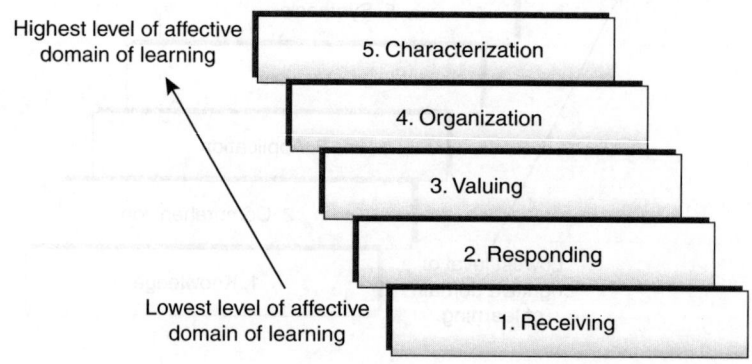

Highest level of affective domain of learning

5. Characterization

4. Organization

3. Valuing

2. Responding

1. Receiving

Lowest level of affective domain of learning

FIGURE 6.13

Categories of affective domain of the educational objectives.

Table 6.2 Description of Categories in Affective Domain with Relevant Examples and Active Verbs

Categories with Description	Examples of Educational Objective	Commonly Used Action Verbs
1. Receiving phenomena: Awareness, willingness to hear, selected attention.	Listen to others with respect Listen for and remember the name of newly introduced people	Asks, chooses, describes, follows, gives, holds, identifies, locates, names, points to, selects, sits, erects, replies, uses
2. Responding to phenomena: Active participation on the part of the learners. Attends and reacts to a particular phenomenon. Learning outcomes may emphasize compliance in responding, willingness to respond or satisfaction in responding (motivation).	Participates in class discussions Questions new ideals, concepts, models, etc., in order to fully understand them	Answers, assists, aids, complies, conforms, discusses, greets, helps, labels, performs, practises, presents, reads, recites, reports, selects, tells, writes
3. Valuing: The worth or value a person attaches to a particular object, phenomenon or behaviour. This ranges from simple acceptance to the more complex state of commitment. Valuing is based on the internalization of a set of specified values, while clues to these values are expressed in the learner's overt behaviour and are often identifiable.	Demonstrates belief in the democratic process Is sensitive towards individual and cultural differences (value diversity)	Completes, demonstrates, differentiates, explains, follows, forms, initiates, invites, joins, justifies, proposes, reads, reports, selects, shares, studies, works
4. Organization: Organizes values into priorities by contrasting different values, resolving conflicts between them and creating a unique value system. The emphasis is on comparing, relating and synthesizing values.	Explains the role of systematic planning in solving problems Accepts professional ethical standards	Adheres, alters, arranges, combines, compares, completes, defends, explains, formulates, generalizes, identifies, integrates, modifies, orders, organizes, prepares, relates, synthesizes
5. Internalizing values (characterization): Has a value system that controls their behaviour. The behaviour is pervasive, consistent, predictable, and most importantly, characteristic of the learner. Instructional objectives are concerned with the student's general patterns of adjustment (personal, social and emotional).	Cooperates in group activities Displays a professional commitment to ethical practice on a daily basis	Acts, discriminates, displays, influences, listens, modifies, performs, practices, proposes, qualifies, questions, revises, serves, solves, verifies

1972; Harrow, 1972) later created the exhaustive subcategories of the psychomotor domain. Simpson's proposed subcategories are as discussed in Fig. 6.14 and Table 6.3.

ACTION VERBS USED FOR WRITING OBJECTIVES

The actions verbs suggested in Tables 6.4, 6.5 and 6.6 should be used for writing objectives in each domain. However, some of these verbs cannot be measured or are redundant and known as *nonfunctional verbs*. They should be *avoided* when writing objectives (Box 6.3).

Text continued on page 206

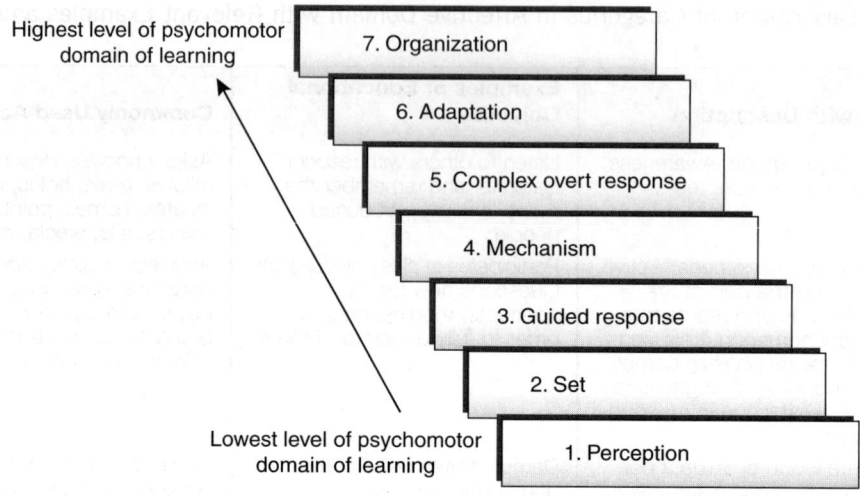

FIGURE 6.14

Categories of psychomotor domain of the educational objectives.

Table 6.3 Description of Categories in Psychomotor Domain with Relevant Examples and Active Verbs

Categories with Description	Examples of Educational Objective	Commonly Used Action Verbs
1. Perception: The ability to use sensory cues to guide motor activity. This ranges from sensory stimulation, through cue selection, to translation.	Detects nonverbal communication cues Adjusts drop rate based on the CVP readings of the patients	Chooses, describes, detects, differentiates, distinguishes, identifies, isolates, relates, selects
2. Set: Readiness to act. It includes mental, physical and emotional sets. These three sets are dispositions that predetermine a person's response to different situations (sometimes called *mindsets*).	Recognize one's abilities and limitations Shows desire to learn a new process	Begins, displays, explains, moves, proceeds, reacts, shows, states, volunteers
3. Guided response: The early stages in learning a complex skill that includes imitation and trial and error. Adequacy of performance is achieved by practising.	Follows instructions to build a model Responds hand signals of instructor while learning to operate a mechanical ventilator	Copies, traces, follows, reacts, reproduces, responds
4. Mechanism: This is the intermediate stage in learning a complex skill. Learned responses have become habitual and the movements can be performed with some confidence and proficiency.	Use a personal computer Operate a mechanical ventilator	Assembles, calibrates, constructs, dismantles, displays, fastens, fixes, grinds, heats, manipulates, measures, mends, mixes, organizes, sketches

Table 6.3 Description of Categories in Psychomotor Domain with Relevant Examples and Active Verbs—cont'd

Categories with Description	Examples of Educational Objective	Commonly Used Action Verbs
5. Complex overt response: The skilful performance of motor acts that involve complex movement patterns. Proficiency is indicated by a quick, accurate and highly coordinated performance, requiring a minimum of energy. This category includes performing without hesitation and automatic performance. For example, players often utter sounds of satisfaction or expletives as soon as they hit a tennis ball or throw a football, because they can tell by the feel of the act what the result will produce.	Operates a computer quickly and accurately Displays competence in performing wound dressing	Assembles, builds, calibrates, constructs, dismantles, displays, fastens, fixes, grinds, heats, manipulates, measures, mends, mixes, organizes, sketches NOTE: The keywords are the same as *mechanism*, but will have adverbs or adjectives that indicate that the performance is quicker, better, more accurate, etc.
6. Adaptation: Skills are well developed and the individual can modify movement patterns to fit special requirements.	Responds effectively to unexpected experiences such as emergency shock case	Adapts, alters, changes, rearranges, reorganizes, revises, varies
7. Organization: Creating new movement patterns to fit a particular situation or specific problem. Learning outcomes emphasize creativity based upon highly developed skills.	Constructs a new nursing theory Develops a new and comprehensive training programming for critical care nurses	Arranges, builds, combines, composes, constructs, creates, designs, initiate, makes, originates

Table 6.4 Active Verbs Used for Writing Objectives in Cognitive Domain

Knowledge	Comprehension	Application	Analysis	Synthesis	Evaluation
Count	Associate	Add	Analyse	Categorize	Appraise
Define	Compute	Apply	Arrange	Combine	Assess
Describe	Convert	Calculate	Breakdown	Compile	Compare
Draw	Defend	Change	Combine	Compose	Conclude
Identify	Discuss	Classify	Design	Create	Contrast
Labels	Distinguish	Complete	Detect	Drive	Criticize
List	Estimate	Compute	Develop	Design	Critique
Match	Explain	Demonstrate	Diagram	Devise	Determine
Name	Extend	Discover	Differentiate	Explain	Grade
Outlines	Extrapolate	Divide	Discriminate	Generate	Interpret
Point out	Generalize	Examine	Illustrate	Integrate	Judge
Quote	Give examples	Graph	Infer	Modify	Justify
Read	Infer	Interpolate	Outline	Order	Measure
Recite	Paraphrase	Manipulate	Relate	Organize	Rank
Recognize	Predict	Modify	Select	Plan	Rate

Continued

Table 6.4 Active Verbs Used for Writing Objectives in Cognitive Domain—cont'd

Knowledge	Comprehension	Application	Analysis	Synthesis	Evaluation
Record	Rewrite	Operate	Separate	Prescribe	Support
Repeat	Summarize	Prepare	Subdivide	Propose	Test
Reproduces		Produce	Utilize	Rearrange	
Selects		Show		Reconstruct	
State		Solve		Reorganize	
Write		Subtract		Revise	
		Translate		Summarize	
		Use		Specify	

Table 6.5 Active Verbs Used for Writing Objectives in Affective Domain

Receiving	Responding	Valuing	Organizing	Characterization by Value
Accept	Agree	Adopt	Anticipate	Act
Acknowledge	Allow	Aid	Collaborate	Administer
Attend (to)	Answer	Care (for)	Consider	Advance
Follow	Ask	Complete	Consult	Advocate
Listen	Assist	Compliment	Coordinator	Challenge
Meet	Choose	Contribute	Design	Change
Observe	Communicate	Delay	Direct	Commit (to)
Receive	Comply	Encourage	Establish	Counsel
	Confront	Endorse	Facilitate	Criticize
	Cooperate	Enforce	Follow	Debate
	Demonstrate	Evaluate	Though	Defend
	Describe	Expedite	Investigate	Disagree
	Discuss	Foster	Judge	Dispute
	Display	Guide	Head	Empathize
	Exhibit	Initiate	Manage	Endeavour
	Follow	Interact	Modify	Enhance
	Give	Join	Organize	Excuse
	Help	Justify	Plan	Forgive
	Identify	Maintain	Qualify	Influence
	Locate	Monitor	Recommend	Motivate
	Notify	Praise	Raise	Negotiate
	Obey	Present	Simplify	Object
	Offer	Propose	Specify	Persist
	Participate (in)	Query	Submit	Praise
	Practice	React	Synthesize	Prompt
	Present	Respect	Test	Reject
	Read	Seek	Vary	Seek

Table 6.5 Active Verbs Used for Writing Objectives in Affective Domain—cont'd

Receiving	Responding	Valuing	Organizing	Characterization by Value
	Reply	Share	Weight	Strive
	Report	Study		
	Respond	Subscribe		
	Select	Suggest		
		Support		
		Uphold		

Table 6.6 Active Verbs Used for Writing Objectives in Psychomotor Domain

Absorb	Cool	Fill	Manoeuvre	Start	Stopper
Add	Correct	Filter	Manipulate	Read	Store
Adsorb	Count	Fractionate	Mark	Record	Suspend
Adjust	Create	Frame	Macerate	Release	Take
Aliquot	Crush	Freeze	Measure	Remove	Test
Apply	Cut	Grade	Mix	Replace	Thaw
Aspirate	Decant	Grasp	Moisten	Resuspend	Thread
Assemble	Demonstrate	Grind	Mount	Retest	Tilt
Balance	Describe	Group	Pack	Rinse	Time
Bind	Design	Guide	Palpate	Roll	Tip
Blend	Dialyse	Handle	Participate	Rotate	Titrate
Build	Differentiate	Heat	Perform	Save	Trim
Calculate	Dilute	Observe	Pick	Scan	Touch
Calibrate	Discard	Obtain	Pipet	Score	Transfer
Centrifuge	Dismantle	Open	Place	Screen	Troubleshoot
Change	Dispense	Hemolyse	Plate	Seal	Turn
Choose	Dispose	Identify	Plot	Select	Type
Classify	Dissect	Illustrate	Position	Sensitize	Use
Clean	Dissolve	Incubate	Pour	Separate	Utilize
Collate	Drain	Inject	Prepare	Set	View
Collect	Draw	Input	Press	Sever	Warm
Combine	Dry	Insert	Process	Shake	Wash
Connect	Elute	Invert	Produce	Sharpen	Watch
Construct	Employ	Investigate	Programme	Ship	Weigh
Control	Estimate	Isolate	Pull	Siphon	Withdraw
Combine	Evacuate	Label	Puncture	Spin	Wipe
Confirm	Examine	Locate	Push	Spread	Wrap
Connect	Expel	Localize	Squeeze	Stick	
Construct	Operate	Maintain	Stain	Stir	
Control	Fasten	Make	Standardize	Stop	

BOX 6.3 ACTION VERBS COMMONLY AVOIDED WHEN WRITING OBJECTIVES

Able to	Familiar with	Learns
Appreciation for	Shows interest in	Memorizes
Awareness of	Knows	Understands
Capable of	Has knowledge of	Will be able to
Comprehend		
Conscious of		

LESSON PLANNING

Lesson planning is an important activity of daily teaching. The lesson plan might include the main points to be covered in the lesson activities for the students to do, questions related to the topic being taught and some form of assessment for the realization of stipulated instructional objectives. It indicates clearly what has already been done, what the students are to do, how the students are to be engaged in various activities and what activities are to be pursued. Lesson planning is the heart of effective teaching. The teacher has to consider the following points while lesson planning:

- Define broader objectives of the subject.
- Define classroom objectives of the lesson.
- Organize the subject matter to be covered to achieve the stipulated objectives.
- Decide on the way of presenting the subject matter, teaching strategies and tactics, and classroom interaction and management.
- Provide appropriate provision for evaluation and feedback.

I. DEFINITIONS OF LESSON PLAN

Lesson plan is the title given to a statement of achievement to be realized and specific meanings by which these are to be attained as a result of the activities engaged during the period.

—N.L. Bossing

Daily lesson planning involves defining the objectives, selecting and arranging the subject matter and determining the method of procedure.

—Bining and Bining

A lesson plan is a teaching outline of the important points of lesson arranged in which they are to be presented. It may include objectives, points to be made, questions to be asked, references to materials, assignments etc.

—Carter V. Good

II. FUNCTIONS OF A LESSON PLAN

- It ensures a definite objective for the day's work and a clear visualization of that objective.
- Lesson planning helps for adequate and appropriate use of resources in an efficient way.

- It keeps the teacher on track to ensure steady progress and a definite outcome of teaching and learning procedures.
- It helps clarify ideas about what, how, where and when and whom to teach.
- Lesson plan directs the teaching–learning process and procedures in the right direction.
- Helps review the subject matter and gives up-to-date knowledge.
- It helps the teacher delimit the teaching.
- When it is planned well, a student's interest can be maintained.
- It provides guidelines for the teacher about classroom instructions.
- It provides sensible framework for a teacher to be taught.
- It provides confidence, self-reliance, ease and freedom to teacher in teaching.

III. SIGNIFICANCE AND IMPORTANCE OF A LESSON PLAN

- In a teaching education programme, the lesson plan provides guidelines to students and the teacher during their teaching–learning practices.
- It helps in achieving the definite objectives.
- It makes teaching systematic, orderly and economical.
- It helps teachers overcome feelings of nervousness and insecurity and gives them confidence to face the class.
- It links new knowledge with previous knowledge acquired by a student.
- It prepares pivotal questions and illustrations.
- It enables the teacher evaluate his work as the lesson proceeds.
- It helps the teacher use a wider variety of teaching materials and learning activities in the classroom through a wider acquaintance with resources.
- It also helps the teacher plan the teaching–learning process per the availability and accessibility of resource materials.

IV. PREREQUISITES OF A LESSON PLAN

- *Knowledge and mastery of subject matter:* The teacher must be a master of his subject. He should have thorough knowledge of the subject matter, materials and activities to be used.
- *Knowledge of student psychology:* The teacher must have knowledge of child psychology, i.e. the teacher should know the standard and individuality of the students and present the subject matter accordingly.
- *Knowledge of methods and techniques:* The teacher should be conversant with the methods and techniques of teaching.
- *Knowledge of aims:* The teacher should have a basic understanding of the aims and objectives of education. He should have the ability and skills to write objectives in behavioural terms and a knowledge of various teaching skills.
- *Knowledge about the student's interests, traits and abilities:* The teacher must have adequate knowledge about the interests, traits and abilities of an individual student. This helps the teacher have an individual customized lesson plan for a specific group of the students.
- *Teacher's competence:* Teacher must have an ability to construct better lesson plans within a short time. In addition, he/she must have the ability to make constructive preparation for cooperative planning of activities with students.

- *Selection and organization of subject matter:* Teaching–learning activities, illustrative material, assignment and evaluation for students, references and bibliography must be planned by the teacher well in advance so that the lesson can be planned and executed in an effective manner.
  - *Learning activities:* The teacher chooses the learning activities. They should be varied sufficiently to allow for individual differences in the group.
  - *Teaching activities:* The teaching techniques that are objective-oriented and cost-effective directly help the teacher to obtain the educational objectives.
  - *Type of illustrative materials:* Audiovisual aids and instruction media.
  - *Assignments:* The plan should use assignments to project the immediate work to the next situation.
  - *Evaluation:* Some type of evaluation should be planned for each lesson.
  - *References and bibliography:* The teacher will have ready references and bibliography to be used indirectly in student assignments.

V. ESSENTIAL CHARACTERISTICS OF A GOOD LESSON PLAN

The essential characteristics of a lesson are discussed below and may also be seen in Box 6.4.

- *Clearly written:* Lesson plans must preferably be in written form. It must be appropriately written and depict who will be taught, who will teach, when will be taught, where the class will be taken, what will be taught, why it will be taught, how it will be taught and what should be expected from students after the lesson.
- *Definite aim and objectives:* A good lesson plan must have clearly defined aim and objectives that very clearly specify the purpose of the lesson and the purpose of each activity included in the lesson plan.
- *Extension of existing knowledge:* The topic of a lesson plan should be planned in a consecutive sequence of the previously taught topics or existing knowledge for better understanding of the topic. It should not be a repetition nor an isolated topic plan.
- *Simple and comprehensive:* Each lesson plan must be simple, lucid, concise and precise and must include all activities that are expected to be carried out by a teacher in classroom during the teaching–learning process comprehensively.

BOX 6.4 ESSENTIAL CHARACTERISTICS OF A GOOD LESSON PLAN

1. Clearly written
2. Definite aim and objectives
3. Extension of existing knowledge
4. Simple and comprehensive
5. Flexible
6. Ensures active teaching–learning process
7. Division with essence of wholesomeness
8. Individualized and customized
9. Feasibility and significance
10. Proceed from general to specific
11. Completeness
12. Inclusion of summary, recapitalization, bibliography and student assignment

---

- *Flexible plan:* A planned lesson must not be rigid; it must be flexible to adopt the changes expected to arise in specific classroom situations. A flexible lesson plan facilities the teacher adapt to specific incidental situations in the classroom.
- *Ensure active teaching–learning process:* A good lesson plan ensures active participation of both the teacher and the student for effective achievement of educational objectives. A passive lesson plan fails to motivate the teacher and/or the student for an effective teaching–learning activity outcome.
- *Division with essence of wholesomeness:* A lesson plan must be divided into subsections for better presentation; however, its wholesomeness must not be distorted. A logical sequence and efficient cohesion of the subsections of the lesson may help in the preservation of the lesson plan's wholesomeness.
- *Individualized and customized:* The content of the lesson plan should be designed according to the needs, interests, abilities and level of the students. This individualized and customized approach helps the teacher achieve the expected aim of a lesson plan.
- *Feasibility and significance:* A lesson plan must be planned in a manner that it is feasible in terms of time and available resources. It must be as practical as possible without overestimations in a hypothetical manner. In addition, a lesson plan must have significance to a particular group of students because nonsignificant topics fail to create interest in learners as well as the teacher. Therefore, the teaching–learning activity may not be fruitful without the significance of a lesson/topic.
- *Proceed from general to specific:* A lesson plan must be planned such that it proceeds from general or basic knowledge to specific knowledge so students can easily understand the lesson.
- *Completeness:* A good lesson plan must be complete in itself without leaving any essential component like topic of the lesson, general and specific objectives, content, teacher–student activity and methods of presentation, audiovisual aids, question to be asked for students, summary, recapitalized and assignment for the students.
- *Inclusion of summary, recapitalization, bibliography and student assignment:* In addition to a basic introductory plan and body of the lesson, the lesson plan must include the summary, recapitalization, bibliography and student assignment.

VI. STEPS OF LESSON PLANNING

1. *Preparation or introduction:* Exploration of the student's knowledge helps to lead them on to the lesson. The teacher needs to prepare the students to receive new knowledge.
2. *Presentation:* The aim of the lesson should be clearly stated before presentation of the subject matter, which helps both the teacher and students have common pursuit.
3. *Comparison or association:* Quote examples and associate facts with two examples so that learners can understand easily and arrive at generalizations on their own.
4. *Generalizations:* The knowledge presented by the teacher should be thought-provoking, innovating and stimulating to assist the students generalize the situation.
5. *Application:* The students should be able to make use of the knowledge acquired and test the validity of the generalization arrived at in theory. It has to apply in the clinical field to make learning more permanent and worthwhile.
6. *Recapitulation:* The teacher has to ask suitable, stimulating and pivotal questions on the topic. The answer will give feedback to the teacher regarding the efficacy of the method of teaching and he can decide whether or not clarification is needed.

VII. TYPE OF APPROACHES TO LESSON PLANNING

Several educational philosophers have suggested a few lesson planning approaches. Some essential approaches of lesson planning have been discussed in the following sections (such as Herbertian approach of lesson planning, Bloom's evaluation approach of lesson planning, Gloverian approach of lesson planning and RCEM approach of lesson planning).

A. Herbertian approach

J.F. Herbart, a German philosopher advocated lesson planning using following five steps:

1. *Preparation:* Preparing means the preparation of the learner's mind to receive new knowledge. Preparation of the learner involves two steps:
   - Previous knowledge testing: Through testing previous knowledge, the teacher becomes familiar with what pupils already know relevant to the topic.
   - Announcement of the aim: An aim will automatically emerge if the lesson has been effectively introduced. The aim should be clear, concise and free from unknown words. J. Welton said, 'To know where the pupils are and where they should try to be are the first two essentials of the teaching'.
2. *Presentation:* It involves a good deal of intellectual activity on the part of the students. A teacher is to put himself into the students' shoes to present things to them. Selected subject matter should be presented according to the needs, interests, abilities and developmental level of the students.
3. *Comparison and abstraction:* Association is linking new ideas with the old ones and with one another into a system. The selected examples or facts are presented before the students and they are asked to carefully observe and compare them with another set of facts to arrive at some conclusion.
4. *Generalization:* Comparison and association helps students find a certain conclusion that enables them to frame general laws, principles or formulas. The teacher's function is to enable the students to draw out the generalization from relevant data.
5. *Application:* Knowledge that is not used will soon fade away from consciousness. Knowledge is power, but it is only when the mind can apply it to practical situation.

Merits

- Avoids unnecessary repetition in teaching
- Simple and easy approach
- Logical and psychological
- Used in achieving the cognitive objective of teaching
- Assists in making the teaching systematic

Demerits

- Highly dominated by the teacher
- More stress on teaching rather than on learning
- Does not consider the learning structure in organizing teaching activities
- Specific objectives are not written in behavioural terms
- Teaching activities are less meaningful and practical

B. Bloom's evaluation approach on lesson planning

B.S. Bloom believed that the teaching–learning process must be objective centric. He considered education as a tripolar process (Fig. 6.15). The three pools are educational objectives, learning experiences and learning outcome or change in the student's behaviour. The major features of this approach of lesson planning are as follows:

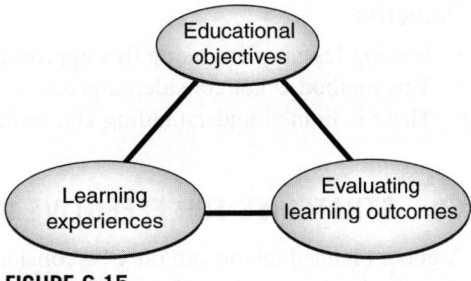

FIGURE 6.15
Bloom's major features of lesson planning.

- Teaching–learning activity is learning objective based rather than content based.
- The expected outcome of the teaching–learning activity is an overall change in behaviour of the student rather than learning specific content.
- The outcome of learning is measured based on predetermined learning objectives, including cognitive, affective and psychomotor learning objective outcome.

Merits

- The objectives are written in behavioural terms.
- The teaching activities are related to learning structures.
- It makes the teaching purposeful and objective centred.
- It is based on psychological and scientific principles.

Demerits

- Gives rise to rigid and mechanical planning which lacks flexibility.
- Does not provide an opportunity for creativity among students.
- It is a highly structured approach and imposes a high demand on the teacher and the student during the teaching–learning process.

C. RCEM approach

RCEM approach was developed by Indian educationists at the Regional College of Education, Mysore, and therefore known as *RCEM approach*. This approach has its roots in the system approach and has defined three main steps of the teaching–learning process: input, process and output.

- *Input:* It includes the identification of objectives. They are also known as expected behavioural outcomes. Input further resembles the preparation steps of the Herbarin approach where the teacher tries to know what students know and what they are expected to know.
- *Process:* The main focus of the process is to create the learning situation. It implies the interaction of teacher and students. It includes teacher and student activities, teaching strategies and audiovisual aids and techniques of motivation.
- *Output:* It is the evaluation phase of the lesson plan. We get desirable behavioural changes among students through the output. These are the real learning outcomes.

Merits

- It is an indigenous method; therefore, more suitable for local teaching–learning pursuits.
- Learning objectives are formulated in the form of measurable student abilities and rational processes.
- The teaching–learning scenario, methods, materials and audiovisual aids are clearly defined.
- This model of teaching can be used to for basic as well advanced learning.
- Theoretical knowledge of teaching concepts can be applied.
- The evaluation aspect of a lesson plan is efficiently and adequately clarified.

Demerits
- Writing lesson plans using this approach is a cumbersome task.
- This method is not considered practical as it is time-consuming.
- There is limited understanding and utilization of this method.

VIII. STRATEGIES FOR EFFECTIVE IMPLEMENTATION OF THE LESSON PLAN

A good, planned lesson can only be considered effective if it implemented in an efficient manner. Some suggested strategies for effective implementation of a planned lesson are as follows:

- The lesson plan must be efficiently written, prepared and designed with a complete sense of confidence.
- The presenter or teacher must be clear about the aim and objectives of the lesson plan. In addition, the presenter must have thorough command on the subject content planned to be delivered to a group of students.
- Use of audiovisual aids must be well planned, judicious and efficient. It is said that the right audiovisual aid at the right time and right place by the right person for the right individuals should be used.
- Efficient classroom management is very important for effective implementation of the lesson plan. It must be ensured that the classroom is well ventilated, clean, optimum temperature and the students are comfortably seated.
- Introduction of the lesson must create interest in the students and they must be well motivated to receive the subject content. This introduction usually takes about the first 5 minutes of the total 45 minutes of class time.
- It is essential to use the right methods of teaching ensuring the active involvement of students and charge their brains to receive and retain the subject content.
- There must be careful use of blackboard and other audiovisual methods. It must be ensured that the content presented on a blackboard or using other audiovisual aids is legible, clear, concise, attractive, lucid and large enough for students to visualize without undue discomfort.
- Questions planned and presented in a lesson plan must be definite, clear, stimulating and thought provoking.
- Content must be delivered in a simple language with a clear and audible voice with complete sense of confidence and using relevant real life examples to promote understanding of the subject content.
- Provide enough time to the students for clarifying their doubts. Confusing content must be clarified and reinforced with simple and relevant examples.
- Individual student attention while taking and giving regular feedback on the understating of subject content is very essential for effective implementation of the lesson plan.
- Efficient time management, appropriate recapitalization of the subject matter and relevant thought provoking questioning and continuous feedback are key aspects of effective implementation of the lesson plan.
- End recapitalization, discussion of reference, bibliography and further reading and expected students exercise assignments are also considered to be important in the success of a lesson plan.

IX. FORMAT OF A LESSON PLAN

An effective lesson must have the following format (refer to a detailed lesson plan in Appendix A).

I. Cover page: This page must include topic of lesson, date of submission, name of supervisor, and name and details of the presenting teacher.

II. First page: This page must include the following basic information:

Basic lesson plan information:

- Subject   : Communication and Education Technology
- Name of topic   : Assessment of learning needs
- Name of student's teacher : Ms Jasveen Kaur
- Name of supervisor   : Dr Suresh K. Sharma
- Date of teaching   : _____
- Time of teaching   : _____
- Venue of teaching   : Lecturer Theater No. 3
- Group   : B.Sc. (N) 2nd year students
- Size of group   : 25
- Method of teaching   : Lecture cum discussion
- Duration   : ___ minutes
- AV Aids   : PowerPoint Presentation

Previous knowledge: The group has some knowledge about the topic: Assessment of learning needs.

General objective: At the end of the class, students will be able to acquire knowledge about assessment of learning needs.

Specific objectives: At the end of teaching, students will be able to

- Define various terms related to assessment of learning needs.
- Explain about historical perspective.
- Enlist types of assessment.
- Enumerate principles of assessment for learning.
- Describe purposes of conducting assessment of learning needs.

III. Main body of lesson plan:

S. No.	Time	Contributory Objective	Content Matter	Teaching–Learning Activities	
				AV Aids	Evaluation

IV. Appendix of lesson plan: This includes giving the assignment to students and recommending further reading, writing the bibliography and references.

CLASSROOM MANAGEMENT

The principal is the head of an institution and a classteacher is the head of a class. Institutional management comes under the preview of the head of the institution but classroom management is the ultimate responsibility of the classteacher. The classteacher is expected to manage his class. Academic success of an institution principally depends on efficient class management by a competent classteacher. A teacher must possess some core qualities for efficient management of a class such as general academic proficiency, professional and managerial efficiency and positive personality traits.

I. DEFINITIONS OF CLASSROOM MANAGEMENT

Classroom management is an organizational function in which tasks are performed in a variety of settings, resulting in the inculcation of certain values such as human respect, personal integrity, self-direction and group cohesion etc.

—Johanson and Brooks

Classroom management is a system of action and activities are managed in classroom to induce learning through teacher–taught relationship. Teacher and students are the basic components for managing classroom activities.

(Operational meaning)

II. DIMENSIONS OF CLASSROOM MANAGEMENT

In behavioural terms, classroom management can be classified in four different dimensions: physical or environmental dimension, psychological dimension, ethical dimension, and social and cultural dimension of classroom management (Fig. 6.16).

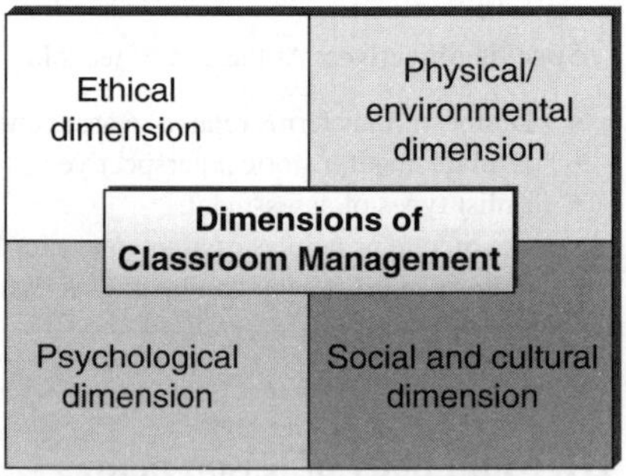

- *Physical/environmental dimension:* Physical or environmental dimension of classroom management includes light and ventilation of the classroom, seating arrangement for students, availability and functioning of blackboard and/or other audio-visual facilities in classroom, offering aesthetic academic environment inside and/or outside classroom. A teacher as a classroom manager should ensure the optimum and efficient management of these physical or environment facilities/services which are essential for overall learning in the students.

- *Psychological dimension:* Psychological dimension of classroom management is considered similar to software of the computer; without its presence mere hardware (physical/environmental dimension) is of no use and vice versa.

Ethical dimension	Physical/environmental dimension
Dimensions of Classroom Management	
Psychological dimension	Social and cultural dimension

FIGURE 6.16

Dimensions of classroom management.

Psychological classroom management includes infusion of motivation in students to promote the learning process. Motivation could be infused verbally or nonverbally through continuous feedback, behavioural reinforcement and positive encouragement in students. Psychological dimension of classroom management plays a pivotal role in the overall management of a classroom.

- *Social and cultural dimension:* A classroom is a miniature replica of an institution as well as of the society. The new society is shaped in the classroom through its desirable social and cultural environment. Classroom management involves the relationship of social and cultural environment in its overall management which depends on certain factors such as the teacher–taught relationship, relationship among students, relationship among teachers, relationship between teachers and the head of the institution. A teacher must know the background of his students and their entering behaviour, learning activities and interests.

- *Ethical dimension:* The ethical dimension of classroom management is concerned with feelings, attitudes, values and ethical aspects of students. A teacher is the manager of the class and an ideal to his students. He should look like and behave like a teacher. Further, the teacher should maintain classroom code and conduct which should be value based or ethics oriented.

III. PRINCIPLES OF THE CLASSROOM MANAGEMENT

Classroom management can primarily be governed by general as well as specific principles discussed below (Box 6.5).

A. General principles of classroom management

General principles can be learned and practised systematically. The general principles can be applied in several situations and provide a strong base to the teachers to manage vivid classroom management related problems. Some of the assumptions related to general principles of the classroom management are as follows:

- *Self-control and role model:* Teachers must follow the principle of self-control and be a role model to the students. This provides a sense of confidence and trust to the students towards their teachers and institution as a whole and effective classroom management can be ensured.
- *Understanding and acceptance:* Teachers must ensure they understand the individual differences of the each student and accept them as they are. This will not only prevent biasness in teachers towards students but also provide each student with an equal opportunity to be a part of the class. This will also promote decreased psychological stress and decreased dissatisfaction in students and ultimately better classroom management.
- *Realistic and practical goals:* Teachers must plan realistic achievable educational goals for their students so undue psychological pressure in students can be avoided and the classroom can be efficiently managed.

BOX 6.5 PRINCIPLES OF CLASSROOM MANAGEMENT

I. *General principles of classroom management*
- Self-control and role model approach of teacher
- Understanding and acceptance of student uniqueness
- Realistic and practical goals of teaching–learning
- Exercising the productive teaching–learning activities
- Understanding student's interest and ability

II. *Specific principles of classroom management*
- Appropriate planning of classroom management
- Encouragement of students
- Giving responsibility to learners
- Minimum disruption of teaching–learning activities
- Clear guidelines of rules for students
- Reward and punishment for student's activities
- Conducive learning environment

- *Productive teaching–learning activities:* Teachers must ensure that learning experiences planned for the students are productive in nature so that classroom academics can be fruitful.
- *Student's interests and ability:* Teaching and learning activities must be planned on the principles of student's interests and ability so that the teaching–learning environment can be goal achieving in nature.

B. Specific principles of classroom management

Specific principles of classroom management can be adapted and used in certain specific situations and can be very helpful for overall classroom management. These are discussed below:

- *Planning:* Plan independent activities as well as organized lessons so students can be motivated to achieve their educational goals.
- *Encouragement:* Encourage effort and cues and reinforce positive and appropriate behaviour so students can be motivated for learning.
- *Responsibility:* Let students assume independent responsibility so they can develop a sense of responsibility and accountability towards their own education.
- *Minimum disruption:* Teachers must ensure that there is minimal disruption in natural learning among the students so they can have uninterrupted natural learning.
- *Clear rules:* The rules established for the students must be crystal clear so that ambiguity can be avoided and following rules and their implementation becomes easy.
- *Reward and punishment:* Students must be rewarded for their behaviour so they can be reinforced for repeating positive behaviour and discouraged from negative behaviour.
- *Conducive learning environment:* It is believed that the environment influences a person more than anything else. Therefore, a conducive teaching–learning environment can help a classteacher achieve the expected positive behaviour in students.

IV. CLASSROOM MANAGEMENT PROBLEMS

- ***Inadequate light and ventilation:*** Effective classroom work can take place only in a congenial classroom atmosphere that includes adequate light and ventilation, temperature, furniture, seats, etc. Inadequate light and ventilation can create problems for the student. It has an adverse effect on their learning as well as health.
- ***Inadequate furniture and lack of conducive seating environment:*** In the absence of proper seating arrangements, the students find themselves uneasy and uncomfortable. They do not feel like working wholeheartedly. They find it difficult to concentrate on learning in the class.
- ***Overcrowded classrooms:*** It is not possible for the teacher to teach effectively in a fully packed classroom. The teacher cannot give individual attention to all students. Therefore, the number of students in a class should not exceed more than 50.
- ***Inadequate apparatus:*** In an overcrowded class, it is difficult to provide adequate equipment to all students affecting their learning.
- ***Lack of routine:*** Breaking a routine creates confusion, chaos, disorder and indiscipline in the class. Routine should be followed in taking roll-calls, performing practicals, entering or leaving the classroom and other activities.
- ***Lack of adequate distance between classrooms:*** Many classrooms are so near each other that the noise of one class disturbs students sitting in other classrooms. This can affect their studies.
- ***Problems of indiscipline:*** Absenteeism among teachers and the taught can also affect classroom teaching.

- *Poor teacher–taught interpersonal relationship:* In ancient times, there was a strong teacher–pupil relationship; however with the present changing cultural values, there is a lack of teacher–taught relationship these days that ultimately affects the teaching–learning outcome in an institution.

V. STRATEGIES FOR CLASSROOM MANAGEMENT

- *Promotion of rhythm in teaching–learning activities:* Rhythm should be introduced in every teaching–learning activity. It guarantees smoothness in the sequence of movements. Routine is essential to rhythm. A chaotic, confusing, disturbing and insecure class is one where routines have been neglected and the sequence of activities has not been followed.
- *Enhancing healthy classroom customs and traditions:* The teacher should develop class traditions in the class. He should encourage the students to play their role well with a sense of responsibility. It will help maintain self-discipline and ensure respect for college authority, self-progress, love for orderliness and development of good character.
- *Promote positivity in teacher's behaviour:* The teacher's verbal and nonverbal behaviour significantly influences student behaviour. The teacher's high character, high moral alertness, courage, practice, love and humility, his love and affection for students, his sense of humour, optimistic and democratic outlook, sympathy and wisdom, justice and impartiality, his resourcefulness, originality, confidence and his emotional and social health can positively influence student behaviour.
- *Infuse motivation in students:* The teaching–learning process is ineffective without proper motivation. The following techniques can be used for motivating students:
  - Goal, ideal and purposeful events
  - Knowledge of results or progress
  - Use of reward or punishment
  - Active participation
  - Use of competition
  - Cooperation
  - Evaluation
  - Audiovisual aids
  - Teacher–pupil relationship
- *Encouraging pupil's participation:* The teacher should encourage students to take part in daily activities and cocurricular activities that suit their interests, abilities and other potentialities such as discussions and declamations. Student participation may also be sought in the following programmes:
  - Development of lessons
  - Activity methods
  - Cocurricular activities

VI. ROLE OF A TEACHER IN CLASSROOM MANAGEMENT

A teacher plays a pivotal role in classroom management because he is the central component of classroom management and has the authority, responsibility and accountability to manage a class. He plays variety of roles such as teacher, manager, philosopher, guide, researcher and leader. Efficient classroom management demands strong interpersonal relationship skills in a teacher, where he/she needs to build strong interpersonal relationship with students, colleagues, head of the institution and even parents of students and society as a whole. The main roles of the teacher in classroom management are as follows (Fig. 6.17):

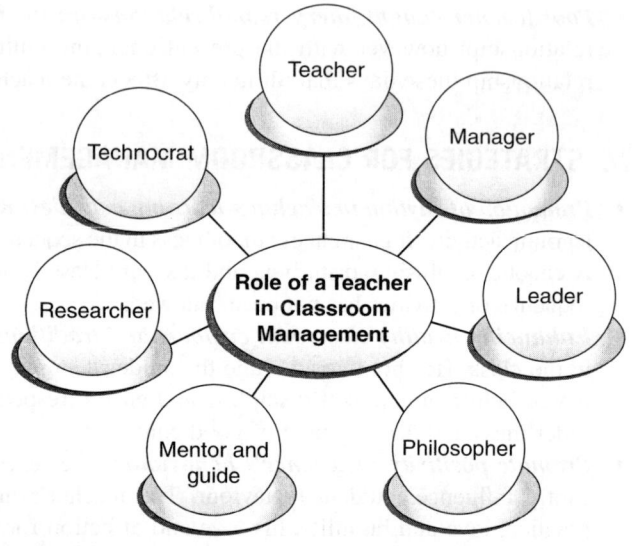

FIGURE 6.17

Role of the teacher in classroom management.

- **Teacher:** The core aim of classroom management is to achieve the expected outcome of the particular teaching–learning process. Therefore, the primary role of the teacher in classroom management is functioning efficiently as a teacher.
- **Manager:** Classroom management demands managerial skills from teachers. They are expected to perform responsibilities of planning, organizing, supervising, directing, coordinating and controlling the teaching–learning process.
- **Leader:** The teacher is expected to lead the class as a classroom manager for its overall functioning and taking desired messages to higher authorities and convincing them with the expected demands.
- **Philosopher:** The teacher is expected to have a strong hold and mastery over the subject content that has to be delivered to students. In addition, a teacher is expected to teach moral values, ethics and discipline to the students.
- **Mentor and guide:** Each of us requires a mentor or guide to help us choose the right path in life. Students also require a mentor or guide to help them take the right decisions for learning activities. Therefore, a teacher is expected to perform the role of a mentor or guide for a particular group of students to solve their personal as well teaching–learning related problems.
- **Researcher:** Solutions for problems are generated through research. A teacher also faces a lot of problems related to classroom management that can be easily solved by generating evidence-based solutions generated through action research. Therefore, a teacher must act as researcher to generate the empirical solutions for classroom management related problems.
- **Technocrat:** Advancement in science and technology has offered a wide range of technologically sophisticated audiovisual aids to the educational institutions. A teacher must be technologically skilled to operate and manage these technologically sophisticated audiovisual aids as and when required.

REVIEW QUESTIONS

Long-Answer Questions

1. Discuss the maxims of teaching.
2. Describe a lesson plan.

3. Discuss the formulation of objectives.
4. Explain problem-based learning.
5. Describe the principles and maxims of teaching.
6. Explain lesson planning.
7. What are the characteristics of learning?
8. Define learning and define its nature.
9. Differentiate between cognitive domain of learning and affective domain of learning.
10. Discuss the principles of learning.
11. Discuss the domains of learning.
12. Discuss the factors influencing learning.
13. Explain the learning process.
14. Describe the principles of teaching.
15. Discuss the dimensions and principles of classroom management.
16. Describe the essential characteristics of lesson planning.
17. Explain taxonomy of educational objectives.
18. Explain the characteristics of educational objectives.
19. Describe the characteristics of good teaching.
20. Discuss the meaning and nature of teaching.
21. Discuss characteristics of learning process.
22. Describe principles of teaching.
23. Explain characteristics of learning. Write principles and maximums of teaching.

Short-Answer Questions

1. Discuss the principles of learning.
2. What are the elements of teaching learning process?
3. State four characteristics of lesion plan.
4. Discuss briefly peer learning.
5. Differentiate between goal and objectives.
6. List down any four qualities of educational objectives.
7. Define lesson plan.

Multiple-Choice Questions (MCQs)

1. Which factors help in measuring learning efficiency?
   (a) Accuracy
   (b) Speed
   (c) Retention
   (d) All of these
2. Average retention rate by a student through practising is about
   (a) 30%
   (b) 75%
   (c) 10%
   (d) 20%

3. Series of steps of learning process include
   (a) Motive of learner ... Establish goals ... Adjustment ... Behaviour change ... Behaviour stabilization
   (b) Motive of learner ... Establish goals ... Adjustment ... Behaviour stabilization ... Behaviour change
   (c) Establish goals ... Motive of learner ... Behaviour change ... Adjustment ... Behaviour stabilization
   (d) Establish goals ... Motive of learner ... Behaviour stabilization ... Behaviour change ... Adjustment

4. Elements of cooperative learning include
   (a) Face-to-face interaction and positive interdependence
   (b) Creativity and professional development
   (c) Continuity and transformation
   (d) Behavioural change and maturity

5. Role plays helps to assess which domain of learning?
   (a) Cognitive
   (b) Affective
   (c) Psychomotor
   (d) All of these

6. _____ domain of learning is evaluated by formal written examinations?
   (a) Cognitive
   (b) Affective
   (c) Psychomotor
   (d) All of these

7. Doing head-to-toe examination in an OPD is an example of which domain of learning?
   (a) Affective
   (b) Psychomotor
   (c) Cognitive
   (d) All of these

8. The international poles of teaching process include
   (a) Teacher, pupil and motivational environment
   (b) Information, knowledge and skills
   (c) Teacher, pupil and subject matter
   (d) Teacher, pupil and communication system

9. Psychological principle of teaching include
   (a) Principle of definite aim
   (b) Principal of activity aim
   (c) Principal of pupil centeredness
   (d) Principle of feedback and reinforcement

10. Educational objectives should be
    (a) Attainable and realistic
    (b) Time bound and unequivocal
    (c) Motivational and professional
    (d) Both (a) and (b)

11. According to the Bloom's taxonomy, educational objectives are classified into how many basic domains?
    (a) Two
    (b) Three
    (c) Four
    (d) Five
12. Characteristics of good lesson plan are
    (a) It should be clearly written
    (b) Simple and comprehensive
    (c) Rigid
    (d) Both (a) and (b)
13. Institutional objectives are also known as
    (a) Behavioural objectives
    (b) Departmental objectives
    (c) Institutional objectives
    (d) General objectives
14. The six main categories of cognitive domain of learning are
    (a) Knowledge, comprehension, application, analysis, synthesis and evaluation
    (b) Knowledge, comprehension, perception, mechanism, synthesis and evaluation
    (c) Knowledge, comprehension, motivation, attitude, coordination, motivation, analysis
    (d) None of these
15. Explaining the role of genetic factors in colorectal cancer is an example of which domain of learning?
    (a) Cognitive
    (b) Affective
    (c) Psychomotor
    (d) All of above

Answers of the Multiple-Choice Questions

1. (d), 2. (b), 3. (a), 4. (a), 5. (b), 6. (a), 7. (b), 8. (c), 9. (d), 10. (d), 11. (b), 12. (d), 13. (a), 14. (a), 15. (a)

FURTHER READING

Abbatt, F. R. (1992). *Teaching for better learning* (2nd ed., p. 183). Geneva: WHO.

Ahrenfelt, J., & Watkin, N. (2006). *100 ideas for essential teaching skills (continuum one hundred)*. New York, NY: Continuum.

Allen, J. D. (1986). Classroom management: students' perspectives, goals, and strategies. *American Educational Research Journal, 23,* 437–459.

Arkoudis, S. (2006). *Teaching international students: Strategies to enhance learning. Centre for the Study of Higher Education.* University of Melbourne.

Baars, B. J., & Gage, N. M. (2007). *Cognition, brain, and consciousness: Introduction to cognitive neuroscience.* London, UK: Elsevier.

Baldwin, G. (2005). *The teaching-research nexus. How research informs and enhances learning and teaching in the University of Melbourne.* Centre for the Study of Higher Education, University of Melbourne.

Barbetta, P., Norona, K., & Bicard, D. (2005). Classroom behavior management: A dozen common mistakes and what to do instead. *Preventing School Failures,* 49(3), 11–19.

Bear, G. G. (2008). Best practices in classroom discipline. In A. Thomas, & J. Grimes (Eds.). *Best practices in school psychology V* (pp. 1403–1420). Bethesda, MD: National Association of School Psychologists.

Bear, G. G., Cavalier, A., & Manning, M. (2005). *Developing self-discipline and preventing and correcting misbehavior.* Boston, MA: Allyn & Bacon.

Berliner, D. C. (1988). Effective classroom management and instruction: A knowledge base for consultation. In J. L. Graden, J. E. Zins, & M. J. Curtis (Eds.). *Alternative educational delivery systems: Enhancing instructional options for all students.* Washington, DC: National Association of School Psychologists.

Bitterman, M. E., Menzel, R., Fietz, A., & Schäfer, S. (1983). Classical conditioning of proboscis extension in honeybees (Apis mellifera). *Journal of Comparative Psychology,* 97, 107–119.

Bloom BS (1956). *Taxonomy of Educational Objectives, the classification of educational goals – Handbook I: Cognitive Domain* New York: McKay.

Brophy, J. E., & Good, T. L. (1986). Teacher behavior and student achievement. In M. C. Wittrock (Ed.), *Handbook of research on teaching* (3rd ed.). New York: Macmillan.

Candy, P. C., Crebert, G., & O'Leary, J. (1994). *Developing lifelong learners through undergraduate education.* National Board of Employment Education and Training, AGPS, Canberra.

Dave, R. (1967). *Psychomotor domain.* Berlin: International Conference of Educational Testing.

Davies, M., & Devlin, M. (2007). *Interdisciplinary higher education: Implications for teaching and learning.* Centre for the Study of Higher Education, University of Melbourne.

Fuchs, A. H., & Milar, K. S. (2003). Psychology as a Science. In Weiner, Irving, & Donald K. Freedheim (Eds.). *Handbook of Psychology.* New York, NY: Wiley.

Gaff, J. G., et al. (1996). *Handbook of the undergraduate curriculum.* San Francisco, CA: Jossey-Bass Publishers.

Gagne, R., & Briggs, L. (1974). *Principles of instructional design.* New York, NY: Holt, Rinehart and Winston.

Gilbert, J. J. (1983). *Educational handbook for health personnel* (6th ed.). New York, NY: WHO.

Gootman, M. E. (2008). The caring teacher's guide to discipline: Helping students learn self-control, responsibility, and respect. *Journal of School Psychology,* 3(6), 36.

Grusec, J. E., & Hastings, P. D. (2007). *Handbook of socialization: Theory and research.* New York: Guilford Press.

Harris, K. L. (2005). *Guide for reviewing assessment. Prompts and guidelines for monitoring and enhancing assessment practices.* Centre for the Study of Higher Education, University of Melbourne.

Harrow, A. (1972). *A taxonomy of the psychomotor domain. A guide for developing behavioral objectives.* New York: McKay.

Heidgerken, L. E. (2004). *Teaching and learning in schools of nursing* (3rd ed., pp. 123–125). New Delhi: Konark Publishers.

Hilgard, E., & Bower, G. (1966). *Theories of learning.* New York, NY: Appleton Century-Crofts.

James, R., Baldwin, G., & McInnis, C. (1999). *Which university? The factors influencing the choices of prospective undergraduates.* Canberra: AGPS.

Kauchak, D., & Eggen, P. (2008). *Introduction to teaching: Becoming a professional* (3rd ed.). Upper Saddle River, NJ: Pearson Education, Inc.

Krathwohl, D. R., Bloom, B. S., & Masia, B. B. (1973). *Taxonomy of educational objectives, the Classification of educational goals. Handbook II: Affective domain.* New York: David McKay.

Laurillard, D. (1993). *Rethinking university teaching: A framework for the effective use of educational technology.* London, UK: Routledge.

Lou, C., & Walter, D. (1978). *The systematic design of instruction.* Glenview, IL: Scott, Foresman.

Marshall, M. (2001). *Discipline without stress, punishments or rewards.* Los Alamitos, CA: Piper Press.

Moskowitz, G., & Hayman, J. L., Jr. (1976). Success strategies of inner-city teachers: A year-long study. *Journal of Educational Research,* 69, 283–289.

Narang, M., & Arora, V. (2005). *Encyclopaedia of techniques of teachings* (vol. 1, pp. 404–405). New Delhi: Anmol Publications.

Pascarella, E., & Terenzini, P. (1998). *How college affects students: Findings and insights from twenty years of research*. San Francisco, CA: Jossey Bass.

Pintrich, P. R., & De Groot, E. V. (1990). Motivational and self-regulated learning components of classroom academic performance. *Journal of Educational Psychology*, 82, 33–40.

Salsbury, D. E., & Schoenfeldt, M. (2008). *Lesson planning: A research-based model for K-12 classrooms*. Alexandria, VA: Prentice Hall.

Sandman, C. A., Wadhwa, P., Hetrick, W., Porto, M., & Peeke, H. V. S. (1997). Human fetal heart rate dishabituation between thirty and thirty-two weeks gestation. *Child Development*, 68, 1031–1040.

Seligman, M. (1970). On the generality of the laws of learning. *Psychological Review*, 77, 406–418.

Serdyukov, P., & Ryan, M. (2008). *Writing effective lesson plans: The 5-star approach*. Boston, MA: Allyn & Bacon.

Simpson, E. (1972). *The classification of educational objectives in the psychomotor domain: The psychomotor domain. Vol. 3*. Washington, DC: Gryphon House.

Skinner, C. E. (1996). *Education psychology* (4th ed., pp. 417–449). London, UK: PHI Publishers.

Skowron, J. (2006). *Powerful lesson planning: Every teachers guide to effective instruction*. Thousand Oaks, CA: Corwin Press.

Tanol, G., Johnson, L., McComas, J., & Cote, E. (2010). Responding to rule violations or rule following: A comparison of two versions of the good behavior game with kindergarten students. *Journal of School Psychology*, 48, 337–355.

Terry, W. S. (2006). *Learning and memory: Basic principles, processes, and procedures*. Boston, MA: Pearson Education, Inc.

Thompson, J. G. (2007). *First year teacher's survival guide: Ready-to-use strategies, tools & activities for meeting the challenges of each school day (J-B Ed: Survival Guides)*. San Francisco, CA: Jossey-Bass.

Thorndike, E. (1932). *The fundamentals of learning*. New York: Teachers College Press.

Thorndike, E. (1999). *Education psychology*. New York: Routledge.

Tileston, D. E. W. (2003). *What Every Teacher Should Know About Instructional Planning*. Thousand Oaks, CA: Corwin Press.

Tingstrom, D. H., Sterling-Turner, H. E., & Wilczynski, S. M. (2006). The good behavior game: 1969–2002. *Behavior Modification*, 30(2), 225–253.

University of Melbourne Curriculum Commission. (2006). *The Melbourne Model: Report of the Curriculum Commission*. University of Melbourne.

Walia, J. S. (2007). *Educational technology*. New Delhi: Ahim Paul Publishers.

Walia, J. S. (2009). *Teaching–learning process*. New Delhi: Ahim Paul Publishers.

Wolfe, S. (2006). *Your best year yet! A guide to purposeful planning and effective classroom organization (teaching strategies)*. New York: Teaching Strategies.

Wood, D. C. (1988). Habituation in Stentor produced by mechanoreceptor channel modification. *Journal of Neuroscience*, 2254(8), 112–116.

Methods of teaching

There is only one good, knowledge, and one evil, ignorance.
—Socrates Wisdom

LEARNING OBJECTIVES

This chapter is designed to enable the reader to

- Define and classify teaching methods
- Describe the purposes, processes, advantages and disadvantages of lecture method, demonstration, group discussion, seminar, symposium and panel discussion as methods of teaching
- Discuss the concept, purposes, processes, advantages and disadvantages of role-play, project method, field trip, workshop, exhibition as method of teaching
- Explain the concept, principles, processes, merits and demerits of programmed instructions, computer-assisted learning, problem-based learning, self-directed learning and problem-solving as method of teaching–learning
- Demonstrate the skills in planning and implementation of micro-teaching
- Appreciate the concept, purposes, principles and processes of clinical nursing teaching methods, such as simulation, nursing clinics, nursing assignment, nursing care conference, nursing rounds and process recording

KEY TERMS

INTRODUCTION

Good teaching is the main criterion of an effective teacher. Every individual is unique and so different teachers adopt different methods and strategies of teaching. The main objective of teaching is to bring about desired changes in the attitude and behaviour of the learner. The selection of the teaching methods depends upon the nature of a task, learning objectives, learner's abilities and student's entering behaviour. Teaching methods, teaching skill and technical competency affect students' learning. Learning the art of teaching is necessary to give systematic attention to methods as well as a mastery over the subject matter.

DEFINITION OF METHOD OF TEACHING

The way or style of the presentation of content in a classroom is called *teaching method*. M. Varma has presented a broad meaning of the term *teaching method*. According to him, content matter is important for determining the teaching method. Teaching methods are classified under three domains: telling method, showing method and doing method (Fig. 7.1).

According to Burton, teaching method is the stimulation, guidance, direction and encouragement of learning.

Teaching method is a broad and general term. It covers both teaching strategies and tactics of teaching. Teaching strategy includes two main concepts, i.e. a generalized plan for a lesson that includes structure and the desired learner behaviour in terms of objectives to be achieved. Teaching tactics,

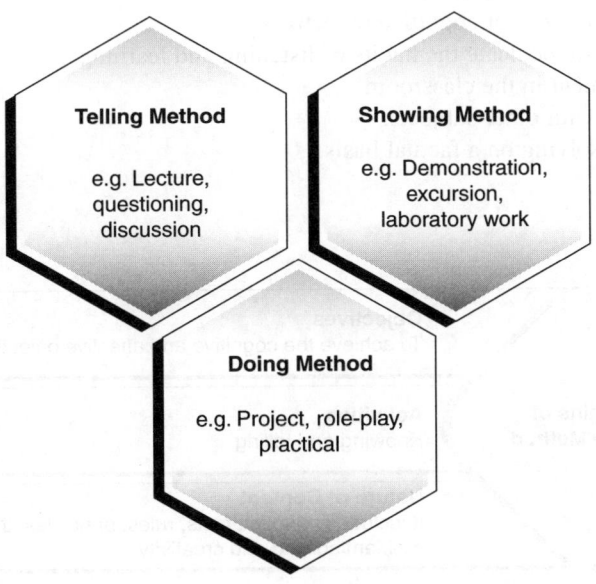

FIGURE 7.1

Domains of teaching methods.

according to E. Stones and E. Moris, are the influencing behaviour of the teacher in the instructional situation to achieve objectives. Tactics may range from nonverbal cues to verbal instructions and the teacher's behaviour. For example, the strategy includes content matter and objectives to be achieved in the lecture method of teaching.

LECTURE METHOD

The lecture method is the oldest method of teaching based on the philosophy of idealism and is an autocratic style of teaching. In this method, the teacher is more active while students are passive listeners. This method is centred on the presentation of content and does not consider the learner's abilities, interests and personality. The purpose of this method is to achieve cognitive and affective objectives. The main focus of this method is on the presentation of content as a whole. The teacher talks continuously to the class and students learn better through listening. This method consists of several special components or domains to be considered (Fig. 7.2). Moreover, several factors related to student, teacher and environment must be considered as depicted in Box 7.1 while planning this method.

> *Lecture method is the teaching procedure comprising the presentation of content, clarification of doubts and explanation of facts, principles and relationships.*

I. PURPOSES OF THE LECTURE METHOD

The main purposes of the lecture method are:

- To stimulate thinking in students.
- To develop concentration in students.
- To achieve a very high order of cognitive objectives.
- To influence learners to inculcate the habits of listening and learning.
- To introduce new content in the classroom.
- To correlate subjects with other subjects.
- To develop problem-solving on a factual basis.

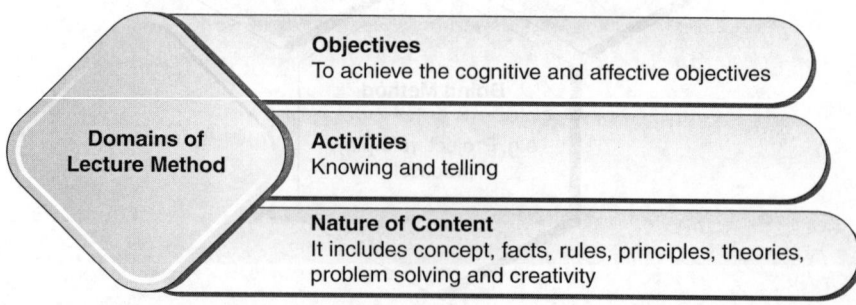

Domains of Lecture Method

Objectives
To achieve the cognitive and affective objectives

Activities
Knowing and telling

Nature of Content
It includes concept, facts, rules, principles, theories, problem solving and creativity

FIGURE 7.2

Domains of lecturer method.

BOX 7.1 FACTORS CONSIDERED WHILE PLANNING THE LECTURE METHOD

Related to Students	Related to Teacher	Related to Environment
Learner's	*Teacher's*	• Time of the day, e.g. morning lecture seems superior to afternoon lectures for recall information
• Capability and ability	• Knowledge and mastery over the subject matter	
• Interest and attitude	• Teaching tactics include voice, gestures, eye contact and manners	• Duration and length, i.e. lecture more than 40 minutes can reduce the absorption and assimilation power of students
• Cognitive level		
• Previous knowledge		
• Type of programme, e.g. ANM, GNM, B.Sc. (N), M.Sc. (N), etc.	• Teacher–learner relationship	
	• Preparation of lecture before presentation	• Use of audiovisual aids
	• Purpose or reason to be taught	• Good light facility

II. COMPONENTS OF THE LECTURE METHOD

Lecture as a teaching method includes the following components:

A. Introduction to the lecture

This is the first component of an effective lecture, and the student's perception and interest depend on this stage. It usually lasts 3–5 minutes. The teacher should provide a general idea and framework for the lecture's content in this stage so that students get familiar with the ongoing topic. It helps the teacher capture the student's attention and stimulate their interest. During the introduction of the lecture, the teacher must ensure the following:

- The teacher should establish good rapport with students. The teacher's tactics and personality should generate interest in students. Establishing friendly communication to provide a positive learning so that students feel comfortable is important.
- In the first meeting with students, teachers should introduce themselves by using an 'ice breaker' and maintain a consistent and affectionate relationship with students so that the students feel comfortable while approaching the teacher.
- Teachers should assess the students' pre-existing knowledge. They should not simply announce the topic. To maintain interest, teachers should disclose the topic in the form of a story, situation or picture or question. For example, a nurse educator may begin a lecture on ventilators while showing pictures of patients on ventilators in the ICU.
- The teacher should relate the student's goals and interest with the topic of lecture. A lecture may also be introduced by describing how it will help the students succeed in their education and careers.
- The teacher should clarify the objectives and purposes of a lecture and describe how it is organized.
- The teacher should introduce the topic by raising some related issues for student participation.

B. The body of the lecture

The body of the lecture covers the content in an organized way. Since this component is allotted the greatest amount of time in a classroom, it includes many more teaching procedures than in introduction and conclusion. The body lays emphasis on the presentation of the content. The teacher is more active, while students are relatively passive participants. The teacher uses question–answer techniques to keep students attentive in class. Teacher controls and plans all student activities. The teacher generally uses maxims of teaching to make the students understand the concept using various examples, situations, etc.

C. Conclusion

Conclusion helps the teacher summarize and re-emphasize the key points of the lecture and also get feedback from the students. The teacher can motivate the students to ask questions by focusing their mind to specific points. Students can also clarify their doubts and raise questions at this stage.

Advantages of the lecture method

- This method develops concentration in students.
- It is an economical teaching strategy. Large subject content may be taught in a relatively small duration.
- Teaching activities are dominated by the teacher.
- It provides current information from many sources.
- It provides a summary or synthesis of information from different sources.

Disadvantages of the lecture method

- The lecturer method lends little emphasis on problem solving, decision making, analytical thinking or transfer of learning.
- It is not conducive to meeting students' individual needs.
- This method brings with it the problems of limited attention span on the part of the learners.
- The lecture does not allow the instructor estimate student understanding easily as the material is covered.

DEMONSTRATION

A teaching method is the stimulation, guidance, direction and encouragement for learning. It inculcates the desire to work with the maximum efficiency one is capable of. The demonstration method is of utmost importance in the teaching of nursing. It teaches by exhibition and explanation and provides opportunities to students to apply their acquired knowledge and skill practically. This method utilizes the patient's bedside as a live teaching field for demonstrations of a variety of nursing care situations. A creative teacher knows how to use the demonstration method to modify concepts and skills and to maximize possibilities for transfer of learning so that students can use previously acquired knowledge in new contexts.

> *Demonstration can be defined as visualized explanation of facts, concepts and procedures. It trains, explains the students in the art of careful observation.*

I. PURPOSES OF DEMONSTRATION

- To show the learner how to perform certain psychomotor skills. The learner must reproduce the behaviour of demonstration exactly.
- To show why things occur. The behaviour is intended only as a strategy to aid the learner's understanding of a concept or principle.

Special purposes in nursing

- Teaches new procedures either at bedside in a ward or in the nursing laboratory on simulators.
- Applies the knowledge of underlying scientific principles to nursing care situations.
- Teaches the uses, functioning and care of new equipment.
- Teaches the application of observation techniques and skills to nursing situations.
- Teach maintenance of health and preventive health care measures to patients and family.

II. CHARACTERISTICS OF DEMONSTRATION

- The demonstrator should understand the entire procedure before attempting to perform.
- All equipment needed should be assembled before demonstration.
- A positive approach should be used.
- Knowledge about the procedure should be given to students.
- The setting for a demonstration should be as real to life as possible.

III. COMPONENTS/STEPS TO DEMONSTRATING

The main components and steps of the demonstration method are as follows.

A. Before demonstration

- Formulate behavioural objectives.
- Perform skill analysis and determine the sequence.
- Assess entry behaviour of learners and determine prerequisites.
- Formulate the lesson plan for demonstration.

B. During demonstration

- State the objectives to the learner.
- Motivate learners by explaining why the skill is required.
- Demonstrate the complete skill at a normal speed.
- Demonstrate each partial skill slowly, in the correct sequence.
- Obtain feedback by questioning and observation of nonverbal behaviour.
- Avoid the use of negative examples and variations in technique.

C. After demonstration

- Provide immediate supervised practice with adequate time allowance.
- Make the environment psychologically safe by providing a friendly atmosphere and constructive criticism.
- Discuss the points for improvement and provide constructive criticism and feedback.

IV. RESPONSIBILITIES OF TEACHERS AND STUDENTS IN THE DEMONSTRATION METHOD

The detailed responsibilities of teachers and students in the demonstration method may be seen from Box 7.2.

Advantages of demonstration
- It provides an opportunity for observational learning.
- It commands interest by using concrete illustrations. Students can not only hear the explanation but also see the process.
- It has a universal appeal because it is understandable to all.
- It is adaptable to both group and individual teaching.
- Return demonstration by the student under the supervision of the teacher provides the opportunity for well-directed practice before the students use the procedure on the ward.
- Questioning forms an important part of demonstration to get feedback from students about their understanding and assimilation.
- Important points and terms are mentioned on the chalkboard. The chalkboard should be behind the teacher and in front of students.
- It activates several senses and increases learning.
- It correlates theory with practice.
- It has a particular reference to student demonstration of procedures already learned.
- It serves as a strong motivational force for students.
- Student's interest is maintained throughout demonstration.

Disadvantages of demonstration
- Only a small group of students can be included in a demonstration.
- Keeps the students in a passive situation.
- Involves a high cost in terms of personnel and time required.
- Difficulty in repeating demonstrations to acquire competence.

GROUP DISCUSSION

Group discussion is an effective method of teaching and considered a learner-centric approach of the teaching–learning process. In a group discussion, a number of learners interact face to face to achieve specific educational objectives. It provides wider interaction among the members of a group and is useful when long-term compliance is involved. Common forms of group discussion are classroom discussions, seminar symposiums, and panel discussions and conferences.

Group discussion is a cooperative, problem-solving activity, which seeks a consensus regarding the solution of a problem.

Group discussion can be defined as three or more participants who have an agreed topic to discuss and share their views in all the aspects and submit/present their views in the form of report to bigger gathering.

I. PURPOSES OF GROUP DISCUSSION

- It provides an opportunity for sharing information among the members of a group.
- Members get an opportunity to attend group consortium to gain and share knowledge necessary to achieve specific educational objectives.
- It develops the skills of group development, group cohesiveness and group socialization in group members under the leadership of teacher.
- A variety of information may be learned in a short time, when a number of people in a group share their own experience and knowledge with others.

II. GUIDELINES TO CONDUCT A GROUP DISCUSSION

A group discussion conducted in an efficient manner using the following guidelines may be one of the best teaching methods because of its richness of vivid content and the ability to get long-lasting memory.

- There must be adequate and effective planning of the topic of discussion, educational objectives to be achieved and environment for group discussion.
- Plenty of time and motivation must be provided to students for preparation on the topic of discussion.
- Group leader and each member should be well aware of their moral and professional responsibilities during group discussion.
- The teacher opens the discussion session with a brief introduction of the topic with specific objectives. This is followed by students who are invited to express their ideas and viewpoints about the topic of discussion.
- During discussion, the teacher assumes the role of the mentor and leader, and students are facilitated to share their viewpoints. Over-talkative students are discouraged and passive students are motivated to participate in the discussion.
- One student from the group is asked to record the proceedings of the discussion.
- During the discussion, the teacher intervenes in case of argumentative and ambiguous discussions and clarifies doubts when required.
- At the end of the discussion, the teacher summarizes the discussion and concludes with a comprehensive note of carry home messages and words of encouragement for the participants.

Advantages of group discussion

- Each group member actively participates in achieving the educational objectives.
- It boosts the self-esteem and morale of students when their viewpoints are accepted and given due regard.
- It helps the students develop a problem-solving approach while working in a group.
- It also offers group members an opportunity to express their viewpoints and ideas in full freedom.
- Individuals in a group develop social skills and feelings of team activity.

Disadvantages of group discussion

- Group discussions are generally time-consuming and are usually not completed in the scheduled time.
- Some members in a group may dominate and some may only be passive listeners.
- Group discussion may not be a very effective method for large groups.
- Adequate preparation is required by each member to have a fruitful discussion; else the discussion may remain polarized.
- Equal participation of group members may not be possible in a group discussion.

SEMINAR

Seminar is a controlled type of discussion. It is a method of teaching where the student's ability to solve problems is increased by way of rational thinking and reasoning. It can be a motivating strategy in nursing, where a learner presents a paper on some aspects of nursing and then participates in a discussion with the group. A seminar can be used in all fields, particularly in colleges or schools to supplement the student learning after they have acquired specific information and experience.

In general, the seminar consists of a scientific approach to the study of a selected problem. It involves a discussion of the problem using a small group of students and a teacher who is an expert in the field of study. The seminar differs from other group discussion methods because of its specific features, i.e. in-depth library research and literature review on presenting problem, systematic writing of seminar report under guidance of teacher or expert and presentation of the report, followed by discussion of the report by the group participants for further analysis, evaluation and drawing conclusions and recommendations. The best distinct feature of the seminar is expert or teacher's significant contribution in planning, presentation and evaluation of teaching–learning activity. A seminar may be a single problem for study by the total group, a problem shared by several group members, or individual subproblems studied by each member and presented as part of the total problem. The nature of the seminar method usually requires a series of sessions for completion of study of the problem.

Seminar is one of the techniques of discussion for small groups, a small group is one in which face to face relationship among participants is there.

Seminars are simply a group of people coming together for the discussion and learning of specific techniques and topics. Usually there are several keynote speakers within each seminar, and these speakers are usually experts in their own fields or topics.

I. SEMINAR AS A METHOD OF TEACHING

- Seminar is a form of a class organization that utilizes a scientific approach for the analysis of a problem chosen for discussion.

- It is an organized, guided discussion with a focus on the discovery of new relationships by the participating individuals. It differs from intellectual initiative. The student's role is active in contrast to the relatively passive role assumed in a lecture.
- The objective of a seminar is to give students the opportunity to participate in methods of scientific analysis and research procedures. Students are expected to do considerable library research and when feasible obtain primary sources of data.
- A seminar group is mainly concerned with academic matters rather than individual students and commonly involves the reading of an essay or paper by one group member followed by a discussion by the total group on the topic.
- It is a discussion method of teaching where an informal group of 10–15 students (not more than 25) participate to solve problems in a scientific approach and analysis. Generally, the duration of a seminar should not be more than 1–2 hours.
- This method gives students the opportunity to participate in methods of scientific analysis and research procedures.
- Students are expected to do considerable library research, and if feasible, obtain primary sources of data. Data is analyzed, critically evaluated and conclusion reached, under the directions of the teacher.
- The teacher should help the students select, formulate and resolve the most significant student problems and suggest the available sources of information.
- As the seminar progresses, the students assume increased responsibilities for preparing the problems and conducting the discussion.

II. CHARACTERISTICS OF THE SEMINAR

- Teacher is the leader (students can also function as leaders in certain selected situations).
- The group generally consists of 10–15 participants.
- An ideal seminar lasts for 1–2 hours. The topic is initially presented by the presenter followed by group discussion.
- The leader should keep the discussion within limits so the focus of discussion can be mentioned.
- In student seminars, students present their data in an informal way under the leadership of the teacher, followed by a teacher-monitored discussion.
- Care should be taken to avoid stereotypes.
- All members take part in discussion in an informal but orderly manner.
- The chairman should be skilled in encouraging timid participants.
- A student secretary may record the problems that came up and the solutions given to them.

III. ORGANIZING A SEMINAR

The establishment of an environment that contributes to the purpose of the seminar is very important and requires a skilled teacher. A motivating learning situation that is not too highly organized or too relaxed is essential. The teacher usually guides the seminar; however, students may carry out this function under the guidance of a teacher. The teacher may decide to be the leader or may delegate leadership to the group.

The basic guidelines for organizing a seminar are:

- To define the purpose of the seminar.
- To relate the topic of seminar and discussion to the main concept or the objectives to be attained.
- To direct and focus the discussion on the topic.

- To help students express their ideas.
- To keep the discussion at a high level of interest so that the students listen attentively to those contributing ideas.
- To plan comments and questions that relate to the subject and also help guide the discussion.
- To set time limitations for each person's contribution.
- To guard against monopoly of the discussion by any member of the seminar.
- To plan for a summary at intervals during the discussion and also at the end and relate the ideas expressed to the purpose of discussion.
- To have the discussion recorded either by a student as a recording secretary or by tape recording.
- To plan for teacher and student self-evaluation of the progress made towards the immediate objectives.

IV. ROLE OF TEACHER IN THE SEMINAR

- Select the topic (giving reasonable time for preparation).
- Remain in the background at the seminar but sit where the whole group can be seen.
- Prepare to help out in the initial stages of using this method in case of long silences.
- See that no essential points are overlooked and that gross inaccuracies are corrected (preferably by another member of the class).
- See that all members have a share in the discussion and that irrelevant discussion is avoided.

Advantages of seminar

- Role of the student is active; it presupposes that the student has background knowledge.
- If properly conducted, the seminar teaches the method of scientific analysis and techniques of research.
- The group as a whole and individual students try to solve problems.
- Exchange of facts and attempts to crystallize group opinion that is sound and workable.
- By participation in the solution of problems, the students develop problem-solving skills.
- By participation in the solution of problems, the students becomes more articulate and develop a more critical point of view and a more organized, scientific approach towards the issue.
- A seminar helps in self-learning and promotes independent thinking.
- Ability to see and solve our own problems is increased because personal difficulties can be compared with those of the group.
- Skilfully directed, the seminar promotes group spirit and cooperativeness.

Disadvantages of seminar

- It is quite a time-consuming process.
- It cannot be applied to new students.
- Timid students cannot improve.
- If subject knowledge is poor, unnecessary discussions arise.
- The approach to problems extends to students' professional and personal activities.

SYMPOSIUM

Symposium technique is a type of discussion where two or more speakers talk for 10–20 minutes, develop individual approaches or solutions to a problem or present aspects of a policy, process or programme. This is a technique of higher learning. It is an instructional technique that is used to achieve higher cognitive and effective objectives.

This technique is also an essential method of teaching and learning. It is useful to achieve high cognitive and effective functioning. This method helps to make a decision about a particular problem or solve the problem. It can help all the students improve their learning skills.

The word *symposium* has several dictionary meanings. Plato used this term for *good dialogue* to present views towards God. Another meaning of the term is intellectual recreation or enjoyment. The main purpose of a symposium is to provide an understanding to students or listeners on the theme or problem specifically to develop certain values and feelings.

Symposium is defined as a teaching technique that serves as an excellent method for informing the audiences, crystallizing their opinion and preparing them for arriving at decision regarding a particular issue or a topic.

I. PURPOSES OF SYMPOSIUM

- To identify and understand various aspects of the theme and problems.
- To develop the ability to come to a decision and provide judgement regarding a problem.
- To develop values and feelings regarding a problem.
- To enable the listeners form policies regarding a theme or problem.
- To provide understanding to the students or listeners on a theme or problem to specifically develop certain values and feelings.
- To investigate a problem from several points of view.
- To boost students' abilities to speak in the group.
- To encourage the students to study independently.

II. CHARACTERISTICS OF SYMPOSIUM

- It provides broad understanding of a topic or problem.
- The listener is provided with an opportunity to take decisions about a problem.
- It is used in higher classes for specific themes and problems.
- It develops feelings of cooperation and adjustment.
- The objectives of synthesis and evaluation are achieved by employing the symposium technique.
- It provides different views on the topic of the symposium.

III. PRINCIPLES OF SYMPOSIUM

- The speeches may be persuasive, argumentative and informative.
- Original presentation is objective and accurate.
- Summary to be always included at conclusion.
- Each speech proceeds without interruption.
- The chairman of the symposium introduces the topic, suggests its importance and sometimes indicates the general approaches.
- All members of the symposium performing group can sit in a straight line behind the table, or in adjoining chairs with the chairman in the middle or to one side of the speakers.

- The symposium presents two conflicting points of view, the reading arrangement can separate the speakers on the platform to indicate differences in opinion or to preserve peace.

IV. GUIDELINES FOR CONDUCTING SYMPOSIUM

- All members of the performing group can sit in a straight line behind a table or in adjoining chairs with the chairman in the middle or to one side of the speakers.
- The chairman of the symposium introduces the topic and suggests something of its importance.
- Two or more speakers talk from 10 to 20 minutes. The speech may be persuasive, argumentative, informative or evocative. Each speech proceeds without interruption.
- The speeches are followed by questions or comments from the audience as in the panel form.

Advantages of symposium

- It is suited to a large group or classes.
- This method can be frequently used to present broad topics for discussion at conventions and organization of meetings.
- Organization is good as speeches are prepared beforehand.
- It gives deeper insight into the topic.
- It directs the students to continuous independent study.
- This method can be used in political meetings.

Disadvantages of symposium

- It provides inadequate opportunity for all students to participate actively.
- The speech is limited to 15–20 minutes.
- It has limited audience participation.
- Questions and answers limited to only 3–4 minutes.
- It has possibility of overlapping of subjects.
- The chairman has no control over the speakers as they have full freedom to prepare the theme for discussion. They can present any aspect of the theme or problem.
- There is a probability of repetition of content. The different aspects of the theme are not prepared separately. It creates difficulty of understanding for the listeners.
- The different aspects of the theme are not presented simultaneously. Therefore the listeners are not able to understand the theme correctly.
- The listeners remain passive in the symposium because they are not given an opportunity to seek clarification and put questions in between the symposium.

PANEL DISCUSSION

All techniques of higher learning require discussion among the participants. The discussion provides equal opportunities in the instructional situation to every participant. This technique was used by Harry A. Ober Street for the first time in 1929. The purpose of the panel is to make use of a small group discussion for the benefit of a large group. Fig. 7.3 depicts a panel discussion in process on the topic of nursing informatics where a group of nursing experts in the presence of a moderator/chairperson are carrying out the discussion in front of a large group of audience.

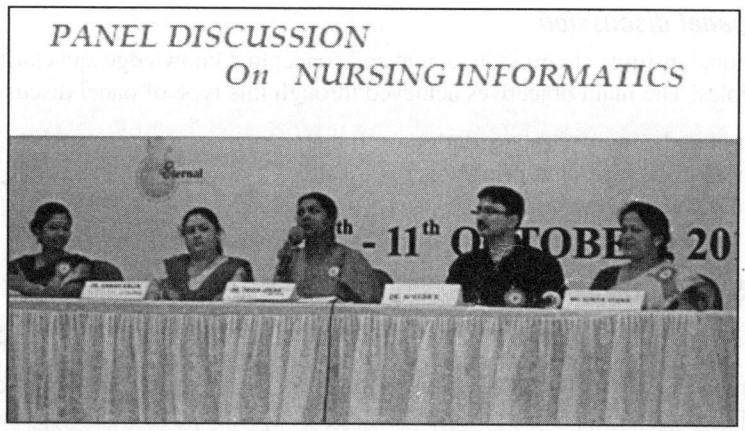

FIGURE 7.3

Panel discussion on nursing informatics.

Panel is a discussion in which a few persons carry out a conversation in front of an audience.

The panel discussion is a method of teaching in which four to six or eight persons or students discuss the assigned topic/issue/problem creatively among themselves in front of an audience which may be too large.

I. PURPOSES OF PANEL DISCUSSION

- To provide information and new facts.
- To analyze the current problem from different angles.
- To identify the values.
- To organize for mental recreation.
- To influence the audience to an open-minded attitude and respect for other's opinion.
- When handled intelligently and creatively, the panel discussion stimulates thought and discussion and clarifies thinking.

II. TYPES OF PANEL DISCUSSION

A. Public panel discussion

This type of panel discussion is organized for the common-man problems. Generally, the public panel discussion is organized through television programmes. The main objectives achieved by this type of panel discussion are:

- To provide factual information regarding current problems.
- To determine social values.
- To recreate the common man.

B. *Educational panel discussion*

It is used in educational institutes to provide factual and conceptual knowledge and clarification of certain theories and principles. The main objectives achieved through this type of panel discussion are:

- To provide factual and conceptual knowledge.
- To raise awareness of theories and principles.
- To provide solutions for certain problems.

III. GUIDELINES FOR CONDUCTING PANEL DISCUSSION

The following guidelines must be kept in mind while organizing and conducting panel discussions:

- Identify or help participants identify an issue or topic that involves an important conflict in values and interests. The issue or topic may be set forth as a topical question, a hypothetical incident, a student experience or an actual case.
- Select panellists who are well informed and have specific points of view regarding the issue or topic. A panel discussion that includes three to five panellists is usually most workable.
- Select a leader or chairperson/moderator of the panel discussion.
- Decide on the format of the panel discussion.
- There should be a rehearsal before the actual panel discussion.

IV. ORGANIZING THE PANEL DISCUSSION

- The panel discussion consists of the chairperson/moderator, the panellists and the audience.
- The panel consists of 4–8 panellists along with a chairperson or moderator seated in a semicircle facing the audience. The chairman or moderator is generally seated in the middle of the panellists.
- The chairperson or moderator should be selected carefully because success of the panel depends on his/her leadership.
- The chairperson must keep the discussion to the subject and see that all members of the panel get an equal opportunity to express their views.
- Further, the chairperson should act as a neutral referee and begin the panel discussion by exploring the whole proceedings.
- The members of the panel are first introduced by name and background of experience. The topic is announced and the limit of discussion is stated.
- The chairperson may start the procedure rolling by making a comment or by directing a question to a particular person.
- The panel discussion should provide a natural setting in which the audience will have the opportunity to ask questions, evaluate replies and make constructive contributions.
- The chairperson coordinates the discussion and makes sure the discussion is carried on in a conversational way.
- The chairperson clarifies an issue or misconception and may also introduce another thought so that the subject is fully covered. Then he/she summarizes the main points presented by the speakers and invites the audience to contribute and ask questions.
- Finally the chairperson sums up the discussion.

Advantages of panel discussion

- Different points of views on the subject are presented by experts.
- The quick exchange of facts, opinions, etc., helps develop critical attitude and better judgement.
- Students learn to discuss a topic in conversational form in a small group in front of a large group.

Disadvantages of panel discussion

- It requires more time for planning, organizing and presentation.
- The discussion may be vague and superficial if the panel members lack mastery.
- The effectiveness of the method depends on:
  - The competency and preparation of the panel members.
  - The competency and leading abilities of the chairperson.
  - Planning, organizing and conducting the panel discussion.

ROLE-PLAY

Role-playing is the spontaneous acting out of a clearly-defined situation by two or more persons for subsequent discussion by the whole class. Role-playing is a teaching method where a group of participants act out the assigned role to deliver the content of topic to be taught to the participants. In a role paying group, the members play the assigned role the way they think the character would act in reality which helps in arousing feelings and elicit emotional responses in learners where cognitive and affective domain learning may be achieved.

According to Karen S. Kesten, role-plays using the SBAR (**S**ituation, **B**ackground, **A**ssessment and **R**ecommendation) technique are helpful to improve observed communication skills in senior nursing students. Skilled communication and respectful interaction between the health care team members are critical to achieve optimization of quality patient care outcomes. Patients in the care of clinically expert professionals suffer medical errors with alarming frequency. The Joint Commission on National Patient Safety Goals strives to improve the effectiveness of communication in caregivers by recommending the implementation of standardized tools known as SBAR. The findings suggest that role-play may have a place in teaching communication skills in nursing schools as well as continuing education and training in hospitals and other health care settings. Interdisciplinary communication training may provide even more effective learning.

> *Role-playing is an educational method in which people spontaneously act out problems of human relations and analyze the enactment with the help of other role players and observers.*

> *Role-playing is a discussion technique that makes it possible to get maximum participation of a group through acting out an example of some problem or idea under discussion.*

Role-play is a spontaneous acting out of roles in the context of human situations. It is a part of two broad methods: sociodrama and psychodrama. Both sociodrama and psychodrama require not only players but also an audience that helps the players interpret their roles.

Sociodrama: It deals with the interactions of people with other individuals or groups like mother, nurse and leader. It always involves situations of more than one person and deals with problems related to a majority of the group.

Psychodrama: It is practised in a group setting, mainly concerned with the unique needs and problems of a particular individual. It should not be attempted except under the guidance of a trained therapist. The audience identifying with roles in a role-playing or critical observation brings about much greater learning than simply passive watching.

I. PURPOSES OF ROLE-PLAY

- To present interpersonal problems.
- To provide emotional and affective stimulus for solving problems.
- To provide awareness about social and psychological issues.
- To develop a situation for an analysis.
- To prevent alternative courses of action.
- To prepare for meeting future situations.
- To develop an understanding of others points of view.
- To convey information to develop specific skills.

II. PRINCIPLES OF ROLE-PLAY

- As a teaching technique, role-play is based on the philosophy that meanings are in people and not in words or symbols. If the philosophy is accurate, we must first of all share the meanings, then clarify our understanding of each other's meanings, and finally, if necessary, change our meanings.
- In the language of phenomenological psychology, this has to do with changing the self-concept. The self-concept is best changed through direct involvement in a realistic and life-related problem situation rather than through hearing about such situations from others.
- Creating teaching situations that can lead to change of self-concept requires a distinct organizational pattern.
- It should be flexible.
- It should be a stimulant to think and should not be an escape from the discipline of learning.
- There is no single best method of selecting the characters; the group may do the assigning.
- It requires rehearsal as an important feature to produce effective outcome and for audience to help players interpret their roles.
- It should be done for a brief period so that the attention of audience may be captured effectively.
- Enough time should be allowed for discussion and analysis of the situation.
- It evaluates the teacher and participants through discussion or follow-up as to specific individual behaviour or sequence of group actions.

III. STEPS IN ROLE-PLAY

The following main steps must be followed while carrying out a role-play.

A. Planning phase

During this phase, the following components must be ensured:

- *Select a problem for role-play*
  - The group leader recognizes a problem that can be used effectively and suggests it to the group.
  - The group can list problems on the blackboard and decide which problem they want to work out.

- *Set up the role-play scene*
  - The group should come to a clear agreement on the chief objectives to be realized in role planning.
  - The group working with the leader must determine:
    - What characters are to be involved.
    - The attitudes and personality of the characters.
    - The setting of the story.
    - The point at which the story should begin.
  - The leader may brief the players on the situation they have decided they want to portray. The leader may arbitrarily assign individuals to take the various roles or members may volunteer to play the different roles.
- *Getting underway in role-play*
  - The role takers usually go out of the room and are given a few minutes to warm up or to get a feeling of the roles they are about to play. Specific names, other than their own, should be used to help them get into their roles.
  - The role-players should attempt to express the attitudes the group has assigned to the various characters as well as achieve the goals decided upon.
  - The story grows out of natural reactions of the characters enacted in role-playing.
  - Those members not involved in the actual role-playing act as observers. They may be assigned to watch particular role-players or to look for important clues that come out of role-playing.
- *Cutting the content and making role-play comprehensive*
  - The leader may cut at a point where enough action has already occurred to provide a basis for discussion.
  - The leader may get immediate reaction of role-players. How they felt in their roles and how they responded to other responses in the scene.
  - The leader may use the role name of each person in the discussion so that the player does not feel he is being evaluated.
  - When role-players succeed in really projecting themselves into the roles assigned to them, they usually give valuable insight into the problem and provide additional material for discussion.

B. Implementation and evaluation phase

The role-play is carried out to convey particular content to the audience and discussion is stimulated.

- *The audience observers*
  - The comments of the audience observers constitute the heart of role-playing as a discussion technique. It may consider:
    - How did the group think the role was handled?
    - What were the good points of the action?
    - What were the poor points or omissions?
- *Role-playing observers*
  - This might be played by different people so that there might be a comparison of the behaviours of different people.
- *Summarize phase*
  - The leader sums up to the group chief points or principles which have come out in role-playing and the comments of the observers that follow.
  - The comments on specific problems should be taken under consideration.

- *Cautions in use of role-playing*
  - Use role-play only when it will be useful and not just for the sake of doing it.
  - Be careful about interpersonal relationships within the group.
  - If there is a popular role, give it to a person with enough status in the group to carry it successfully. If necessary, the leader might play it to spare the feelings of others.
  - Avoid uncovering deep seated personal problems that require professional help.

Advantages of role-play

- Develop real communication skills in leadership, interviewing and social interaction and obtain constructive feedback from peers. For example, learning how to put another case, how to listen, how to lead a discussion and how to be a member of the team responsible for patient care.
- Develop sensitivity to another's feelings by having the opportunity to put oneself in another's place, by noting there is a difference between what a person says and what a person does and develop empathy and understanding.
- Develop skills in group problem solving. For example, the group works as a whole to develop concerns for the group, develop the situation, identify critical issues and come to some mutual agreement.
- Develop an ability to observe and analyze situations. For example, discussion following role planning provides the opportunity to identify critical issues, suggest alternatives to deal with a situation and to appraise the actor's concept of role.
- Practice selected behaviours in a real-life situation without the stress of making a mistake. A person is more appropriate to permit true feelings to be expressed when it is a safe role. For example, the student is exposed to reaching to and having others react to her pointing up strengths and weakness with dramatic impact retained, but she is working with others in a similar situation.
- In a teaching–learning situation, role-play provides the opportunity to:
  - Note individual student needs by observing and analysing student needs in a simulated real life situation.
  - Assist the students in meeting their own needs by either giving them or encouraging group members to give them on the spot suggestions.
  - Encourage independent thinking and action by stepping aside or giving indirect guidance as emphasis is on the students helping themselves.

Disadvantages of role-play

- Role-playing is a means, not an end.
- It requires expert guidance and leadership.
- Participants may sometimes feel threatened.
- It is used as an education technique, not as a therapeutic one, strongly dependent on student's imagination.
- It is time-consuming in developing group readiness, should not be used when time constraints are present.
- It is limited only by the teacher's ingenuity and realistic use.

PROJECT METHOD

The project method has been recognized as a teaching technique since many years; it has its primary inception in the field of agriculture sciences where students carried out some planned creative activities in a natural environment or a planned work field to produce certain products. Later it was used in vocational education programmes. The essential characteristics of the project method are planned activity of the individual and production of tangible results.

This method is a teaching method where students learn to work individually or in a group to achieve preplanned learning objectives. Williams H. Kilpartric viewed the project method as a vivid educational activity where several types of learning activities included enhancing the learning over already learned behaviour or knowledge. He also emphasized on the importance of the learner's activity and attitude while working in an environment rather than just considering the educational objectives to be achieved. Therefore, true creative thinking and true mental activity is essential to the project method and ultimately there will be a production of some physical or mental products and acquisition of the ability to handle real life problems.

- According to Prof. Ballard, *'a project is a bit of real life that has been imparted into the school, further in project method, learning by living; this life has spontaneity, purpose, significance and interest, freedom'*.
- According to Williams Kilpartrick, *'project method is a whole-hearted, purposeful activity proceeding in a social environment'*.
- According to Stevenson, *'a project method is a problematic act carried to completion in its natural setting'*.
- Stevenson also mentioned that to be a project method, the learning activity must be:
  - Problematic in nature.
  - Aimed at a definite, attainable goal.
  - Purposeful, natural and lifelike in its procedure to attain the goal.
  - Directed and planned by the student.
  - Practical in nature with an emphasis on a single, resulting in a concrete achievement. The undertaking must be complete in itself and the goal must be definite and objectively measurable.
- Project method involves all types of mental and manipulative activities according to the purpose and objectives by which the learning activities are unified and shaped.

I. CHARACTERISTICS OF A GOOD PROJECT METHOD

- The method aims at teaching the learner to get the best out of life.
- An attempt to use experience, trust and the best master whose lessons are unforgettable.
- The project method gives an opportunity for self-expression.
- The experiments of the project method want to reset the whole curriculum and break all barriers of the subject matter.
- The project matter proposes the whole sequence of activities involved in complete understanding.
- A project can be a large unit of appreciational learning or of attitude development that increases motor skills and technical knowledge.
- A project is a play activity and learners are engaged in carrying out the activity.
- The project method is a complete surrender to the learner's point of view.
- In the project method the procedure of the school is liable to be determined by the technique of a workshop because the individual learns much better from his own activity than by constant instruction.
- An attempt is made to establish a positive relation with life.

- The project method lends itself naturally to group work.
- It is a large unit plan of teaching.
- The method seeks to have individuals see and understand life in its unity.

II. TYPES OF PROJECTS

According to Williams Kilpartrick, project method is classified in the following four categories (Fig. 7.4):

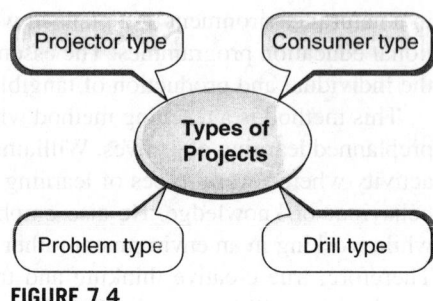

FIGURE 7.4

Types of projects used as a teaching method.

- *Projector type:* Projects where students are getting to something like building a house or a garden or planning to execute a model of a textile factory are called *projector type projects*.
- *Consumer type:* Projects where students set and enjoy the direct experience with their future expected consumers. *For example*, a master level community health nursing student may be given a consumer type project to carry out the home visits and make the assessment of most common primary health problems of elderly residing in urban communities and suggest the best possible solution for the identified problems based on locally available resources. In such a project, nursing student will get direct experience and will enjoy working with his future expected consumers of his services.
- *Problem type:* Projects where a solution to a problem is to be found out.
- *Drill type:* The drill type projects involve an activity that aims at acquiring greater skill. *For example*, a nursing student may be given a project to obtain competency skills in specific nursing procedures such as mouth care, back care, enema administration, intramuscular injection, suctioning and so on.

III. ESSENTIALS OF A GOOD PROJECT

- The project should stress present and future values and experiences that supplement and extend rather than duplicate learning acquired outside the school.
- The projects must have a bearing on a great number of subjects and the knowledge acquired through it may be applied in a variety of ways.
- The project should be timely.
- The project should be challenging.
- The project should be feasible.

IV. ORGANIZING A PROJECT

- The teacher must exercise guidance in the selection of a project.
- Whole-hearted acceptance of the project, almost every student must be secured if the teacher wants to ensure its success.
- Good planning should be done by the students beforehand. It may be in the form of a drawing or a list of steps to be followed, materials to be used, a picture to be prepared or other specific indications of what is to be done.

- The project is an activity to accomplish certain purposes.
- Sufficient preparations must be made to avoid interruptions and delays later.
- During the execution of the project, the teacher should carefully supervise the students in manipulative skills to prevent a waste of materials and to guard against accidents.
- The relation between chalked-out plans and the developing project should be constantly checked.
- The evaluation of a project should be done by both—the students and the teacher.

V. THE ROLE OF TEACHER IN THE PROJECT METHOD

- The teacher has to skilfully guide in the selection.
- The student has to be given help when required.
- The teacher should be good prompter.
- The relations of the teacher and students should be much closer and informal than in ordinary classroom teaching.
- The teacher is like a friend with rich and mature experience.
- The teacher acts as a director, i.e. the teacher's psychological knowledge must be thorough and specific.
- The teacher must be a keen observer and a true sympathizer.
- The teacher should be a store house of information and knowledge.

Advantages of the project method

- It follows the psychological laws of learning:
  - Law of readiness.
  - Law of exercise.
  - Law of effect.
- It gives freedom to the students.
- It suited to the psychological concept of maturation.
- It drives social values.
- It trains for social adjustments.
- It saves children from insincerity and superficiality.
- It trains for a democratic way of life.
- It promotes learning through practical problem saving.
- It helps the students and teachers grow. The student stimulated by and encouraged in his exploration of many materials will ultimately approach other areas of learning in a similar manner. The teacher will grow in his or her understanding of a child's creative developments.
- It confers on school work a much needed sense of reality.
- It sets up an intrinsic standard of evaluation.
- It leads to satisfaction of completing the whole task.
- It is economical; the students take more interest and learn in the shortest possible time.
- It is ideal for science work, handicrafts and practical geography and dramatic work literature.

Disadvantages of the project method

- The role of communication is subordinated to the glorification of active learning.
- The practical difficulties of covering a syllabus rule out the project method as the basis of teaching in most schools.

- It is time-consuming and limited by availability and cost of materials.
- It is most valuable in students with lesser academic interest, for it provides an opportunity for the practical enthusiast.
- It leaves gaps in student knowledge.
- It may be too ambitious: beyond a student's capacity.
- Opportunity for the correlation with the academic subjects is extremely limited.
- In this method instructions are more planned; therefore it may disturb the regular instructional schedule.
- It involves difficulty to ensure any kind of systematic progress in instructions.
- A complete reorganization of the school is needed for a new teacher.
- Children may ignore maxims, working from simple to complex.
- Time-bound projects are introduced artificially and may require more than necessary help.
- Projects may be adopted or abandoned at will.
- The project approach often results in an incomplete mastery of the tools of learning, which are essential to student education later.

FIELD TRIP

An educational trip is defined as an educational procedure by which the students obtain first-hand information by observing places, objects, phenomena and processes in their natural setting to further learning.

I. PURPOSES OF FIELD TRIP

The main purposes of the field trip are:

- To provide real-life situations for first-hand information.
- To supplement classroom instruction, to secure definite information for a specific lesson.
- To serve as a preview of a lesson and gather instructional material.
- To verify previous information, class discussion and conclusion of individual experiments.
- To create situational teaching for cultivating observation, keenness and discovery.
- To serve as a means to develop positive attitudes, values and specific skills.

II. GUIDELINES FOR USING FIELD TRIP AS A TEACHING METHOD

- The field trip must be planned to meet specific educational objectives rather than merely a picnic activity.
- Plan the field trip with a specific checklist such as prior permissions, arrangement of transpiration, booking boarding facility, parental notification and safety and emergency arrangements.
- Plan a schedule and route plan for the field trip. Further, identify a main leader of the group and subleaders of the small groups.
- Assign different responsibilities to different individuals and make every individual understand the overall schedule and route plan of the field trip.
- Have a list of all the candidates, contact numbers of the people in case of an emergency or special needs.

- During a field trip, individuals must be provided with opportunities to achieve educational objectives of the field trip.
- Post the field trip, a review and presentation along with a report must be made to the institutional head and other target group of the institution.

Advantages of field trip

- Classroom experiences could be further enriched with field trip experiences.
- Field trips provide the opportunity for learners to get first-hand information from natural settings.
- The monotony and boredom of classroom teaching may be supplemented with natural, interesting and exciting teaching methods.
- Field trips give natural stimulation that motivates and makes learners interactive and creative.
- Field trips help the learners learn things very quickly and remember them for a longer period.
- They provide an opportunity to solve the individual's problems by interacting with a group in a natural setting.

WORKSHOP

The word *workshop* is related to any area that provides both space and tools required for the manufacture and repair of goods. Similarly, in educational workshops, experts provide knowledge and skills to deal with problems. It is a teaching method organized to develop the psychomotor aspects of the learner regarding the practices of new innovations in education, where persons are trained to use new practices in their teaching learning process.

Workshop is a meeting during which experienced people in responsible positions come together with experts and consultants to find solutions for the problems that cropped up in the course of their work and they have had difficulty in dealing with on their own. It is a large group discussion method.

Workshop is defined as assembled group of 10–25 persons who share a common interest or problem. They meet together to improve their individual skill of a subject through intensive study, research, practice and discussion.

I. ESSENTIAL FEATURES OF WORKSHOP

- Complete active involvement by the participants.
- The whole point of attention is to work and learn from practical experiences.
- Participants may have to work as reporters or a leader.
- Workshop offers each member an opportunity to make his own contribution.

II. PRINCIPLES OF WORKSHOP

- Allowing the participants to prepare and select objectives to be reached will increase the participant's motivation.
- Giving the participant an active role will make teaching more effective.

- Improve a person's attitude towards other people.
- Learn better human relations.
- Every individual has worth and contributes to the common goals.
- Cooperation is a technique and a way of life that is superior to competition and is a primary factor to be allowed.

iii. OBJECTIVES OF THE WORKSHOP

An educational process has two aspects: *theoretical and practical*. The objective of a workshop is to achieve higher cognitive objectives and develop psychomotor skills (Box 7.3).

IV. PREPARATION OF A WORKSHOP

The success of a workshop will depend largely on the way it is planned and on the arrangements made before the opening session. The following activities have to be carried out (Fig. 7.5):

- *Opening a file:* A suitable system might be a loose leaf with the following subdivisions: budget, workshop sitting arrangements, selection of participants, documentation and equipment checklist, publicity press and evaluation.
- *Formulation of aims and objectives:* Aims and objectives of the workshop should be formulated for the participants as well as the organizers. At the first stage of the workshop, theoretical aspects are discussed by experts on the theme of the workshop.
- *Arrangement of funds:* The whole programme and schedule is prepared by the organizer. He has to arrange for the funds needed for boarding and lodging facilities for participants as well as experts.
- *Choosing the date and place:* For the first day of the workshop, a nonworking day is usually selected. Ensure that at least one working day precedes the opening of the workshop. While selecting a place, it should be kept in mind that the place should enable the participants to take part in all activities without interruption.
- *Identifying the experts or resource persons:* In organizing a workshop, resource persons play an important role in providing theoretical and practical aspects of the theme. They provide guidance to participants at every stage and train them to perform the task effectively.

BOX 7.3 OBJECTIVES OF THE WORKSHOP

Cognitive Objectives	Psychomotor Objectives
• To learn the new innovations and practices of education. • To solve problems in the area of teaching education. • To provide a broad understanding of a topic and theme. • To provide a rationalized and philosophical background for instructional and teaching situation.	• To put people in a situation where they will evaluate their own efforts. • To develop the proficiency for planning and organizing teaching and instructional activities. • To provide an opportunity for personal growth through accepting and working towards a goal held in common with others.

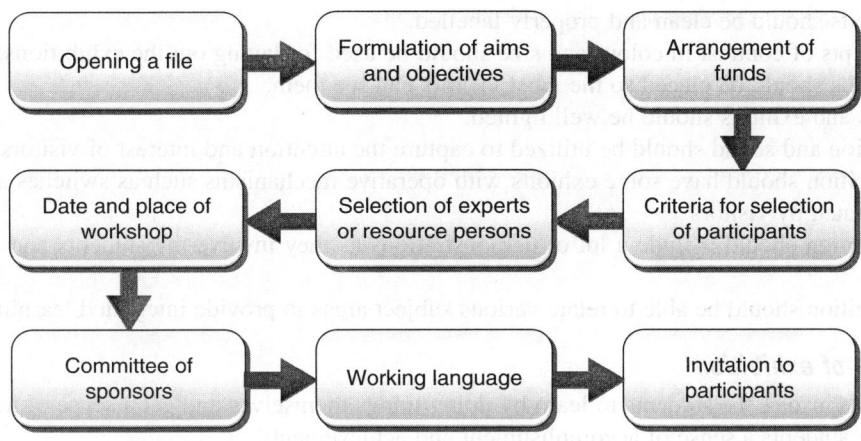

FIGURE 7.5

Steps in preparation of a workshop.

- *Selection of participants:* The participants should be keen or interested in the theme of the workshop. Number of participants, type of participants and voluntary participation should be specified.
- *Identifying the sponsors:* People in administrative positions should be represented as committees that will be called on to apply the selection criteria defined earlier.
- *Working language:* The workshop is usually carried out in a national language or preferred one.
- *Invitation to the participants:* A personal letter should be sent to the participants selected with the following points:
  - Aims of the workshop
  - What is implied by the workshop
  - Working methods of the workshop
  - Theme of the workshop

V. OUTCOMES OF THE WORKSHOP

- Widening specified knowledge
- Professional and personal growth
- Friendships, team spirit and human relations

EXHIBITION

Many times in the school, a department of the school or a class puts up their work for showing it to people outside the school and such a show is called *exhibition*. The pieces of work done by students for an exhibition are called *exhibit*.

I. BASIC CHARACTERISTICS OF EXHIBITION

- The exhibition should have a central theme with a few subthemes to focus attention on a particular concept.

- The exhibits should be clean and properly labelled.
- The concepts of contrast in colour and size should be used for laying out the exhibitions.
- The exhibits should be placed so the most visitors can see them.
- The place and exhibits should be well lighted.
- Both motion and sound should be utilized to capture the attention and interest of visitors.
- The exhibition should have some exhibits with operative mechanisms such as switches and handles to be operated by visitors.
- The exhibition should include a lot of demonstrations as they involve the students and the visitors deeply.
- The exhibition should be able to relate various subject areas to provide integrated learning.

Advantages of exhibition

- Exhibitions inspire the students to learn by doing things themselves and get a sense of involvement.
- They give students a sense of accomplishment and achievement.
- They develop social skills of communication, cooperation and coordination.
- They foster better school community relations and make community members conscious about the school.
- They couple information with pleasure.
- They foster creativity in students.

Disadvantages of exhibition

- It requires thorough preparation.
- It is a time-consuming process.
- It requires a large amount of funds or budget.

PROGRAMMED INSTRUCTIONS

The instructions provided by a teaching machine or programmed textbook are referred to as *programmed instructions*.

- According to J.E. Espich and Bill Williams, 'programmed instruction is a planned sequence of experiences, leading to proficiency, in terms of stimulus–response relationship that have proven to be effective'.
- According to Susan Markle (1969), 'programmed instruction is a method of designing reproducible sequence of instructional events to produce a measurable consistent effect on a behaviour of each and every acceptable student'.

I. CHARACTERISTICS OF PROGRAMMED INSTRUCTIONS

- The subject matter is broken down into small steps called *frames* and arranged sequentially.
- Frequent response of the student is required.
- There is an immediate confirmation of the right answer or correction of wrong answers given by the learners, i.e. 'self-correcting feature'.
- The content and sequence of the frames are subjected to actual try out by students and are revised on the basis of data gathered by the programmer, i.e. 'diagnostic feature'.

- Each student progresses at his own pace without any threat of being exposed to any humiliation in a heterogeneous class.
- The assumption about the learner is clearly stated in the programmed learning materials.
- The objectives underlying programming instructions are defined explicitly and in operational terms so that the terminal behaviour is made observable and measurable.
- The interaction between the learner and the programme is emphasized in programmed learning.
- In a programmed material, continuous evaluation is possible by recording the student's response.
- The strategy provides sufficient situations for teaching the students to discriminate between a range of possibilities and reduce generalizations.

II. TYPES OF PROGRAMMING

Programming can be divided into the following two categories.

A. LINEAR PROGRAMMING

In a linear programme, the learner's responses are controlled externally by the programmer sitting at a distant place. A linear programme is called a *straight line programme* as the learner starts from his initial behaviour to the terminal behaviour following a straight line. The student proceeds from one frame to the next until he completes the programme. The basic characteristics of linear programming are as follows:

- Linear programmes are exposed to a small amount of information and proceed from one frame or one item of information to the next in an orderly fashion.
- They respond overtly so their correct responses can be rewarded and incorrect responses can be corrected.
- They are informed immediately about whether or not their response is correct (feedback).
- They proceed at their own pace (self-pacing).

Scope of linear programming

- *Elementary education:* Generally there are single-teacher schools where a teacher is required to teach all subjects. This strategy will help the teachers.
- *Secondary education:* In secondary education, the diversity of interest and curriculum necessitates this method. It may be used as a remedial teaching method. Classroom teaching may be helpful for nonscience teachers to prepare for science, a compulsory subject up to high school.
- *Correspondence education*
  (a) *For high school students:* It is necessary to realize that the self-instruction could be made possible if the correspondence lessons are programmed.
  (b) *For school teachers:* When new course is being introduced, programmed instruction will equip them with content and new methods of teaching.
  (c) *For university education:* This will help the students who are under correspondence to learn and bring them at par with regular students. Thus, they can maintain the standards of higher education. In the medical and health education field, there are rapid advancements in medical education and hence in these circumstances, programmed learning will help the health care team.

Principles of linear programming

- *Principle of small steps:* A student can proceed from knowing very little about a subject to mastery over the subject by going through a programme.
- *Principle of active responding:* Another way to say 'learning by doing'; people learn by active responding.
- *Conformation:* It is a type of reinforcement to work on the programme or to learn. A student who must wait two weeks for the test results probably will not learn as properly as the student whose test is scored immediately.
- *Principle of self-pacing:* The student can work each step as slowly or as quickly as he chooses. If the pace of classroom is too fast or too slow for a child, he will probably not learn as properly as going at his own pace.
- *Student testing or evaluation:* This provides a detailed record of the student and is the basis for revising the programme.

Types of linear programming

The main types of linear programming are as follows:

- *Construct response:* Skinnerian type where the learner has to construct responses while going through such formats of programme text.
- *Multiple-choice questions:* Sydney L. Pressy selected a response on each frame and is presented in the discrimination frame sequence type of programme.
- *Conventional chaining:* In this type of format by John Barlow, each frame is connected to the second frame which becomes a part of the stimulus of the third and so on down the line.
- *Skip linear:* It uses the skipping device for solving problems of review and over review where a bright student may skip the simple programme.
- *Criterion frames:* This is used to direct the learner along the linear path according to their responses at those critical situations. The creation frames decide whether the student should go through a particular sequence or not.
- *Ruleg system:* The content is organized in terms of rules first and then the examples. The rule is given a complete form and the examples are in incomplete form. A learner has to construct responses to complete the example.
- *Egrule system:* It is just the opposite of the Ruleg system. The content is organized in terms of examples and then the rules. The examples are given in complete form and the rules in incomplete form.

B. BRANCHING OR INTRINSIC STYLE PROGRAMMING

Norman Crowder, a contemporary of Skinner, was working independently for the armed services on programmed instructions. He felt a programme was a form of communication between a programmer and a user. Like any communication, the programme must be directed to the individual. Unlike Skinner, Crowder was not working from a psychological perspective, but from a communications point of view. In an intrinsic or branching programme, each frame presents more text than the average linear frame. After reading, the user responds to an adjunct question, usually in a multiple-option format.

Principles of the branching programme

- *Principle of exposition:* Here the whole concept is presented to the student so that he can learn the complete information better which is provided in the home page. It serves two purposes: teaching and diagnosis.
- *Principle of diagnosis:* Here the weakness of the learner is identified after exposition and it is assessed whether the learner could learn what the causes are, and then it can be modified.
- *Principles of remediation:* If a learner chooses the wrong alternative, the learner has to move to a wrong page where a remedial instruction is provided and the student is directed to return to the home page and he/she is asked to choose the right answer.

Structure of a branching programme

The programmed text is called *scrambled text* and consists of two types of pages: home page and wrong page.

Home page: This page consists of content or concept and followed by multiple-choice questions, which involve four aspects:

- *Teaching:* The learner goes through the instruction to comprehend the concept or information.
- *Response:* At the end of the instruction, multiple choice is given to the learner to choose the correct response, which the learner has to discriminate. The response is intrinsic.
- *Diagnosis:* If the learner chooses the wrong response, he has to move to the wrong page. If he chooses the right response, he moves to the next home page, where the next unit is presented.
- *Reinforcement:* The response is reinforced by confirming it at the beginning of the home page; hence the learner is encouraged through verbal approval or praise.

Wrong page: Wrong page or remedial frame involves:

- Repeating student response.
- Negative confirmation.
- Reason to why he/she is wrong.
- Further explanation in a single language.
- Direction as to where the learner should go next.

Technique of the branching programme

- *Backward branching:* If the learner makes an error, he has to take to the remedial frame where he is given some more help in understanding the concept and solving the problem. He is then directed to the original frame number one. So the learner goes through the same frame twice, once before the remedial material is referred by him.
- *Forward branching:* When the learner gives a correct or wrong response, he goes to the next or new page. If he makes a wrong choice, he is directed to the remedial frame where his mistakes are fully explained, followed by another parallel question from which he goes to the next frame in the main stream.

C. COMPUTER-ASSISTED INSTRUCTION

It consists of individual learning booths, each with a console. It has a television screen for displaying information. A complete package of information is stored in the system and is presented sequentially. The student may question the computer and feed the answer into it. It helps determine subsequent activities in the learning situations.

III. **DEVELOPMENT OF A PROGRAMMED INSTRUCTION**

The main phases or steps for the development of a programmed instruction (Fig. 7.6) are as follows.

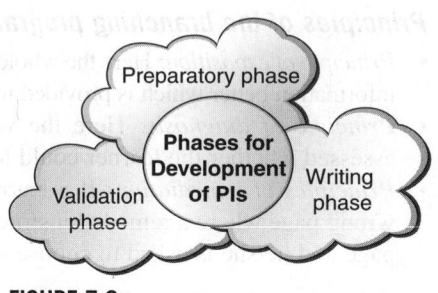

I. Preparatory phase: It involves the following steps:

- Viewing the programme on any topic.
- Deciding to prepare a programme.
- Selecting a topic.
- Preparing a content outline.
- Specification of objectives in behavioural terms.
- Specifications (assumptions about learner).
- Entering behaviour. Prerequisite skills.
- Preparation of pretest.
- Terminal behaviour. Expected performance of the learner at the end of a course.
- Preparation of post-test, i.e. preferably criterion test.

FIGURE 7.6

Phases of programmed instructions.

II. Writing phase: The writing of a programme involves five steps:

- *Present the material in frames*
  - A frame is a small segment of information that calls for particular student response.
  - The task of a programmer is to provide the stimulus necessary to evoke student response.
  - The acquisition of these responses is a step towards terminal behaviour.
  - You should also note that each frame presents a relatively small segment of material.
  - The programmer should present only enough material to elicit a single response.
- *Require active student response*
  - An essential part of the frame is the response the student is asked to make.
  - The responses in programmed material should be overt or covert.
  - Students who make overt responses should write down their answers on sheets of paper.
  - Student who make covert responses should mentally compose the responses to each blank in the frame before turning the page to the correct answers.
- *Provide answers for confirmation or correction of student responses*
  - Providing the correct response with which students can compare their own responses is a standard characteristic of programmed instruction.
  - Students come to know their responses are correct or incorrect.
- *Use prompts to guide student response*
  - Prompts are provided in the programme frame to guide the student to the correct response.
  - Prompts are supplementary stimuli; they are added to a frame to make the frame easier but are not sufficient in themselves to produce the responses.
- *Provide careful sequencing of the frames*

The sequence or order the frames appear in depends on two factors:

- The description and analysis of the behaviours the programme intends to teach.
- The conditions necessary for the learning required by the various tasks.

It is even possible to develop frames that engage the student in problem solving and discovery learning.

- All the basic learning conditions—discrimination, generalization, contiguity, practice and reinforcement—can be embodied in the frame sequence.
- Frame sequence can also provide for review and testing whenever these are necessary.

III. Validation phase: It involves:

- Tryout and revision.
- Individual tryout.
- Small group tryout.
- Master validation.
- Editing, reviewing, revising and modifying the programme for final preparation based on fruits of tryout.

Advantages of programmed instructions

- Programmed instructions are more successful in critical sagacity (discernment) of the logic of various subjects and inspiring students' creative thinking and judgement.
- Good teachers are freed from the humdrum of routine classroom activity and they are in a position to devote their time to more creative activities.
- Some educationists fear that the programmed instructions will deteriorate the quality of instruction. On the other hand, their use has improved the quality of education in general.
- The use of programmed instructions has brought a revolution in the social setting of the classroom. Many emotional and social problems have been eliminated and problems of discipline have been solved automatically.
- Programmed instruction is a great thrust in the direction of individualized instruction. A well-organized programmed instructional device is tailored to cater to the needs of individual students of the class.
- It helps the teacher diagnose the problems of the individual learner.
- By presenting the material in small segments of information, i.e. frames, it makes learning an interesting game in which the learner is challenged by his own capabilities.

Disadvantages of programmed instructions

- Programmed instruction does not eliminate competition or grades as often claimed.
- Mere manipulation of machine is not rewarding to children as Skinner seems to think. Once the novelty wears and if, at the start, too many errors appear, the students lose interest and motivation. Later reinforcements often do not accelerate learning.
- Programmed instructions restrict the learner's freedom of choice resulting in cramping of his imagination and initiative.
- Operant conditioning is found successful only with some students in some cases and not in all. Programmed instructions ignore or make inadequate provisions for variables like cognitive, personality and motivational variables.
- The teacher–pupil contact, which is so vital for development of human personality and relationship, is completely lost.
- In language learning, speech is equally important as development of reading and comprehension skills. There is no scope for providing this experience.

COMPUTER-ASSISTED LEARNING

The word *computer* is derived from the word *compute*, which means to calculate justifying its usefulness. A computer is an electronic machine, which works under the control of a stored programme, automatically accepting processing of data to producing designed results. Computer-assisted learning (CAL) is also known as *computer-assisted* instruction (CAI).

Computer-assisted instruction or learning refers to the introduction or remediation presented on a computer. Many educational computer programmes are available online from computer stores and textbook companies. They enhance the teacher's instruction in several ways.

Computer-assisted learning or computer-assisted instructions facilitate access to information with infinite patience, accuracy and provide an opportunity to all learners. It provides complete individualizing instruction.

CAI mechanizes human brain and human beings are converted into machines.

I. TYPES OF COMPUTER-ASSISTED LEARNING

* *Logo:* This system was developed by Feurzing and Papart. Logo is a simple programming language, which can be taught to children. The programme provides instructions that can be used to produce pictures on an oscilloscope or make a little mechanical robot. The children who learn logo make up their own programmes to draw flowers or faces or generate designs on the screen.
* *Stimulation:* This language enables students to mount an experiment in a symbolic form.
* *Controlled learning:* Controlled learning involves the use of interesting adaptive strategies. It includes both drill and practice. Drill and practice programmes are supplementary to the regular curriculum followed by the classroom teacher.

II. COMPUTER-ASSISTED WRITING INSTRUCTIONS

A computer programme for writing helps students with developing ideas, organizing, outlining and brainstorming. A template provides the framework and reduces the physical effort spent on writing so that students can pay attention to organization and content.

Computer programmes for writing

* *Word prediction*
    * Speech: Specific programmes that identify words students use repeatedly; when a student types the first few letters, the programme lists the frequently used words that start with those letters.
    * Speeds up the typing process.
* *Speech-to-text*
    * Students speak into a microphone and the programme types the words.
    * Programme must be 'trained' to the student's word pronunciation and speech style.
    * Students must be taught how to use the programme.
    * Increased speed from voice to text.
* *Text-to-speech*
    * Students can hear what they have typed to check if it says what they want it to say.
    * Good for editing.
* *Spellchecker*
    * Helps students identify misspelled words.
    * Automatically corrects words if the teacher sets to the programme that way.

III. EXPERTS NEEDED IN COMPUTER-ASSISTED LEARNING

* Computer engineer
* Lesson writer
* System operator

IV. ROLE OF A TEACHER IN COMPUTER-ASSISTED LEARNING

- The teacher will be liberated from his routine duty.
- The computer-assisted instruction can complete the language data accurately and rapidly.

Disadvantages of computer-assisted learning

- Inadequate training of teachers and inadequacy of instructional material.
- The computer fails to appreciate the students' emotions. The warm emotional climate created by the teacher in classroom interaction with the students is lacking in CAL.
- CAL fails to develop essential features of language competency.
- CAL is a mechanical approach to education.
- The peripheral equipment puts constraints in the ways a student can interact with the computer.

APPLICATION OF COMPUTERS IN NURSING

The main areas for the application of computers in nursing are as follows.

I. EDUCATION

- Knowledge of computers can be applied to prepare slides in MS PowerPoint on the topics to be taught to students.
- Knowledge of multimedia helps the nursing teachers and students teach effectively.
- Education through internet and CAL has simplified education in nursing schools.
- A computer aids in learning and instructions:
  - By providing information and instructions.
  - By asking questions.
  - By doing difficult calculations.
  - By being tireless and repetitive.
  - By simulated process.
  - By selecting the right speed for providing information to individual learners.

II. ADMINISTRATION

- Preparing records of nursing students by lecturers and nursing superintendent.
- Preparing and maintaining records of assessment and results.
- Preparing duty rosters that saves time.
- Preparing drafts of a plan annually, monthly and weekly.

III. HOSPITAL

- Computers keep records of patient's health status during hospital stay and OPD.
- Hospital information management system (HIMS) helps to have access to the patient treatment chart, operation list or anaesthetic record; this is possible with computer knowledge.
- Computer helps nurses manage routine documents in a fraction of a time, which may otherwise take up a lot of time manually.

- It increases productivity of nurses.
- Other functions in hospitals, i.e. automatic generation of reminder letters, determination of milestones, are performed with the help of appropriate softwares.

Features of HIMS

- Data is retrieved quickly and easily.
- Entry of data is easy.
- It has a high degree of security of data.
- Data validation is stringent.

Benefits of HIMS

- Improvement in the doctor's productivity.
- Reduced patient waiting time.
- Eliminating wastage of stationary.
- Prompt medical attention.
- Accuracy and timeliness of data.
- Eliminating any possibility of mixing of blood samples.
- Authorization check and accuracy of billing.
- Prompt issue of medication for patients.
- Maintaining inventory of medication.
- Safe recording of data and saving the time that has to be spent in the medical record department.
- Carrying legal value.
- Prescribing diet from the ward through a computer.
- Giving secret code to prevent manipulation for security reasons.
- Blood bank module for donor registration and certification helps make referrals within the hospital, prepare duty rosters, OT scheduling, diagnostic appointments and patient records.

IV. RESEARCH WORK

- Computers are used to get information on the research works being carried out via the internet.
- They help support research findings with other research that has been carried out.
- Knowledge of computers helps nurses increase their productivity and provide the best patient centred care. A knowledge of computers reduces the time taken to for documentation which usually takes time when done manually.

MICRO-TEACHING

The idea of micro-teaching originated for the first time at Stanford University, USA, when an experimental project on the identification of teaching skills was in progress under the guidance and supervision of faculty members. The team of experts was assigned the development of testing and evaluation tools to measure the attainment of teaching skills. A research worker was investigating the utility of video tape recorders in the development of technical teaching skills. This instrument could be used for recording class interaction and behaviours of the trainees vividly and accurately, which led to the development of a systematic and accurate method of providing feedback to teacher trainees. All the steps of the micro-teaching technique, i.e. *Teach → Feedback → Re-plan → Re-teach → Re-feedback*, were formulated. The term *micro-teaching* was coined for this method of developing teaching skills in 1963. Since then this technique has been widely used in almost all colleges and universities. It is being used with great emphasis in all teacher training programmes for developing teaching skills and competencies in teacher trainees.

Micro-teaching is a teacher training technique that helps the teacher trainee to master the teaching skills. It requires the teacher trainee:

- To teach a single concept of content.
- Use a specified teaching skill.
- Teach for a short time.
- Teach to a very small number of students.

In this way the teacher trainee practices the teaching skill in terms of definable, observable, measurable and controllable form with repeated cycles till he attains a mastery in the use of that skill.

I. ASSUMPTIONS OF MICRO-TEACHING

From the foregoing discussion about the concept of micro-teaching, the basic assumption on which it is based is the premise that teaching can be analyzed into various teaching skills that can be practised and evaluated.

- Micro-teaching seems to be based on Skinner's theory of operant condition. This theory is the very basis of feedback session. Skinner's theory of shaping a successive approximation can be applied to explain the acquisition of new patterns of behaviour in the *teach → feedback → re-teach* pattern in micro-teaching.
- Teaching is a complex process but can be analyzed into simple skills.
- Teaching skills can be practised one by one up to the mastery level under specific and simplified situations.
- Appropriate feedback, if systematically given, proves very significant for obtaining a mastery level in each skill.
- When all skills have been mastered, taken one by one, they can be integrated for real classroom teaching.
- Skill training can be conveniently transferred from a simulated teaching situation to the actual classroom teaching situation.
- Teaching skill is the set of behaviours or acts of the teacher that facilitate students' learning.
- Teaching is observable, definable, measurable and demonstrable and can be developed through training.
- Micro-teaching is a teacher training technique that plays a significant role in developing teaching skills in the student teachers.
- The procedure of micro-teaching involves the following steps: *Plan → Teach → Feedback → Re-plan → Re-teach → Re-feedback*. These steps are repeated till the student teacher attains mastery in the use of the skill.
- The micro-teaching cycle consists of all the essential steps of basic teaching.
- For practising teaching skills, the setting of micro-teaching involves:
  - A single skill for practice.
  - One concept of content for teaching.

- A class of 5–10 students.
- 5–10 minutes of practice time.
- Systematic use of feedback plays a significant role in the acquisition of the skill up to the mastery level.
- After the acquisition of the core skills, it is possible to integrate them for effective teaching in actual classroom situations.

II. BENEFITS OF MICRO-TEACHING

- Visual feedback (through watching a recorded lesson) has been found to provide one of the most effective means of evaluating teaching strengths and identifying areas of improvement.
- Micro-teaching enables both intrinsic (self-assessment) and extrinsic (peer-review) assessment of teaching behaviours.
- Through micro-teaching, one can seek to identify and improve these observable teaching skills and behaviours. Some such skills and observable teaching behaviours include:
  - Oral presentation skills (voice modulation and articulation, enthusiasm, gestures, nonverbal cues, clarity of explanations and examples)
  - Organization skills (structure of lessons, strong opening and closing, good transitions between sections, clear learning objectives, effective use of time and good pacing)
  - Relating to the student (speaker engages audience, material is audience-appropriate, effective questioning and use of real-life examples)
  - Effective use of teaching aids (handouts, blackboard, presentation software, overhead transparencies, props and charts, etc.).
- Aside from helping to identify teaching skills to be improved as well as teaching strengths, micro-teaching sessions can also provide an opportunity for the following:
  - Practising a part of a lecture or running an activity or explaining a procedure before you have to deliver a course or demonstrate a lab for the first time.
  - Practising a guest lecture you have been asked to deliver in someone else's course.
  - Practising a job talk before you visit a campus when applying for jobs.
  - Practising public speaking skills before you address students for the first time.
  - Polishing your questioning techniques or your opening and closing skills, if you are already an experienced instructor.

III. STEPS OF MICRO-TEACHING

It is also known as the *micro-teaching cycle* and includes the following six steps (Fig. 7.7):

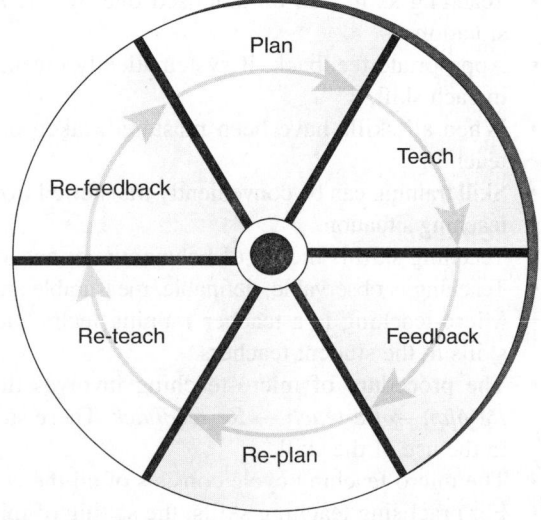

FIGURE 7.7

Micro-teaching cycle.

A. Plan

- This involves the selection of the topic and related content of a nature in which the use of components of the skill under practice may be made easily and conveniently.
- The topic is analyzed into different activities of the teacher and the students.
- The activities are planned in a logical sequence such that the maximum application of the components of a skill is possible.

B. Teach

- This involves the attempts of the teacher trainee to use the components of the skill in suitable situations in the process of teaching–learning per his or her planning of activities.
- If the situation is different and not as visualized in the planning of the activities, the teacher should modify his or her behaviour per the demand of the situation in the class.
- The teacher should have the courage and confidence to handle the situations arising in the class effectively.

C. Feedback

- This term refers to giving information to the teacher trainee about his performance.
- The information includes the points of strength as well as weakness relating to his or her performance.
- This helps the teacher trainee improve his or her performance in the desired direction.

D. Re-plan

The teacher trainee re-plans his lesson incorporating the points of strength and removing the points not skilfully handled during teaching in the previous attempt either on the same topic or on another topic suiting the teacher trainee for improvement.

E. Re-teach

- This involves teaching the same group of students if the topic is changed or a different group of students if the topic is the same.
- This is done to remove boredom or monotony in the students.
- The teacher trainee teaches the class with renewed courage and confidence to perform better than the previous attempt.

F. Re-feedback

This is the most important component of micro-teaching for behaviour modification of the teacher trainee in the desired direction in each and every skill practice.

IV. PHASES OF MICRO-TEACHING

There are three phases of the micro-teaching procedure and they are (Fig. 7.8):

- *Knowledge acquisition phase:* In this phase, the teacher trainee learns about the skill and its components through

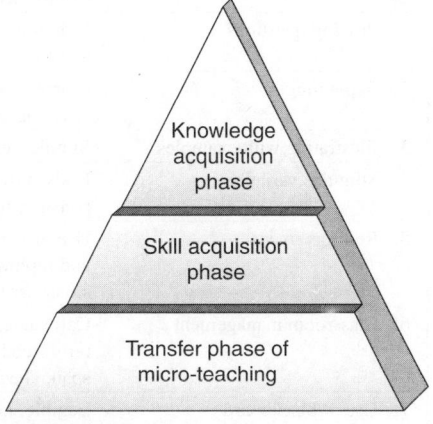

FIGURE 7.8

Phases of micro-teaching.

discussion, illustrations and demonstration of the skill given by the expert. He learns about the purpose of the skill and the condition under which it proves useful in the teaching–learning process. The teacher trainee's analysis of the skill into components leads to various types of behaviours to be practised. The teacher trainee tries to gain the skill from the demonstration given by the expert. He discusses and clarifies each and every aspect of the skill.

- *Skill acquisition phase:* On the basis of the demonstration presented by the expert, the teacher trainee plans a micro-lesson for practicing the demonstrated skill. He practices the teaching skill through the micro-teaching cycle and continues his efforts till he attains the mastery level. The feedback component of micro-teaching contributes significantly towards the mastery level acquisition of the skill. On the basis of the performance of teacher trainee in teaching, feedback is provided for the purpose of change in behaviour of the teacher trainee in the desired direction. These skills are called *core skills* because of their extensive use in classroom teaching. The specifications of these skills are given in Box 7.4.

- *Transfer phase of micro-teaching:* After attaining mastery and command over each of the skills, the teacher trainee integrates all these skills and transfers to actual classroom teaching during this transfer phase.

V. ORGANIZATION OF THE MICRO-TEACHING SESSION

- It is not easy and workable to get actual students practice the skill because of administrative reasons so a simulated class of peers has been found suitable and useful for this purpose. How to organize the micro-teaching cycle for 10 teacher trainees who have come prepared with planned micro-lessons for the practice of a particular skill? Allot roll numbers to teacher trainees from 1 to 10 and prepare the following plan (Box 7.5).

BOX 7.4 TEACHING SKILLS AND THEIR SPECIFICATIONS

Skill	Components
1. Probing questions	Prompting, seeking further information, redirection, focusing, increasing critical awareness
2. Explaining	Clarity, continuity, relevance to content using beginning and concluding statements, covering essential points
3. Illustrating with examples	Simple, relevant and interesting examples and use of appropriate media
4. Stimulus variation	Body movements, gestures, changes in speech pattern, changes in style of interaction, pausing, focusing, oral–visual switching
5. Reinforcement	Use of words and statements of praise, accepting and using students' ideas, repeating and rephrasing, extra vertical cues, use of pleasant and approving gestures and expressions, writing students' answers on the blackboard
6. Classroom management	Call students by names, make norms of classroom behaviour, attending behaviour reinforced, clarity of direction, check nonattending behaviour, keep students in eye span, check inappropriate behaviour immediately
7. Use of blackboard	Legible, neat and adequate with reference to content covered

BOX 7.5 ORGANIZATION MATRIX OF A MICRO-TEACHING SESSION

Teacher (Roll No.)	Students (Roll No.)	Supervisor (Roll No.)	Feedback (Roll No.)	Re-plan (Roll No.)
1	3, 4, 5, 6, 7, 8, 9, 10	2	–	–
3	5, 6, 7, 8, 9, 10	4	2 to 1	–
5	2, 7, 8, 9, 10	6	4 to 3	1
7	1, 2, 4, 9, 10	8	6 to 5	3
9	1, 2, 3, 4, 6	10	8 to 7	5
2	3, 4, 6, 5, 8	1	10 to 9	7
4	5, 6, 7, 8, 10	3	1 to 2	9
6	1, 7, 8, 9, 10	5	3 to 4	2
8	1, 2, 3, 9, 10	7	5 to 6	4
10	1, 2, 3, 4, 5	9	7 to 8	6

PROBLEM-BASED LEARNING

Problem-based learning is a student-centric instructional strategy where students collaboratively solve problems and reflect on their experiences. It is an inquiry-based method of instruction that guides students to solutions of real-world problems through cooperative group work and builds critical thinking skills.

- According to D.J. Boud (1985), 'the principal idea behind problem-based learning is that the starting point should be a problem, a query, or a puzzle that the learner wishes to solve'.
- According to John Dewey (1916), 'a careful inspection of methods which are permanently successful in formal education. Problem based learning will reveal that they depend for their efficiency upon the fact that they go back to the type of situation which causes reflection out of school in ordinary life. They give pupils something to do, not something to learn; and if the doing is of such a nature as to demand thinking naturally results'.

Problem-based learning is a process of acquiring understanding, knowledge, skills and attitudes in the context of an unfamiliar situation and applying this learning to that situation. Problem-based learning includes the following components:

- Nonlecture format with the teacher as a facilitator.
- The presentation of real world situation or problems that expand on previous learning.
- Student group work and discussion.
- Student-directed solution of the problem.

Problem-based learning is guided by a constructivist framework that emphasizes problem solving should occur in the same environment as the problem, the presence of a problem is what starts and guides the learning process and determines how the problem is solved, and knowledge is expanded through group discussion and collaboration.

I. USE OF PROBLEM-BASED LEARNING

Problem-based learning is introduced and continued for many reasons including:

- Acquiring subject matter knowledge.
- Motivating students to learn.
- Helping students with retention.
- Developing students' thinking skills.
- Developing students' key skills relevant to employment such as interpersonal communication skills.
- Fostering professional competence and confidence together with professional identity.
- Mirroring the interdisciplinary team process graduates will use in work and research.
- Facilitating students how to learn.
- Encouraging students to integrate knowledge from different subjects, disciplines and sources.
- Linking theory and practice.
- Having a sense of belonging and friendship.
- Having a sense of fun while learning.
- Expressing in operational form a philosophy of learning that is student-centric and problem focused.

II. COMMON FEATURES OF PROBLEM-BASED LEARNING

The main features of problem-based learning are:

- Learning is initiated by a problem.
- Problems are based on complex, real-world situations.
- All information needed to solve the problem is not given initially.
- Students identify, find and use appropriate resources.
- Students work in a permanent group.
- Learning is active, integrated, cumulative and connected.

III. PROCESS OF PROBLEM-BASED LEARNING

The main steps in the process of problem-based learning are (Fig. 7.9):

- Presentation of problem.
- Organize ideas and prior knowledge.
- Pose questions.
- Assign responsibilities for questions and discuss resources.
- Research questions, summarize and analyze findings.
- Reconvene and report on research.
- Integrate new information and refine questions.
- Resolution of problem.

IV. THE PROBLEM-BASED LEARNING CYCLE

Problem-based learning consists of the following steps (Fig. 7.10):

Kenneth J. Oja conducted a study on using problem-based learning in the clinical setting to improve nursing students' critical thinking. In today's arena, new graduate nurses are exposed to increasingly

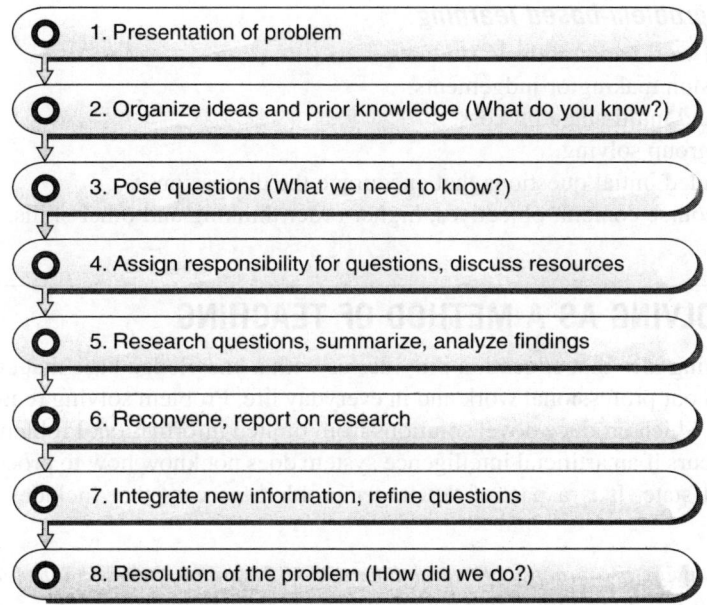

FIGURE 7.9

Steps of the problem-based learning process.

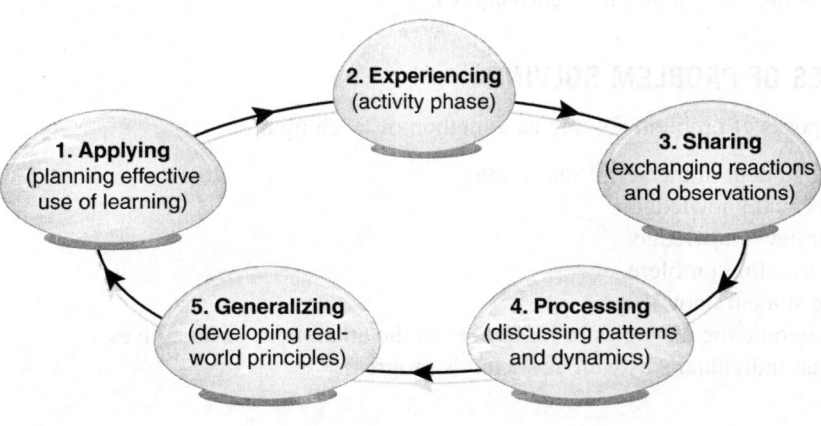

FIGURE 7.10

Steps of the problem-based cycle.

demanding and complex acute care environments that require an ability to effectively think and reason to provide quality patient care. So there is a need to demonstrate critical thinking skills to the new graduate students. Problem-based learning is a method of education designed to encourage critical thinking. The studies reviewed a positive relationship between problem-based learning and improved critical thinking in nursing students.

Advantages of problem-based learning

- Relates to real world and motivate students.
- Requires decision making or judgements.
- A multipage and multi-stage process.
- Designed for group solving.
- Poses open-ended initial questions that encourage the discussion.
- Incorporates course content, objectives, higher-order thinking and other skills.

PROBLEM SOLVING AS A METHOD OF TEACHING

There is a prevailing idea that education provides us with a knowledge base that enables us to deal with life's problems in our professional work and in everyday life. Problem solving requires an integrated use of thinking skills which produce novel solutions from limited information. Problem solving forms a part of thinking. It occurs if an artificial intelligence system does not know how to proceed from a given state to a desired goal state. It is a part of the larger problem process that includes problem finding and shaping.

> *The problem solving is a process of overcoming difficulties that appears to interfere with the attainment of goal. It is a procedure of making adjustment in spite of interferences.*
>
> **—Skinner**

> *Problem solving is a method of organization of subject matter in such a way that it can be dealt with through the study of problems encountered.*

I. PURPOSES OF PROBLEM SOLVING

The main proposes of problem solving as a method of teaching are:

- To train the student in the act of reasoning.
- To give practical knowledge.
- To discover new knowledge.
- To solve a puzzling problem.
- To improve student knowledge.
- To help overcome the obstacles or inferences in the attainment of objectives.
- To help in an individual's as well as society's progress.

II. ESSENTIAL FEATURES OF PROBLEM SOLVING

The main features of problem solving as a method of teaching are:

- The problem should be meaningful, interesting and worthwhile.
- It should have correlation with life.
- It should arise out of the real needs of students.
- Students must possess some background knowledge of the problem.
- The problem should be clearly defined.
- The solution of the problem should be found out by the students under the guidance of the teacher.

III. STEPS IN PROBLEM SOLVING

The main steps followed in the problem-solving process are (Fig. 7.11):

- Recognizing the problem.
- Defining the problem.
- Collecting relevant data and information.
- Organizing conclusion.
- Drawing and testing conclusion.

IV. METHODS/APPROACHES TO PROBLEM SOLVING

- *Inductive method:* The inductive method is a method of development. The student is led to discover the truth about him. It includes:
  - Observation of the given material
  - Discrimination and analysis noting differences and similarities.
  - Classification.
  - Abstraction and generalization.
  - Application or verification.
- *Deductive method:* In the deductive method rules, generalizations and principles are provided to students and they are asked to verify them with the help of particular examples.
- *Combination of deductive and inductive method:* Induction is followed by deduction and deduction is followed by induction. According to Miller, induction is the making of the tools of thought and deduction is the using of tools.

V. ROLE OF TEACHER IN PROBLEM SOLVING

The major roles of a teacher in problem solving as a method of teaching are:

- To get the students to define the problem clearly.
- To aid them to keep the problem in mind.
- To get them to make suggestions by encouraging them.

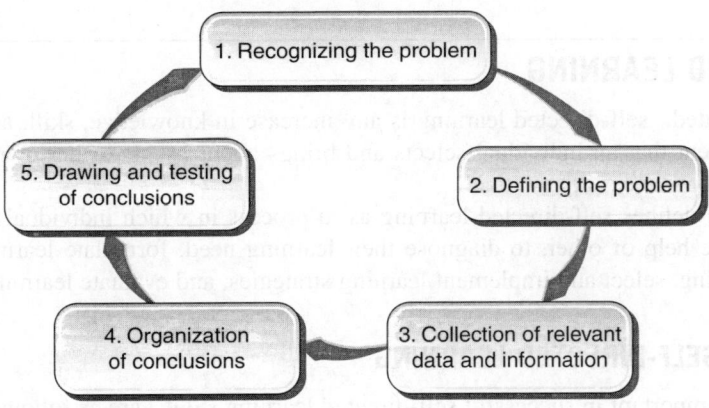

1. Recognizing the problem
2. Defining the problem
3. Collection of relevant data and information
4. Organization of conclusions
5. Drawing and testing of conclusions

FIGURE 7.11

Steps in problem solving.

- To give them time to evaluate each suggestion carefully.
- To give them time to organize material.
- To set up an atmosphere of freedom in the class.

Advantages of problem solving

- Improves problem-solving abilities.
- Is student-centric rather than teacher-centric.
- Is an activity of collaboration.
- Helps in the development of constructivism.
- Allows for multiple intelligence development.
- Offers opportunity of extended time frames.
- Provides a deeper understanding of knowledge.
- Other advantages of problem solving as a method of teaching:
  - It helps in developing good study habits.
  - It affords opportunities for participation in social activities.
  - The students learn to be self-dependent.
  - Discussions help develop the power of expressions of students.
  - It provides opportunities to the teachers to know their students in detail.
  - Students learn facts that are meaningful and have been discovered by their own efforts.
  - It helps in the maintenance of discipline.
  - Learning becomes more interesting in place of dread.
  - It gives the power of critical judgement.
  - It helps verify an option.
  - It satisfies curiosity.
  - It helps learn how to act in a new situation.

Disadvantages of problem solving

- Problem solving involves mental activity only. There is less body activity.
- There is a lack of suitable references and source books for students.
- It involves a lot of time and teachers find it difficult to cover the prescribed syllabus.
- Problem-solving methods need very capable teachers to provide effective guidance.

SELF-DIRECTED LEARNING

Gibbons (2002) stated, 'self-directed learning is any increase in knowledge, skill, accomplishment, or personal development that an individual selects and brings about by his or her own efforts using any method in any circumstances at any time'.

Knowles (1975) defines self-directed learning as 'a process in which individual take the initiative, with or without the help of other, to diagnose their learning need, formulate learning goals, identify resources for learning, select and implement learning strategies, and evaluate learning outcomes'.

I. SKILLS FOR SELF-DIRECTED LEARNING

Skills particularly important in successful self-directed learning (SDL) are as follows (Fig. 7.12):

- Goal-oriented skills.
- Information-processing skills.

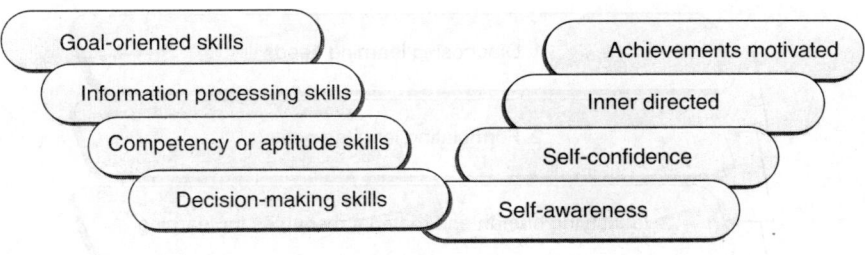

FIGURE 7.12

Skills for self-directed learning.

- Competency and aptitude skills.
- Decision-making skills.
- Self-awareness.
- Self-confidence.
- Inner direction.
- Achievement motivated.

II. PRINCIPLES OF SELF-DIRECTED LEARNING

The basic principles of self-directed learning as a method of teaching:

- Self-directed learning should be congruent with lifelong, natural and individual learning drives.
- It should be adapted to the maturation, transformations and transitions experienced by students.
- It should be concerned with all aspects of a full life.
- It should employ a full range of human capacities, including senses, emotion and action as well as intellects.
- The self-directed learning activities should be conducted in settings suited to their development.

III. PROCESS OF SELF-DIRECTED LEARNING

Knowles has given the five-step model for the process of self-directed learning. His five-step model of self-directed learning is illustrated in Fig. 7.13.

IV. ROLE OF TEACHER IN SELF-DIRECTED LEARNING

The principal responsibilities of a teacher using self-directed learning as a method of teaching are:

- To teach inquiry skills, decision making, personal developments and self-evaluation of work.
- To help learners develop positive attitudes and feelings of independence related to learning.
- To help learners acquire the needs and assessment techniques necessary to discover what objectives they should set.
- To help the learners identify the starting point for a learning project and understand the relevant modes of examination and reporting.
- To create a partnership with the learner by negotiating a learning contact for goals, strategies and evaluation criteria.

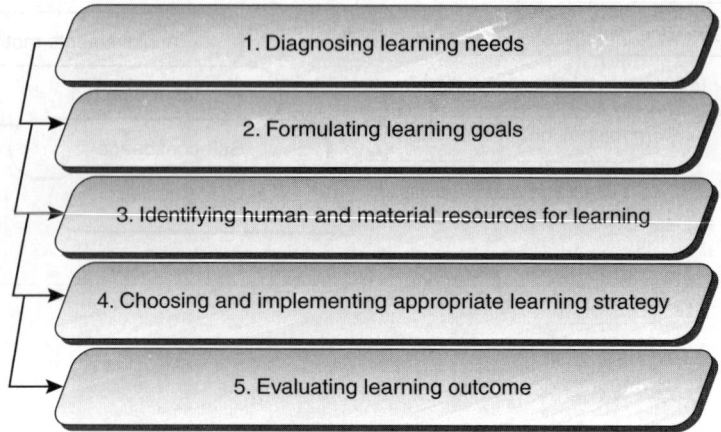

1. Diagnosing learning needs

2. Formulating learning goals

3. Identifying human and material resources for learning

4. Choosing and implementing appropriate learning strategy

5. Evaluating learning outcome

FIGURE 7.13

Process of self-directed learning.

- To make sure that learners are aware of the objectives, learning strategies, resources and evaluation criteria once they are decided.
- To teach inquiry skills, decision making, personal development and self-evaluation of work.
- To act as advocates for educationally underserved populations to facilitate their access to resources.
- To help match resources to the needs of the learners.
- To help learners locate resources.
- To encourage critical thinking skills.
- To create an atmosphere of openness and trust to promote better performance.

Advantages of self-directed learning
- Self-directed learning allows learners to be more effective learners.
- It helps the learner develop a sense of responsibility.
- It can encourage students to develop their own rules and leadership patterns.
- It helps the learners to be motivated and persistent, independent, self-disciplined, self-confident and goal oriented.

Disadvantages of self-directed learning
- Learners can easily be distracted by their own needs, assumptions, values and misperceptions.
- Research has shown that some adults are unable to engage in self-directed learning because they lack independence, confidence or resources.
- Self-directed learning needs to be combined with other learning methods for content to be fully learned.

SIMULATION

Simulation is a newer pedagogical approach that has recently got much of popularity because it facilitates to provide the learning experiences in the controlled environment that enhances the patient safety and students' confidence and comfort. Simulation is role-playing where the process of teaching is displayed artificially and an effort to practice some important skills is made. The teacher and students simulate an actual life situation or a person's actual role.

As defined in Wikipedia encyclopedia 'Simulation is the imitation of the operation of a real-world process or system over time. The act of simulating something first requires that a model be developed; this model represents the key characteristics or behaviors/functions of the selected physical or abstract system or process'.

Simulation as a method of clinical teaching is rapidly recognized as an effective method to supplement and enhance clinical learning in nursing education. Simulation is a method of clinical teaching, where real-life clinical scenarios are simulated for leaning and practicing new clinical skills without involving real patients. The level and sophistication of simulation vary from simple skill training model to computerized full body mannequins with all possible control and responses, which are as close to real patients. The emerging research evidence has proven the importance of simulations in nursing education. However, it must be integrated into curriculum in such a way that there is clarity on transition of clinical skill learnt through simulation to the real patients.

Recently, use of simulation in nursing education has increased because of (i) increased awareness about availability and usefulness of simulators in nursing education; (ii) shortage of clinical facilities for real patient care experiences for the nursing students; (iii) decreasing cost of simulators; (iv) increased felt need of patient safety and (v) support of empirical evidences about usefulness of simulators in skill building among nurses.

I. TYPES OF SIMULATORS

Based on the simulator's ability to be realistic as close to the real patient and its ability to simulate the real patient scenario, the simulators may be classified into three broad categories, i.e. low fidelity, moderate fidelity and high fidelity. The term fidelity is used for simulator to describe the extent of accuracy of system being used to produce the clinical scenario as close as to the real one.

- *Low-fidelity simulators:* The low-fidelity simulators are static, lack the realism, vitality and they just structurally resemble to the actual part or whole body. For example, foam made intramuscular model or a patient care dummy.
- *Moderate-fidelity simulator:* Moderate-fidelity simulators are relatively more complex than low-fidelity simulators, where learner may get feedback from the simulator. They may also provide limited opportunity to experience airway, breathing, chest movements, pulse, breath or heart sounds, etc. but will not be as sophisticated as high-fidelity simulators. An example of this is a feedback-oriented basic life support mannequin.
- *High-fidelity simulator:* High-fidelity simulator may produce the most realistic simulated patient experiences. They have ability to react as close as to real patient, when the students are interacting or practicing the nursing procedures. In addition, nursing faculty also has opportunity to control the different scenarios using remote computer device. They cosmetically also looks and give feel of as real as an actual patient. An example of this is advanced level ACLS simulator. The high-fidelity simulators are relatively more expensive than the moderate and low-fidelity simulators. These simulators do have the facility of simultaneous video recording, which is useful in debriefing conference to give feedback to the students.

II. PRINCIPLES OF SIMULATION

- The simulators are representative of the real patients and then make decisions in response to their assessment of the setting they find themselves in.
- The experiences simulated are consequences that relate to their decisions and general performance.
- Monitoring the results of their actions to reflect upon the relationship between their own decisions and the resultant consequences.

III. PURPOSES OF THE SIMULATION

- Enables the learner to learn directly from simulated experience which are as close to as real one.
- Promotes a high level of skills and critical thinking.
- Develops in the students an understanding of the problems may be encounter in real situation and ability of decision-making.
- Enables the individual to empathize with the real life situations.
- Provides feedback to the learners on the consequences of actions and decision made.
- Motivates the students by making real life situations exciting and interesting.
- Enables teachers and learners to assess the realism of the situation by uncovering misconceptions.

IV. MODES OF SIMULATION

There are a variety of ways to simulate the clinical environment as discussed below:

- *Full-body mannequins:* These simulators physically look like a patient; however, the complexity of full-body simulators varies from just being physically like a patient to be a sophisticated electronically controlled simulator, which has ability to provide most of the physiological or pathological responses when remotely controlled through computer device.
- *Part-task trainers:* The part-task trainers are the models that are primarily used for practicing the technical nursing skills, e.g. a gluteal intramuscular injection model or airway trainer model or an intravenous arm. These models are available as the specific part rather than the full body, which make them more cost-effective and easy to handle and store.
- *Simulated patients:* They are popularly known as 'patient actors' or 'standardized patients'; they are also called as clinical teaching associates who are especially trained to behave like a particular patient to create an artificial clinical scenario. They are especially used for the situations that are sensitive in nature or require a real individual vital signs monitoring, physical examination, breast examination, etc.
- *Computer-generated simulators:* The computer-generated simulators may be as simple as computer programme, which demonstrates the steps of equipment functioning, e.g. a mechanical ventilator. They may be as complex as a three-dimensional virtual clinical environment, where student gets an opportunity to virtually interact with virtual patient and healthcare team.
- *Hybrid simulators:* They are the combination of standardized patient and the part-task trainer to make clinical learning more real. For example, a gravid uterus is worn by a simulated or standardized patient, where students may have more close to realist experience of the clinical skills, communication skills and professional behaviour. The specific electronic devices, such as modified stethoscope,

may be used to create the desired physiological or pathological responses such as adventitious respiratory sounds or abnormal heart sounds.

Advantages of simulation

- Simulation establishes a setting where theory and practice can be combined.
- Simulation requires the teacher to be an active participant in the process.
- Patient safety can be ensured. The decisions are made and carried out without physical or psychological harm to real patients.
- It is possible to have a very good control over clinical teaching environment.
- Simulation is a teaching technique that motivates and involves students. It changes teacher behaviour and introduces novelty in the whole learning process. The level of freshness and novelty is maintained throughout the learning session.
- Students are not expected to identify the group time and follow it. Every student is expected to have experiences that are different from the usual laboratory type experiences common to all.
- It stimulates the students for the acquisition of purposeful activities and they feel keenly interested.
- It removes the student–teacher polarization. Simulations are self-monitoring. Participants recognize their aim progress by various feedback methods. Students are involved in decision-making. They observe their own evaluation of these consequences, which influence their future actions. Personal tensions in the teaching situation are likely to be reduced by the process of self-monitoring. The teacher's role may be as an interpreter of the simulation and as a guide, but he does not have to pose as an expert or as a judge.
- It develops decision-making skills into action. It develops various skills in students in an increasing order or difficulty.
- It provides an integrated view and is a vehicle for free interdisciplinary communication.
- It provides dynamic framework.
- Simulation works to bridge the gap between unreal and real. Students enact real situations and learning becomes more interesting and lively than purely theoretical.

Disadvantages of simulation

- It is not possible to simulate each and every scenario in all subjects of the curriculum.
- Inadequately designed simulated scenario may convey the unintended message to the learners.
- Simulators may not provide some of the realistic clinical presentations, such as sweating, skin colours, which lead to the habit of ignoring these presentations in real-life situations.
- In simulations, generally shortcuts are used such as not obtaining consent, using safety precautions, lack of complete communication, use of opened IV fluid, expired drugs and not wearing gloves lead to habit of unsafe behaviour/practice in real-life clinical setting.
- It is also a problem in simulation that students get habitual of artificial communication rather than realistic communication skills.
- Simulation cannot be conveniently used in the case of isolated simpler tasks because mechanism is too difficult for them to follow.
- It requires a lot of preparation on the part of teachers; very few teachers are prepared to take up the extra work which is required to make this technique as a success.
- Learning is a serious activity which is highly individualized and needs concentration on the part of the learner. Simulation reduces the seriousness of learning.
- It has difficulty in using analytic approach.
- Many simulators are needed sometimes, which may not be practically possible sometimes.

CLINICAL TEACHING METHODS

Nurses need learning in three domains i.e. cognitive, affective and psychomotor. However, psychomotor domain of learning is most essential in nursing discipline because nurses need to have hands-on skills to provide best quality nursing care to their patients or clients. Therefore, it is essential for nurse educators to provide clinical teaching through most robust and advanced methods, so that nursing students can swiftly learn the real-life clinical knowledge and clinical skills.

According to Schweer (1972), 'clinical teaching is a vehicle that provides students with the opportunity to translate basic theoretical knowledge into the learning of a variety of intellectual and psychomotor skills needed to provide patient centred quality nursing care'.

Clinical teaching is a time-bound process in which the teacher and the student create a partnership within a shared environment in such a way that the teacher's primary operational frame of reference is maintained as the legitimate means for affecting the student's behaviour towards intended purposes.

A teacher's core activity in the clinical setting is clinical instruction and guidance. The teacher must guide, support, stimulate and facilitate learning. He/she can facilitate learning by designing appropriate activity in appropriate setting and allowing the student to experience that learning. The main responsibilities and qualities of a clinical teacher are presented in Box 7.6.

BOX 7.6 RESPONSIBILITIES AND QUALITIES OF A CLINICAL TEACHER

I. Responsibilities of clinical teacher
1. Plan and implement the clinical learning experiences through most effective methods of clinical teaching.
2. Plan and prepare required clinical area and needed resources for effective clinical experiences.
3. Orient the new group of students to the clinical environment to promote their adaptation to the new clinical setting.
4. Facilitate in arranging all the essential resources required for the clinical learning.
5. Demonstrating clinical nursing skills and motivating the students to carryout return demonstrations to ensure that they have acquired the required clinical learning.
6. Helping the students to gradually become independent in performing the learned clinical knowledge and skills.
7. Assessing the students to ensure that they have achieved optimum level of desired learning in the particular clinical field/area.
8. Keep himself/herself updated with most advanced and effective methods of clinical teaching.

II. Qualities of a good clinical teacher
1. Available, approachable and nonthreatening.
2. Resourceful.
3. Clinically competent.
4. Nonjudgmental.
5. Enthusiastic and passionate in clinical teaching and learning.
6. Empathetic and tolerant.
7. Three 'A' for qualities of clinical teacher are
   - Ability (attitude, knowledge and clinical skills).
   - Availability (physical presence of teacher in clinical setting/bedside).
   - Affability (approachable, affectionate, gentle, gracious and friendly).

BOX 7.7 TYPES OF CLINICAL TEACHING METHODS

Type of Clinical Teaching Method	Concept/Meaning
1. Nursing case study	Nursing case study is in-depth study and analysis of progress of a patient with specific disease, who received nursing care for an extended period ranging between 7 and 10 days. In the case study, students get an opportunity to understand the effects of particular nursing interventions on specific nursing problems/diagnoses.
2. Nursing case presentation	Nursing case presentation refers to a formal discussion of a particular patient in details regarding medical diagnosis, clinical features, diagnostic tests, medical/surgical treatment, nursing assessment findings, identified nursing problems and best possible planned nursing care interventions considering best recommended practices.
3. Nursing rounds	It is a clinical teaching method in which a group of nursing students are taken for a selected patient's bedside visit by one or more nursing faculties to discuss about the progress of the patient and further plan of care, which provides the students first-hand clinical learning experiences.
4. Bedside nursing clinics	Bedside nursing clinic is a method of clinical teaching, which is also called as bedside teaching where a small group of students are taught about a disease condition or nursing care practices directly on a real patient at bedside, which provides rich opportunity of visual, auditory, tactile and olfactory experiences.
5. Nursing assignments	Nursing assignment refers to the assignment of particular patient or nursing task of the patient to the nursing students under the direct supervision of nursing teacher, where he/she gets an opportunity to obtain direct clinical learning experiences.
6. Nursing care conferences	Conference is the act of coming together of two or more nursing individuals in a formal meeting for the purpose of giving or exchanging ideas or in a formal discussion of problems and their possible solutions. It could be a group or individual activity based on the needs and purposes of conference.
7. Health team conference	Health team conference is a multidisciplinary team activity, where professionals from different discipline formally meet together to discuss particular case or issue of the common interest.
8. Process recording	Process recording is a method of clinical teaching in which students get an opportunity to directly interact with patient in the supervision of clinical faculty where he/she gets a chance to obtain skills of communication, history taking, critical thinking and recording of interaction.
9. Field visits	Field visit is defined as a planned activity to take the students out of classroom for an observation of particular place, persons, organization or situation to obtain first-hand experiences.

I. TYPES OF CLINICAL TEACHING METHODS

The brief description of types of clinical teaching methods are presented in box. 7.7.

II. GUIDELINES FOR SELECTION OF CLINICAL TEACHING METHODS

The selected method for the clinical teaching must be in

- Concurrence with the educational objectives and desired behavioural changes of learner.
- Accordance with the principles of teaching and learning.

- Accordance with the capacity and capabilities of the learner.
- Accordance with the availability of resources.
- Accordance with the teacher's ability to use it effectively and creatively.

CASE METHOD/CASE STUDY

Nursing case study is the blueprint of nursing care rendered by a nursing student to a selected patient, for a particular period by following nursing process approach, with an intention to develop comprehensive nursing care abilities.

I. PURPOSES OF CASE STUDY

- It provides an opportunity to the student to learn nursing skills using the problem solving approach.
- Students learn to identify and define a patient's problem.
- It trains the students to locate, gather and process the information required to solve the patient's problem.
- It develops a sense of accomplishment from providing individualized comprehensive care.
- It helps the student solve the patient's problems by critical and reflective thinking.
- It emphasizes the facts that the patient is an individual personality with unique problems.
- It accentuates the health and social aspects of nursing.
- It points out the relationship and cooperation of the various agencies interested in the patient's problems and welfare such as social service and public health nursing.

II. PRINCIPLES OF CASE STUDY

- The students should be able to make their nursing care study on a patient for whose nursing care they are responsible for.
- The selection of patients can be done by coordination between the clinical instructor and students.
- With the help of a case study, the student should be able to study the patient's state of health and self-help abilities, his cultural background, his economic level, hobbies and interests, as an understanding of all these factors will contribute to the patient's welfare.
- The first part of the study should be concerned with information and facts about the patient, his disease condition and his social and personal history, and how this knowledge is applied in providing nursing care to the patient.
- The second part of the nursing study takes in the responsibilities and the activities the nursing student will be concerned with in giving complete comprehensive nursing care to the patient.
- It should emphasize on the individual needs of a patient and how they are met.
- Special emphasis should be made on patient learning.
- If outpatient experience and home nursing is included in the study, it helps in better evaluation of the patient's recovery and his ability to maintain healthy health habits.
- It should serve as an excellent tool to demonstrate nursing skills, scientific knowledge, and sociological or psychological insight into the problems of the patient.
- It should encourage critical evaluation of solutions presented by others. The student is presented with the whole situation so that she may visualize it completely.

III. FORMS AND PRESENTATION OF CASE STUDY

- Written
- Verbal/oral

Advantages of case study
Written case study

- It provides for individual differences of the student.
- It provides an opportunity for self-expression in writing.
- It provides experience in organizing and writing a paper in a scientific manner.
- It provides a source of material for future reference.

Oral case study

- It provides an opportunity for the instructor to direct student thinking into new channels and to correct errors of information.
- It serves as a basis for better personal understanding and relationship between the instructor and the student.
- It is time-saving, and does not require lengthy recopying of the notes to acceptable forms.
- It offers an opportunity for a public-speaking experience.
- If discussion is invited after presentation, the case becomes cooperative and everyone involved benefits from the study. This is a source of motivation to the student because she shares the benefits of her study with other students.
- The student feels the thrill of achievement in presenting her study to others.

Disadvantages of case study
Written case study

- It gives no opportunity to branch out and incorporate new ideas once the study is completed.
- It requires a great deal of time to rewrite to an acceptable form.

Oral case study

- It does not offer an opportunity for writing and other creative expressions, since only notes are used for the presentation.
- It leaves no records that may be kept for future reference as it is used generally.

NURSING CASE PRESENTATION

It is also an important method of clinical teaching for the students in healthcare disciplines in which a patient with unique clinical condition is allotted to a student, who study the patient in detail including detailed health assessment, diagnostic test, medical-surgical management and nursing management and present it in a peer group under the supervision of clinical faculty.

'Nursing case presentation refers to a formal discussion of a particular patient in details regarding medical diagnosis, clinical features, diagnostic tests, medical/surgical treatment, nursing assessment findings, identified nursing problems and best possible planned nursing care interventions considering best recommended practices'.

I. PURPOSES OF CASE PRESENTATION

- It provides opportunity for the students to understand a unique clinical condition in real patient.
- It helps the students to compare the patient's clinical presentation, diagnostic tests carried out, medical-surgical management done with the existing literature and evidence.
- It also facilitates the students to develop the assessment skill, writing and presentation skills.
- The case presentation also helps to orient the group of students with the different rare clinical conditions through peer presentation.

II. PROCESS OF CASE PRESENTATION

- First a patient with a unique clinical condition is chosen by the student.
- Then student collects the detailed information about clinical features, health assessment findings, reports of diagnostics tests and planned treatment. This information is collected as either a first-hand information or observation from patient or referring case sheet already written by the healthcare team members.
- The case details are compared with existing literature/evidence and a written report is prepared or case may be presented orally without a written report of case.
- During case presentation, the peer group may also ask questions from the presenter.
- Finally, the supervising clinical teacher should do debriefing of the case and clarify any doubts of the group.

III. ADVANTAGES OF CASE PRESENTATION

- It provides student an opportunity to understand a particular disease condition in a real situation and solve the nursing problems encountered in particular patient.
- It also provides opportunity for the students to speak in a group and answer the questions raised by the students in the group.
- Students also get an opportunity to integrate the knowledge to different subjects, such as anatomy, physiology, microbiology, pathophysiology, pharmacology, diagnostic test, medical, surgical and nursing interventions for particular case or disease condition.
- Students get an opportunity to relate the existing scientific literature with the real disease condition/patient.

IV. DISADVANTAGES OF CASE PRESENTATION

- Good command over language, expression and presentation are required for case presentation; therefore, in absence of these qualities it is difficult to achieve the better outcome of learning with this method of clinical teaching.
- It is difficult to get the ideal patient at right time to teach through case presentation without bothering the patient much for this purpose.

NURSING ROUNDS

Nursing rounds is an excursion into the patient's area involving the student's learning experiences. Generally, a small group of nursing professionals such as nursing faculty, ward nurse manager, bedside nurses and nursing students assemble on the patient's bedside to discuss the routine nursing care provided to patients so that efficient nursing care be ensured. Meanwhile, nursing students can also be taught about nursing care.

A nursing round is a tour into the patients' ward to provide the student a learning experience. In this clinical teaching method, a group of nurses visit all or selected patients at their bedside in a particular ward with directly or indirectly contributing into clinical teaching.

I. PURPOSES OF NURSING ROUNDS

- To acquaint the staff and students with all the patients admitted in the ward including their disease condition, diagnostic test, ongoing treatment and nursing care provided.
- To demonstrate the specific clinical features of particular disease condition, which are important for planning the nursing care interventions.
- To clarify the terminology studied.
- To compare a patient's reaction to disease and study the disease condition.
- To demonstrate effects of the drugs.
- To plan and illustrate skilful nursing care.
- To promote team spirit and professionalism among nurses.
- It also facilitates in building the skills of handing over and taking over of patients by nurses at change of shift.
- The students develop an ability to categorize patients into high-risk, moderate-risk and low-risk patients, depending on severity of the disease condition of particular patients.

II. ADVANTAGES OF NURSING ROUNDS

- This method provides opportunity to learn about the patient's progress through the highly experienced nursing experts.
- Nursing rounds provide an opportunity for students to learn about the effect of different drugs, treatment modalities and nursing interventions and change in the plan of medical and nursing management based on the progress of patient.
- This method facilitates to learn about more patients in short time through nursing rounds.

III. DISADVANTAGES OF NURSING ROUNDS

- It is not a suitable method of teaching for a bigger group of students.
- The bedside discussion about patient during nursing rounds may be discomforting and uncomfortable for patient and it may be a cause of anxiety.
- It may be wastage of time for nurses who are not directly involved in care of particular patient.

BEDSIDE NURSING CLINICS

The nursing clinic is a group discussion that utilizes the presence of a selected patient, whereby nursing aspects are presented and discussed. Ahmed M. (2002) described bedside teaching as 'a rich visual auditory, tactile and olfactory experience'. Bedside clinic, also called bedside teaching, is a teacher-centred method where a small group of students are taught in the presence of the patient. This method enables learners to acquire skills in observation, recording of health history, communication and physical examination, knowledge of clinical ethics and professionalism. Depending on the patient's convenience, the nursing clinic can be conducted at the patient's bedside or in a clinical teaching/conference room.

I. PURPOSES OF BEDSIDE NURSING CLINICS

- To apply theory into actual practice by observing, interviewing and studying a patient.
- To apply knowledge and experience to real-life situations.
- To highlight the uniqueness of each individual patient, this can give deeper insight into their individualized nursing problems.
- To understand certain types of apparatus used for particular patient care.
- To improve quality nursing care.

II. ADVANTAGES OF BEDSIDE NURSING CLINICS

- Bedside nursing clinics provide an opportunity for the learner or actively participate in real-life situation learning, thereby building close relationship between theory and practice.
- It provides opportunity for the nursing students to learn how to interact with patient, develop rapport, empathy, self-confidence and develop qualities of observation and decision-making.
- Nursing clinics facilitate the students to relive their anxieties, while learning through directly interacting with patient in the presence of the clinical nursing teacher.

III. DISADVANTAGES OF BEDSIDE NURSING CLINICS

- It is not a suitable clinical teaching method for the large group of students.
- It may not be convenient and confortable for a patient, when he/she is used an object of bedside teaching.
- Sometimes bedside nursing clinics may disrupt the routine care of patient or vice versa.
- Bedside teaching–learning environment may not be always conducive for student, teacher, patient and neighbouring patient and healthcare workers of a particular ward.

NURSING ASSIGNMENT

It is that part of learning experience where students are assigned with patients or other activities concerning patients in the clinical ward/laboratory. It is through the assignment that the teacher is able to arouse interest, stimulate right mental promotional attitudes and sets forth good study habits. The students carryout nursing care for the assigned patient under the supervision of clinical teacher, where they utilize nursing care plan for planning and implementation of nursing care. A nursing care plan is a road map or blueprint of nursing activities and patient care for a patient, family and community, which includes five systematic and logical phases i.e. nursing assessment, diagnosis, expected outcome, intervention and evaluation. In this, student gets an opportunity to master the nursing assessment skills, identification of nursing problems, planning and implementation of nursing interventions and evaluation.

I. CRITERIA FOR EFFECTIVE ASSIGNMENT

- Students are informed about the objectives of their assignment to a particular ward or unit of the hospital.
- Students are to be oriented to the new clinical area.
- Students are given facilities to practice nursing according to principles taught.
- Assignments have to be assigned according to the consistent level of learning the students have reached or attained ranging from the particular nursing procedure to the complete care of an assigned patient.
- Proper guidance and supervision has to be provided to students during their clinical experience.
- Students should be given opportunities for working in a team.
- Student performance should be evaluated and discussed with the students for their improvement, correction, etc.

II. ADVANTAGES OF NURSING ASSIGNMENT

- Students get an opportunity to practice the learned theory of nursing procedures in real patient scenario.
- Students are able to achieve much realistic confidence and competence in performance of nursing skills and care.

III. DISADVANTAGES OF NURSING ASSIGNMENT

- It is not a suitable method for beginners because direct exposure of real patient may cause undue anxiety and stress among students.
- The constant supervision by the nursing teachers is required in this method of clinical teaching, otherwise students may not feel comfortable or it may not be safe for the patient.

NURSING CARE CONFERENCE

Nursing care conference is a method of teaching that provides an opportunity for an informal discussion of a problem and free exchange of knowledge and experiences about the common interest. It consists of a group discussion using problem-solving techniques of the nursing process. It is a method of teaching where a teacher meets a small group of students for the purpose of accomplishing clinical learning objectives.

Advantages of a nursing care conference

- It helps the students collect information in a creative way.
- It provides a real practical learning environment to students.
- It provides free opportunity to think.

Disadvantages of a nursing care conference

- It will be of little use if the students are not accustomed to such situations.
- There are chances of using these conference hours for classroom teaching.

INDIVIDUAL CONFERENCE

Individual conference is sometimes described as a conversation with a purpose or more simply as an interview. The teacher may introduce the students to new fields of knowledge, imparting information to them regarding this field and strive to motivate them in the acquisition. Individual conference may be organized for apprising the several purposes, such as giving directions, obtaining progress report, suggesting the solutions for the specific problems or discussing a specific patient, which are specifically important for the particular student.

Individual conference may be defined as a teaching tool, which primarily gives an opportunity to discuss a student's professional problems privately.

I. PURPOSES OF INDIVIDUAL CONFERENCE

- To clarify the personal and professional doubts of the student and provide him/her educational guidance.
- To answer queries and clarify doubts of students individually.
- To discover the interests, needs and problems of students individually.
- To help the students help themselves and achieve self-development.
- To also help in supplementing the clinical instructions provided.

II. ADVANTAGES OF INDIVIDUAL CONFERENCE

- Individual conference offers the teacher opportunity to know the student as a unique individual and understand his/her strength and weakness.
- The student gets an opportunity to know about his/her progress and achievements and gains encouragement to do better in future.
- It provides a useful avenue and opportunity for individual teaching and guidance.
- The student feels more secure in the learning environment when his/her problem and difficulties are discussed confidentially and guidance is provided.
- It provides excellent opportunity for individual learning.

III. DISADVANTAGES OF INDIVIDUAL CONFERENCE

- If a teacher has any prejudice or bias towards a student, the individual conference may provide an opportunity for its demonstration.
- The students may not convey his/her entire problems to the teacher.
- Facing teacher alone without the support of other group members may create anxiety in the student.

GROUP CONFERENCE

Group conference may be defined as meeting of a group of professionals in the presence of expert teacher or a senior person in a group to discuss a topic of common interest. The group nursing conference can be easily observed in the clinical settings as a method of teaching or solve a particular clinical problem. The main purpose of group nursing conference is to communicate the common message face to face in short time, where group also gets an opportunity to seek the clarifications.

I. PURPOSES OF GROUP CONFERENCE

- To communicate a message of common interest to large groups in short-time period.
- A unique clinical problem or nursing issues may be discussed by an expert to a common group.
- To obtain the inputs from the each member of group so that the best accepted and recognized solution can be drawn for a particular problem of clinical interest.
- To help students in developing problem-solving and critical thinking skills.

II. PRINCIPLES OF GROUP CONFERENCE

- The essential principles of the group conference are that there must be common objective or common topic of interest in the conference.
- There must be an expert team leader to conduct the conference and clarify the doubts of the group.
- In addition, teacher leader must motivate each member to participate in the discussion so that fruitful results of the group conference may be achieved.
- The topic, place, time of conference must be decided and communicated to all the group members well in advance so that they may come prepared to discuss on the topic.
- The topic of conference must have unique and latest clinical topic of common interest to achieve the objectives of clinical learning.

III. ADVANTAGES OF GROUP CONFERENCE

- Group conference facilitates to teach a clinical topic to a group of students, which helps in creating open-mindedness and cooperation in group.
- It also provides an opportunity to each student to actively participate in group activity, which enables to create a conducive social-learning environment in clinical setting.
- It helps students in developing problem-solving and team-building skills as well as the ability to express their ideas assertively.

IV. DISADVANTAGES OF GROUP CONFERENCE

- It is not suitable for the beginning level of students because they hardly can contribute in the discussion of unique new clinical cases.
- Students may not always come prepared to group conference to share their own ideas, and purpose of group conference is defeated.
- The suggestions that come forth from the discussion may not be realistic, applicable and acceptable.
- It requires lots of efforts and time in planning and implementation of group conference activity.

HEALTH TEAM CONFERENCE

Health team conference is a group of health professionals involved in accomplishing common goals for the purpose of interchanging ideas and solving problems which are centred around the patient. It provides a useful tool for building and maintaining mutual understanding through which it is possible to attain and maintain optimum emotional, physical and social health of a patient.

Health team conference may be defined as group-integrated clinical teaching method, where multidisciplinary health professionals meet to discuss a topic to enhance the mutual understanding of all the dimensions of care and management of a patient. In which, students from different disciplines get an opportunity to understand the role of own discipline and other disciplines in care and management of a patient.

I. PRINCIPLES OF HEALTH TEAM CONFERENCES

- There must be an objective or a purpose that is to be accomplished.
- Prior announcement of time, place, purpose and duration of conferences to all concerned promotes the assembly of a group that is well prepared and ready to focus attention on the purposes of the conference.
- Obtaining the most recent data available prior to a conference assures the leader that the imparted information is pertinent and accurate.
- Interaction of conference's members on an equal basis encourages active participation and leads to usable solutions to the objective.
- Sharing feelings through conferences unifies and integrates membership and allows progress.

II. ADVANTAGES OF HEALTH TEAM CONFERENCE

- It is the most modern method of clinical teaching, where in a short time students from different disciplines may be obtaining the clinical learning from experts of multidisciplinary team.
- The compartmentalized clinical learning may be avoided.
- Students get an opportunity to learn the latest advancements in the other related disciplines from the experts of particular.
- It is the most useful method in nursing, where students may be largely benefited from the involvement and inputs of experts from the medical disciplines.

III. DISADVANTAGES OF HEALTH TEAM CONFERENCE

- Sometimes, the students may not be interested in learning the clinical informations of other related disciplines.
- It may be wastage of time and resources while covering the topic vertically and horizontally integrated with multidisciplinary approach.

PROCESS RECORDING

Process recording refers to as a systemically written formal report of a therapeutic conversation, occurred between patient and healthcare provider. According to Walker, 'the process recording is a verbatim account of a visit for purpose of bringing out the interplay between nurse and the patient in relation to the common objectives'. In other words, process recording may be defined as 'a written account or verbalism recording of a conversation that occurred between a patient and the professional nurse, when they are working together towards a common therapeutic objective, which is recorded during and immediately following the nurse–patient interaction'.

I. FEATURES OF PROCESS RECORDING

- It is written during and immediately after the therapeutic nurse–patient interaction.
- Process recording also can be used as an excellent clinical teaching method.
- It also has therapeutic purposes, where recorded conversation is used to understand the patient's behaviour and problem in depth.

II. USES OF PROCESS RECORDING

- As a teaching–learning tool.
- As an evaluation tool.
- As a therapeutic tool.

III. PURPOSES OF PROCESS RECORDING

- Assists the nurse gain competency in interpreting and synthesising raw data under supervision.
- Helps to consciously apply theory to practice.
- Helps the students develop an increased awareness of their habitual, verbal and nonverbal communication pattern.
- Helps the nurse to learn to identify thoughts and feelings in relation to self and others.
- Helps to increase observation skills as there is a conscious process involved in thinking, sorting and classifying the interaction under the various headings.

IV. ADVANTAGES OF PROCESS RECORDING

- It is the most suitable method of teaching to develop competency in interpreting and synthesizing the abstract concepts.
- It also provides opportunities for students to develop the good communication skills through practice of process recording.
- Process recording also helps to develop the keen observation skills and critical thinking.

V. DISADVANTAGES OF PROCESS RECORDING

- The process recording as a method of teaching is very time-consuming.
- It is not a suitable method of clinical teaching for an average IQ student because it is a highly complex process.
- The students with poor communication skills cannot be benefited with this method of clinical teaching.
- Sometimes patients do not offer the cooperation with this complex process of clinical teaching.

FIELD VISIT

Naturalistic philosophy of education believes that direct experience in natural environment with the learning material, object, situation or a phenomenon is one of the best ways of learning. The filed visit is one of the methods of teaching, which is strongly recommended in the naturalistic philosophy of education. The research evidence has also proved the field visit as one of the best methods of teaching and learning, where students directly encounter with the particulate learning experience in real environment under the supervision of an expert, who may answer his/her questions or clarify the doubts.

The field visit or field trip may be referred to as an educational procedure by which the students undertake a first-hand experience and exploration of material, object, situation or phenomenon in their natural environment.

A field visit entails a visit to a place outside the regular classroom and is designed to meet certain objectives that cannot be achieved by other methods of teaching. It provides a learner an opportunity to come out of formal classroom and obtain direct new experience in natural environment. The principal features of a field visit are (i) to facilitate learning of an abstract concept, (ii) to enhance students' interest and curiosity and (iii) to increase social interaction of students and develop social awareness among them.

I. PURPOSES OF FIELD VISIT

- To make learning more meaningful and memorable.
- To provide an opportunity to learn from actual hands-on experiences rather than by simply reading or hearing about something.
- To supplement the regular classroom instructions and establish a connection between reality and literature.
- To give students experiential learning environment.
- Field visit is also useful in developing the concrete skills, such as note taking and public speaking.
- To help the students to appreciate the relevance and importance of what they have learnt in the classroom.
- To provide authentic learning experience by involving five senses in the learning experiences i.e. vision, touch, feel, smell and test.

II. ADVANTAGES OF FIELD VISIT

- Field visit is a first-hand source of knowledge and information and supplements and enriches the classroom instructions.
- It integrates the classroom learning with real-life situations, which in turn help the students to develop a sympathetic understanding of problems as well as enable them to recognize the contribution of other organizations in patient care.
- Students develop a better understanding of the natural history of the disease and aetiological factors like housing, sanitation and socioeconomic conditions.
- It helps students to develop keen observation skills to study problems/situations.
- Field trip provides realistic resource material for study; thus arouse the interest and motivation among learners.

III. DISADVANTAGES OF FIELD VISIT

- Most field visits are more time-consuming, which necessitates adjustment of other classes' time schedule.
- The field visit has to be planned as per the convenience of the organizations, which are to be visited.

- Students may not have the necessary data or sufficient background information and understanding to obtain the maximum learning benefit from field visits.
- Transportation may prove to be an inconvenience, if it is not readily available with particular department or organization.
- Field visits are more effective for smaller groups; however, large group is very difficult to supervise and control during field visit.
- It is difficult to create the ideal teaching–learning environment in field setting, which affects the outcome of learning.

REVIEW QUESTIONS

Long-Answer Questions

1. Explain simulation as teaching methods.
2. Disucss the advantages of nursing care studies.
3. Explain the demonstration method.
4. Explain the advantages and disadvantages of micro-teaching.
5. Explain the various methods of clinical teaching.
6. Discuss field trips.
7. Explain panel discussions.
8. Discuss the lecturer method.
9. Discuss the project method.
10. Discuss a symposium.
11. Discuss role-plays.
12. Write in detail about nursing rounds as teaching method.
13. Describe principles of using clinical teaching methods.

Short-Answer Questions

1. List down the four clinical teaching methods.
2. Discuss briefly the four purposes of laboratory methods.
3. Mention the four limitations in field trip.
4. Discuss in brief any four advantages of lecturer method.
5. Enumerate the advantages of problem-based learning.
6. Mention two differences between seminar and symposium.
7. Mention four clinical teaching methods.

Short Notes

Write short notes on the following:

1. Bedside clinics.
2. Workshop as a method of teaching.

Multiple-Choice Questions (MCQs)

1. An important aim of lecture method of teaching should be to
   (a) Make students memorize
   (b) Tell and explain
   (c) Use audio visual aids
   (d) Stimulate thinking

2. Demonstration method strives to achieve the following type of objectives
   (a) Cognitive
   (b) Affective
   (c) Psychomotor
   (d) Observation

3. A nurse educator is interested to teach neonatal assessment to nursing students. The best suitable method would be
   (a) Lecture
   (b) Demonstration
   (c) Project
   (d) Bedside clinic

4. The essential principle behind effective group discussion is
   (a) Formulation of educational objectives
   (b) Timely preparation and execution
   (c) Well-defined responsibility of each group member
   (d) Record of proceedings of discussion

5. Group discussion techniques are best suitable for achievement of
   (a) Complex learning outcomes
   (b) Defined discussion
   (c) Conflicting view points
   (d) Independent learning

6. The topic for panel discussion should be
   (a) Current
   (b) Debatable
   (c) Interesting
   (d) All of these

7. Chances of overlapping of content material are minimal in
   (a) Panel discussion
   (b) Seminar
   (c) Symposium
   (d) Group discussion

8. The teaching technique that has the ability to connect with the audience at an emotional level is
   (a) Role-play
   (b) Demonstration
   (c) Seminar
   (d) Panel discussion

9. The skills of problem solving, analysis and synthesis are best developed by
   (a) Lecture method
   (b) Demonstration method

(c) Project method
(d) Role-play method

10. Field trip can be made different from a usual picnic by
    (a) Proper planning and arrangement
    (b) Assigning defined responsibilities to group members
    (c) Seeking prior permission
    (d) Defined educational objectives

11. In which of the following techniques, participants are actively engaged in problem solving?
    (a) Panel discussion
    (b) Workshop
    (c) Exhibition
    (d) Seminar

12. In which of the following method subject matter is broken down into small frames and arranged sequentially?
    (a) Programmed instruction
    (b) Role-play
    (c) Field trip
    (d) Simulation

13. All are types of programme instruction except
    (a) Linear programming
    (b) Branching programming
    (c) Selective programming
    (d) Computer-assisted programming

14. The main aim of micro-teaching is
    (a) Effective teaching
    (b) Developing specific teaching skills
    (c) Seeking feedback
    (d) Teach a small topic

15. The correct sequence of steps of micro-teaching is
    (a) Teach → feedback → replan → reteach → refeedback
    (b) Teach → plan → replan → reteach → refeedback
    (c) Teach → feedback → reteach → replan → refeedback
    (d) Teach → feedback → replan → reteach → replan

Answers of the Multiple-Choice Questions

1. (d), 2. (c), 3. (b), 4. (c), 5. (a), 6. (d), 7. (b), 8. (a), 9. (c), 10. (d), 11. (b), 12. (a), 13. (c), 14. (b), 15. (a)

FURTHER READING

Agnew, P. W., Kellerman, A. S., & Meyer, J. (1996). *Multimedia in the classroom*. Boston, MA: Allyn and Bacon.

Ahmed, M. (2002). What is happening to bedside clinical teaching? *Medical Education, 36*, 1185-1188.

Alberto, P., & Troutman, A. (2003). *Applied behavior analysis for teachers* (6th ed.). Columbus, OH: Prentice-Hall-Merrill.

Alley, C. (1972). *Classroom*. Boston, MA: Allyn and Bacon.

Boud, D., & Feletti, G. (1999). *The challenge of problem-based learning* (2nd ed.). London, UK: Kogan Page.

Boud, D. (1985) *Reflection: Turning Experience into Learning*. London: Kogan Page.

BPP. (2000). *Success in your research and analysis project*. London, UK: BPP.

Cano, F. (2005). Epistemological beliefs and approaches to learning: Their change through secondary school and their influence on academic performance. *British Journal of Educational Psychology*, 75, 203–21.

Clark, D. (2010). *Bloom's taxonomy of learning domains*. Retrieved from http://www.nwlink.com/~donclark/hrd/bloom.html. Retrieved 1 March 2012.

Dewey, J. (1910). *How we think*. New York: D.C. Heath & Co.

Dewey J. (1916). *Democracy & Education*. New York: The MacMillian company.

Everett, D. M. (1926). *The Meaning of a liberal education*. New York: W. W. Norton & Co.

Farrell, J. P., & Oliveira, T. (1993). *Teachers in developing countries: Improving effectiveness and managing costs*. Washington, DC: World Bank.

Gibbons, P. (n.d.). *Scaffolding language, scaffolding learning: Teaching Second Language learning in the Mainstream Classroom*. Portsmouth, USA: Heinemann

Halpern, D. F. (1998). Teaching critical thinking for transfer across domains. *American Psychologist*, 53, 449–55.

Hofstetter, F. T. (1995). *Multimedia literacy*. New York: McGraw-Hill.

James, W. (1983). *Talks to teachers on psychology and to students on some of life's ideals*. Cambridge, MA: Harvard University Press. (Original work published 1899).

Jonassen, D. H., Peck, K. L., & Wilson, B. G. (1999). *Learning with technology: A constructivist perspective*. Upper Saddle River, NJ: Merrill/Prentice Hall.

Knowles, M. (1975). *Self-Directed Learning*. Chicago, IL: Follet.

Lieberman, A. (2004). *Teacher leadership*. San Francisco, CA: Jossey-Bass.

Lindstrom, R. (1994). *The business week guide to multimedia presentations: Create dynamic presentations that inspire*. New York: McGraw-Hill.

Lucas, J. L., Blazek, M. A., & Riley, A. B. (2005). The lack of representation of educational psychology and school psychology in introductory psychology textbooks. *Educational Psychology*, 25, 347–351.

Markel Susan M. (1969). *Good Frames and Bad: a Programmar of Frame Writing*. New York: Wiley.

Monroe, P. (1915). *A text-Book in the history of education*. New York: Macmillan.

Nordlund, C. Y. (2006). *Art experiences in Waldorf education* (PhD Dissertation). University of Missouri-Columbia.

Schweer, J. E. (1972). *Creating Teaching in Clinical Nursing*. St. Louis: Mosby.

Tapscott, D. (1998). *Growing up digital: The rise of the net generation*. New York: McGraw-Hill.

Taylor, J. (2002). *A different kind of teacher: Solving the crisis of American schooling*. Berkeley, CA: Berkeley Hills Books.

Teo, R., & Wong, A. (2000, December 4-7). Does problem based learning create a better student: A reflection? In *Proceedings at the 2nd Asia Pacific Conference on Problem-Based Learning: Education Across Disciplines*. Singapore.

Thorndike, E. L. (1912). *Education: A first book*. New York: MacMillan.

Vaughan, T. (1998). *Multimedia: Making it work* (4th ed.). Berkeley, CA: Osborne/McGraw-Hill.

Vives, J., & Watson, F. (1913). *On education: A translation of the de tradendis disciplinis of Juan Luis Vives*. Cambridge, MA: Cambridge University Press.

Woolfolk, A. E., Winne, P. H., & Perry, N. E. (2006). *Educational psychology* (3rd Canadian ed.). Toronto, Canada: Pearson.

Educational media

People everywhere like to learn through pictures and graphics instead of text because when content of text travels through audiovisual media it becomes incredibly interesting, which promotes the purpose of learning.
—**Reena Sharma**

LEARNING OBJECTIVES

This chapter is designed to enable the reader to

- Define audiovisual aids
- Understand the concept, importance, purposes, characteristics, sources and principles of audiovisual aids
- Classify the types of audiovisual aids
- Describe the concept, characteristics, purposes, types and guidelines for preparation and uses, advantages and disadvantages of different graphic audiovisual aids, such as chalkboard, charts, graphs, poster, flashcards, flannel board, bulletin board and cartoons
- Discuss the concept, characteristics, purposes, types and guidelines for preparation and uses, advantages and disadvantages of different three-dimensional audiovisual aids, such as objects/specimens, models, puppets, exhibitions, museum and dioramas
- Explain the concept, characteristics, purposes, types and guidelines for preparation and uses, advantages and disadvantages of different printed audiovisual aids, such as pamphlets and leaflets
- Appraise the concept, characteristics, purposes, types and guidelines for preparation and uses, advantages and disadvantages of different projected audiovisual aids, such as slide projector, overhead projector, opaque projector, filmstrips, television, video cassette recorder player, camera, microscope and LCD projector
- Explore the concept, characteristics, purposes, types and guidelines for preparation and uses, advantages and disadvantages of different audio/audiovisual aids, such as tape recorder, public address system and computer
- Recognize the guidelines for effective use of audiovisual aids

KEY TERMS

INTRODUCTION

The educational media are the objects that help in teaching and learning activities and enhance the delivery of knowledge to the learners. In other words, educational media are learning devices that help the teacher clarify, establish, correlate and coordinate accurate concepts and interpretation to make learning more concrete, effective, interesting, meaningful and vivid. Audiovisual aids, audiovisual materials, audiovisual media, communication technology, educational or instructional media or learning resources are interchangeably used terms. Broadly speaking, however, all of them have the same meaning.

AUDIOVISUAL AIDS

Scientifically, it is believed that during the communicative process, the sensory register of the memory acts as a filter. The working short-term memory functions are limited by both time and capacity. Therefore, it is essential that the information be arranged in useful bits or chunks for effective coding, rehearsal or recording, and audiovisual aids best suit this function. Therefore, audiovisual aids in the classroom can enhance teaching methods and improve student comprehension. Today's technology offers many choices to the educator who wishes to capitalize on the new generation's appetite for multimedia presentations. An efficient lesson plan that incorporates the use of audiovisual aids consistent with curriculum objectives may do miracles in the achievement of purposes of the teaching–learning process.

I. DEFINITIONS OF AUDIOVISUAL AIDS

Audio-visual aids are those sensory objects or images which initiates or stimulate and reinforce learning.

—**Burton**

Audio-visual aids are those devices by the use of which communication of ideas between persons and group in various teaching and training situation is helped. These are also termed as multi sensory materials.

—**Edgar Dale**

Audio-visual aids are anything by means of which learning process may be encouraged or carried on through the sense of hearing or sense of sight.

—Good's Dictionary of education

Audio-visual aids are devices which can be used to make the learning experience more concrete, more realistic and more dynamic.

—Kinder S. James

Audio-visual aids are supplementary devices by which the teacher through the utilization of more than one sensory channel is able to clarify, establish and correlate concepts, interpretations and appreciations.

—Mckown and Roberts

Audio-visual aids are those aids which help in completing the triangular process of learning i.e. motivation, classification and stimulation.

—Carter V. Good

An audio-visual aid is an instructional device in which the message can be heard as well as seen.

II. CONCEPT OF AUDIOVISUAL AIDS

Audiovisual aids are planned teaching aids that appeal to the senses of people and enhance clear understanding and improve quick learning among learners. A Chinese proverb proves the importance of audiovisual aids in the teaching–learning process:

'*I hear, I forget*'
'*I see, I remember*'
'*I do, I understand*'

It is generally believed that the best learning can be achieved through doing things but good learning can also be achieved through the use of appropriate audiovisual aids. Furthermore, audiovisual aids help in the completion of the triangular process of learning, enhance motivation, stimulation and improve the clarity of understanding in learners as depicted in Fig. 8.1. It can be inferred that the presentation of content with verbal and audiovisual aids motivates and stimulates the learner, reinforces the learning and enhances the clarity of the content.

Research has shown that oral presentations that use visuals are more persuasive, more interesting, more credible, more professional and more effective than presentations without such aids particularly when the presentation is long (about 20 minutes or more); the audiovisual aids can help the audience follow ideas easily and with fewer lapses in attention. In addition, Edwards and Mercer found in their research study that visual perception contributes about 90% to all human learning. Moreover, audiovisual aids:

- Help to maintain a high level of interest in the lesson and to create interest in the group.
- Help to get students to use the language, especially at the beginning stages.

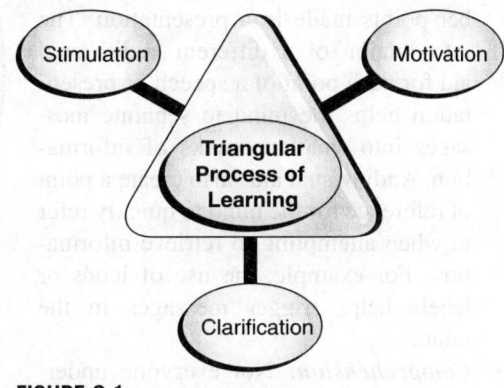

FIGURE 8.1

Triangular process of learning.

- Help to promote greater student participation.
- Can be used at all levels of learning.
- Supplement and enrich the teachers' own teaching to make the teaching–learning process more concrete.
- Serve an instructional role in itself.
- Make teaching an effective interactive process.

III. IMPORTANCE OF AUDIOVISUAL AIDS

Effective communication can be quite challenging, especially when making a presentation or giving a speech. For communication to be effective, one must keep the attention of the listeners and deliver information in such a way that it is fully understood. Audiovisual aids are one of the most effective ways to get the message across and make it memorable. Joey Papa suggested the following benefits of audiovisual aids (Fig. 8.2):

- *Memory retention:* The Office of Training and Education of the United States Occupational Safety and Health Administration has reported that psychologists and educators have found the use of audiovisual tools led to retention of information for three days after a meeting or other event. This is six times more than when information is presented by spoken word alone. Visual aids allow the speaker to use verbal and nonverbal communication to solidify the message and provide a point of reference for the mind.
- *Improved attention span:* Everyone has a limited attention span. Once this capacity is spent, the mind decreases its ability to retain information and listen effectively. Using audiovisual aids refreshes the mind and engages it in a different way, renewing the attention span. Visual aids keep the mind entertained and therefore sharp and ready to receive information.
- *Organizing communication:* Audiovisual aids can be used to organize communication making it easier to remember points made in a presentation. The introduction of a different audiovisual aid for each point of a speech or presentation helps the mind to separate messages into smaller chunks of information. Audiovisual aids also create a point of reference for the mind to quickly refer to when attempting to retrieve information. For example, the use of icons or labels helps trigger messages in the mind.
- *Comprehension:* Not everyone understands concepts and information at the same rate. Some people can understand

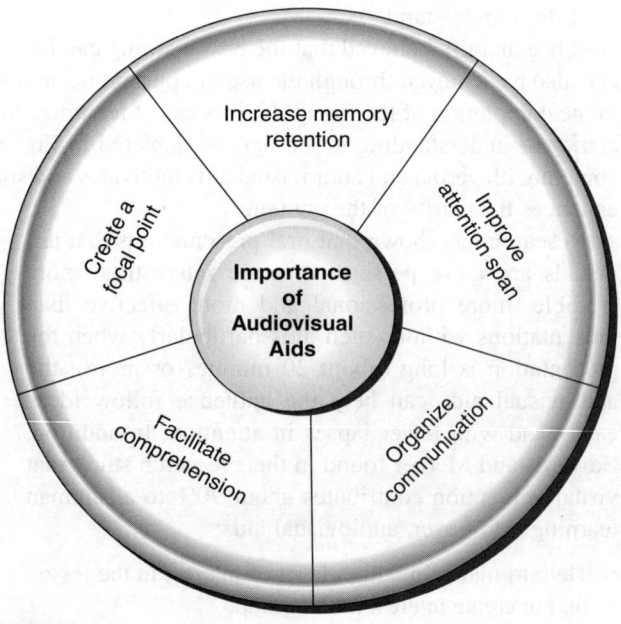

FIGURE 8.2
Importance of audiovisual aids.

messages quickly while others need help to grasp what is being said. Audiovisual aids are a way of further explanation. If some people are more visual than audio learners, the visual aids may be necessary for comprehension. Audiovisual aids create repetition and the more repetition in communication, the greater the chances are that your audience will understand and remember effectively.

- *Create a focal point:* Audiovisual aids help a speaker stay on track. If there is one central visual aid that the speaker can use, then the speaker's thoughts and the audience's attention will stay on course. There is nothing worse than listening to a speaker ramble and lose the audience. Audiovisual aids assist in avoiding such a scenario.

IV. PURPOSES OF AUDIOVISUAL AIDS

Audiovisual aids enhance clarity in communication, provide diversity in the methods of teaching and increase the forcefulness of the subjects being learned or taught. Furthermore, students get direct experience of real-life situations or direct sensory experiences or symbolic experiences through the use of audiovisual aids. Moreover, some essential purposes of the audiovisual aids are as follows:

- They help in effective perceptual and conceptual learning.
- They are helpful in capturing and sustaining the attention of students.
- They are helpful in new learning. New things are interpreted in terms of past experiences.
- Imagery helps preserve and clarify past experiences and provides near realistic experience.
- They increase and sustain attention, concentration and the personal involvement of students in actual learning.
- They create interest, secure attention and motivate students to learn.
- It is easier to understand any given concept through the use of sensory aids.
- They help in saving energy and time of both the teachers and students.
- They give the student an opportunity to touch, feel and see a model, map, picture or specimen and provide a sensory stimulus to enhance learning.
- They provide for purposeful self-activity and student participation.
- They help provide concreteness, realism and lifelikeness in the teaching–learning process.
- Pictures are helpful in studying concrete reality to gain actual meaning.
- They help explicate and increase the meaningfulness of abstract concepts.
- Concrete experience helps combat the tendency to abstractness.
- Visual materials give definite meaning to words.
- They bring remote events of either space or time into the classroom.
- They serve as an open window through which the student can view the world or its entire phenomenon.
- They introduce an opportunity for situational or field type of learning as contrasted with the linear order verbal and written communication.
- It provides direct experience to the student in the clinical setting and observation experience through field trips or such other media.
- They provide, facilitate and advance the process of applying what is learned to realistic performance and life situations.
- They can meet individual demands.
- They are useful for the education of masses.

V. CHARACTERISTICS OF A GOOD AUDIOVISUAL AID

An audiovisual aid must posses the following basic characteristics to be an effective aid for the teaching–learning process:

- *Meaningful and purposeful:* An audiovisual aid can be only considered good if it is meaningful and purposeful for the particular teaching–learning process. Very attractive and expensive teaching aids may not have any value until and unless they are meaningful and purposeful for the teacher–taught activity. For example, a tiny tot can be taught the preliminary things with real-life specimens easily rather than with expensive computerized teaching tools.
- *Motivate the learners:* A good audiovisual aid must sufficiently motivate the learner so that he can achieve learning swiftly, quickly and promptly. Until and unless an audiovisual aid motivates the learner; it cannot be considered effective in spite of all its other appealing characteristics.
- *Accurate in every aspect:* Each audiovisual aid has its peculiar characteristics and must follow some set of rules and principles in preparation and use during the teaching–learning process. Thus, audiovisual aids can only be considered good if they encompass all the essential characteristics and are accurate in all the aspects.
- *Simple and cheap:* Along with all the essential characteristics, one of the most essential characteristics of audiovisual aids is their simplicity and cost-effectiveness. The simplicity of an audiovisual aid promotes broader popularity and more adaptability among teachers and learners. In addition, cost-effectiveness of audiovisual aids enhances its acceptability and practicability.
- *Appropriate size:* Audiovisual aids used in the teaching–learning process must not be too large or too small. Very large tools create problems of handling and transpiration, while very small tools may not enhance learning because of a poor sense triggering ability due to their small size.
- *Up to date:* Science and technology is an ever-progressing field where things are developing and progressing everyday and old products are becoming outdated. The field of educational media and technology has also revolutionized to a great extent in the last few years. Therefore, educationists must ensure that audiovisual aids are continuously updated so that a pace can be maintained with other fields. An audiovisual aid can only be considered good if it is up to date with reference to technology and new principles of practice.
- *Easily portable:* A good audiovisual tool must have a characteristic of easy portability so that it can be easily handled and transported where required. Easy portability increases the access of audiovisual aids as well as prevents damage and discomfort during handling and transportation.
- *Customized to the type of educational materials:* Every tool does not fit all the educational material to be delivered. Therefore, educationists must predetermine which tool will be appropriate for a particular type of teaching content. Appropriately customized and adapted tools promote the teaching–learning process.
- *Suitable to the mental level of learners:* While deciding on a tool to be used for teaching a particular group of students, their intellectual ability must be considered so that the objective of the teaching–learning process can be achieved.
- *Variety:* A teaching aid may be considered good, if it is providing a variety of experiences to the learner so that actual learning can be achieved more swiftly and promptly.

VI. SOURCES OF AUDIOVISUAL AIDS

The development and distribution of audiovisual aids is done by a variety of organizations such as government, premier educational institutions, professional organizations, nongovernment organizations

(NGOs), national and international voluntary organizations and commercial industry. Government, premier educational institutions, professional organizations, NGOs, national and international voluntary organizations are generally involved in the preparation and distribution of the audiovisual aids used for mass communication and education. However, for the educational institutions audiovisual aids are generally supplied by the government, premier educational institutions and commercial companies producing the audiovisual aids. A brief discussion of each of these sources is given below (Fig. 8.3).

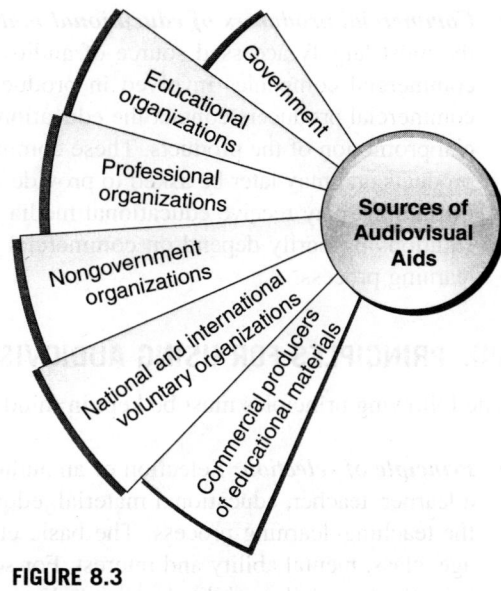

FIGURE 8.3

Sources of audiovisual aids.

- *Government:* The central or state government has two main departments: department of communication, broadcasting and mass media and the department of education, regularly involved in the development and distribution of audiovisual aids for different purposes. The department of communication, broadcasting and mass media is generally planning, preparing and disseminating the audiovisual aids required for mass communication rather than educational institutional media. On the other hand, the department of education has its focus on planning, preparing, developing and disseminating the educational material and media to educational institutions. The experts in these departments make use of latest research and technology developments for designing and disseminating educational aids to the different departments and educational institutions.
- *Educational organizations:* Some premier educational institutions have experts involved in regular research and development for generating new empirical evidences for the effectiveness of different teaching tools. These institutions are given the responsibility to use the latest innovations in the development of teaching aids and distribute them to the educational institutions as required.
- *Professional organizations:* Some professional organizations involved in using the latest technology towards the development of the most technocratic audiovisual aids may be a source of supply of audiovisual aids. These institutions are involved in the research and development of the most suitable audiovisual aids using technology that meets the latest requirements of educational institutions.
- *NGOs:* Some NGOs are also acting as a good source of developing and supplying the educational media. However, these NGOs are usually involved in developing and distributing the educational media to organizations engaged in providing mass education but they may also be a source of educational media for educational institutions.
- *National and international voluntary organizations:* Some national and international voluntary organizations provide funds to the educational institutions for direct purchase of the audiovisual aids or voluntary organizations themselves may supply the audiovisual aids to these educational institutions to promote the teaching–learning process. Therefore, educational institutions in need of audiovisual aids may contact these national and international voluntary organizations such as World Health Organization and World Bank.

- *Commercial producers of educational materials:* Commercial producers of educational media are the most largely accessed source of audiovisual aids. There are a lot of national and international commercial companies involved in producing and supplying educational media. Generally, these commercial producers contact the educational institutions themselves or may advertise for commercial promotion of the products. These commercial companies may be contacted to demonstrate their products and may later be asked to provide quotations for buying products. Government educational institutions may receive educational media from different sources; however, private educational institutions primarily depend on commercial suppliers for buying audiovisual aids for the teaching–learning process.

VII. PRINCIPLES FOR USING AUDIOVISUAL AIDS

The following principles must be kept in mind for the effective use of audiovisual aids.

- *Principle of selection:* Selection of an audiovisual aid must be based on the basic characteristics of a learner, teacher, educational material, educational institution and the philosophy and objectives of the teaching–learning process. The basic characteristics of a learner that should be considered are age, class, mental ability and interest. For selecting a teaching tool, it must be ensured that teachers have the knowledge, ability and attitude to use a specific audiovisual aid. Furthermore, educational media must be selected according to the type of educational content delivered, resources and readiness of the educational institution. Moreover, educational media must be the best substitute for the real-life experience.
- *Principle of preparation:* To promote the efficient use of audiovisual aids, sound preparation is required in special reference to infrastructure, training of teachers and money for the preparation and maintenance of audiovisual aids. Primarily, self-made, cost-effective, locally available and teacher–taught friendly audiovisual aids must be used.
- *Principle of physical control:* For the efficient use and durability of audiovisual aids, it is necessary to have an appropriate control of the physical environment, e.g. a proper place for storage, appropriate environmental temperature, proper cleanliness. An appropriate physical control for audiovisual aids in the classroom and institution promotes the working, durability and hindrance-free use of the audiovisual aids.
- *Principle of proper presentation:* The presentation of the teaching aid is the operation stage. The teachers must carefully ensure that the audiovisual aid is in good working condition. They should acquaint themselves with all the operating systems so that aids can be handled without any undue discomfort. Furthermore, teaching aids must be presented in a manner that every student can visualize them with the greatest comfort and it should catch the attention of students and ultimately enhance learning in the learners.
- *Principle of response:* Teachers must ensure that students respond to the stimulus provided by the audiovisual aids so that they can judge the effectiveness of the audiovisual aid in promoting learning in students. In absence of students' response, teachers will not be able to evaluate the effectiveness of the teaching aids in the achievement of educational objectives.
- *Principle of evaluation:* Evaluation is one of the most essential principles because it conveys the efficacy of a particular teaching aid. The teachers can modify their plans of audiovisual aids used in light of the results of evaluation of a particular audiovisual aid. Evaluation of audiovisual aids should be made a regular and continuous process so that timely action can be taken and educational objectives can be achieved without any undue inconvenience and delay.

- *Other miscellaneous principles:* Some additional miscellaneous principles for the use of audiovisual aids are as follows:
  - Audiovisual materials should be utilized as an integral part of the educational programme.
  - Educational aids should be central to the teaching–learning process, under special direction and leadership in educational objectives.
  - An advisory committee must be consulted in the selection and utilization of audiovisual materials for different group of students.
  - Educational aids and educational materials must be mutually flexible so they can be adapted based on the needs.
  - Ethical and legal aspects should be considered in the production and the utilization of educational communication media.

VIII. TYPES OF AUDIOVISUAL AIDS

Edgar Dalt's cone of experience is the most fundamental explanation to understand the types of audiovisual aids (Fig. 8.4). A basic classification of the types of different audiovisual aids is given below. Furthermore, a comprehensive description of selected types of audiovisual aids with guidelines for effective use is presented in a later section (page 345; Table 8.1).

A. Comprehensive Classification Based on the Mode of Presentation

I. Auditory aids

– Radio	– Tape and disc recordings	– Mike (public address system)
– Phonograms	– Megaphone	– Microphone
– Gramophone	– Language laboratories	– Tape recorder

II. Nonprojected/Unprojected visual aids: included both graphical and display aids

– Models	– Pictures	– Charts
– Flannel boards	– Graphs	– Chalkboards
– Cartoons and comics	– Maps	– Photographs
– Flash cards	– Illustrations	– Posters and printed media

III. Projected visual aids

– Epidiascope	– Slide projector	– Overhead projector
– Film projector	– Opaque projector	– LCD (liquid crystal display)

IV. Audiovisual aids

– Television, VCR/VCD	– Video and camera	– Sound-motion pictures

V. Activity aid

– Field trips	– Model making	– Collection of material
– Exhibition	– Demonstration	– Computer-assisted instructions
		– Programmed instructions

VI. Traditional media

– Puppets	– Dramas	– Folk songs and folk dance

B. Microscopic Divisional Classification Based on the Mode of Presentation

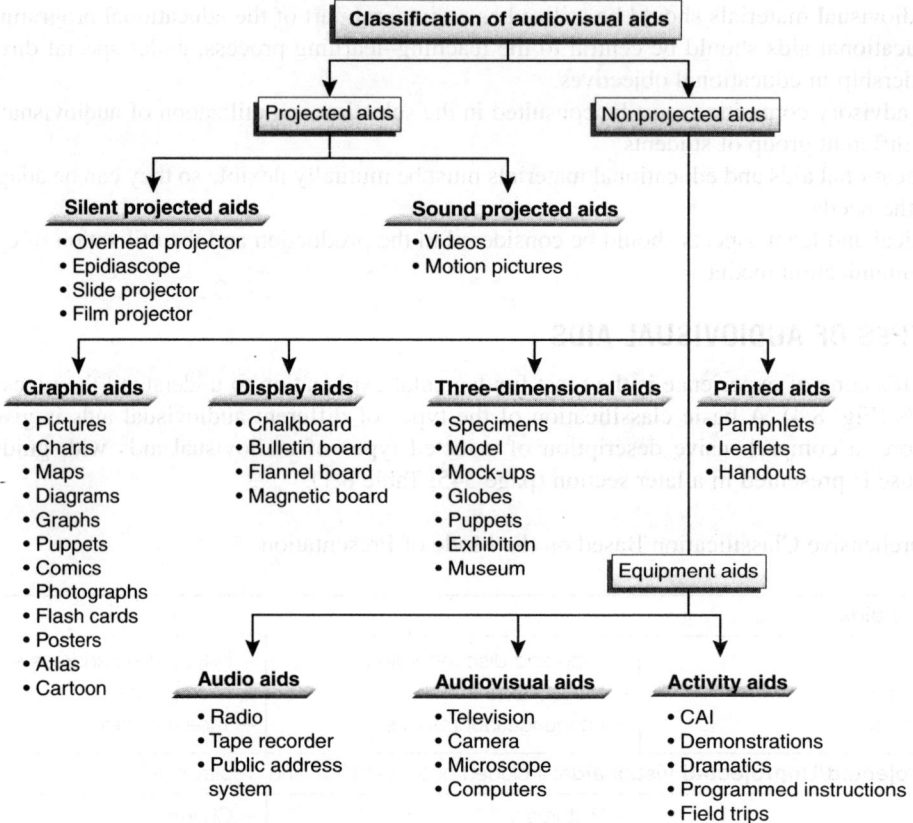

C. Types of Audiovisual Aids Based on the Size of Media

Big Media	Little Media
– Computer	– Radio, filmstrips
– VCR/VCD	– Graphic, audio cassettes
– Television	– And other visuals

GRAPHICAL TEACHING AIDS

The word *graphics* is derived from the Greek word *graphikos* that means visual presentations on some surface such as a wall, canvas, computer screen, paper or stone to brand, inform, illustrate or entertain. Graphics can be functional or artistic. The latter can be a recorded version, such as a photograph, or an interpretation by a scientist to highlight the essential features, or an artist, in which case the distinction with imaginary graphics may become blurred.

The use of graphic aids in the classroom has become an important teaching strategy in education. As educators learn more about how to reach all types of learners, the use of graphic aids assists in differentiating

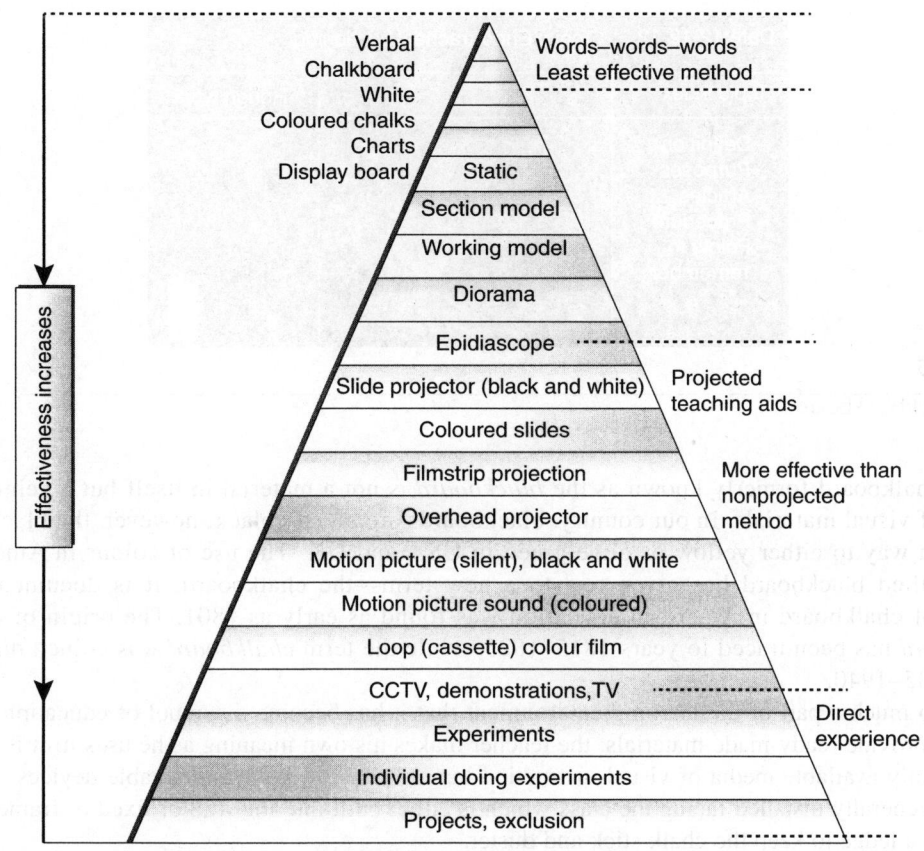

FIGURE 8.4

Edgar Dalt's cone of experience in audiovisual aids.

instructions, giving students greater access to content and helping students achieve greater comprehension of new information. There are multiple graphic aids that can be used in today's classroom and motivate students to learn. The most commonly used graphical teaching aids include chalkboard, chart, graphs, posters, flash cards, flannel board, bulletin board and cartoons, which are discussed below.

I. CHALKBOARD/BLACKBOARD

A blackboard is any dark-coloured, flat, smooth surface on which one can write or draw with a chalk (Fig. 8.5). It is one of the oldest and simplest visual aids. A chalkboard is also known as a *blackboard* that is a dark-coloured writing surface especially black or green in colour used for classroom teaching by writing or drawing illustrations using sticks of chalks. Originally, chalkboards were prepared using smooth, thin sheets of slate or stone of black or dark grey colour. However, in the new era, green coloured blackboards are becoming more popular because of their better compatibility viewers' vision.

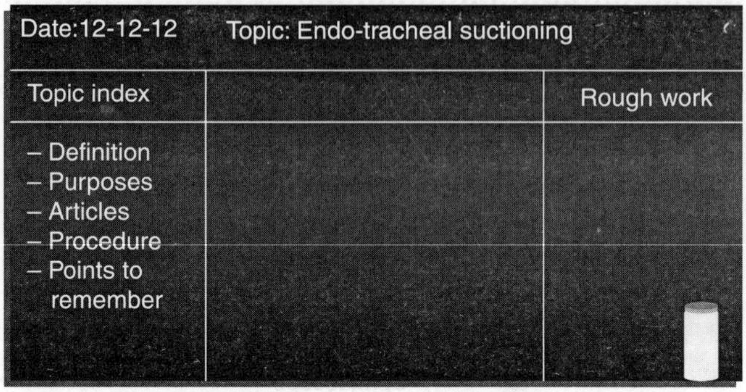

FIGURE 8.5

Chalkboard/blackboard.

The chalkboard formerly known as the *blackboard* is not a material in itself but a vehicle for a variety of visual materials. In our country, blackboards are mostly black; however, the black colour has given way to either yellow or olive green in USA and UK. The use of colour in America for the so-called blackboard has given rise to a new term—the chalkboard. It is documented that the use of chalkboard in American education was found as early as 1801. The origin of the term *blackboard* has been traced to years 1815–1825, while the term *chalkboard* was coined during the years 1935–1940.

It is so much a part of the learning environment that it has become a symbol of education itself. It does not provide ready-made materials; the teacher makes his own meaning as he uses it. It is not only a universally available media of visual instruction but also one of the most valuable devices. A chalkboard is generally installed facing the class which is either built into the wall or fixed or framed on the wall with a ledge to keep the chalk stick and duster.

A. Basic characteristics of a chalkboard

The recommended size of chalkboard is 5 × 6 m. For effective use of the chalkboard, the following characteristics should be considered:

- Surface should be rough enough to hold the chalk particles used for writing on the board.
- Surface should be dull enough to eliminate the glare that hampers the visibility of the writing board.
- Surface should be such that chalk can be easily removed with a cloth or foam duster.
- Surface should be mounted on appropriate height within the reach of teacher and visibility of students.

B. Purposes of a chalkboard

The main purposes of the blackboard are as follows:

- It makes group instruction more concrete and understandable.
- It can set standards of neatness, accuracy and speed, if used properly.
- It can restore the attention of the group.
- It helps in avoiding many vague statements that can be clarified by drawing sketches, outlines, diagrams, directions and summaries.

- It initiates aural and visual sensations and helps in learning.
- It can be a means of motivation and interest.
- It can be used for recording the progress and status.
- It provides many educational opportunities in all curricular and cocurricular activities. The teacher can present facts, principles, processes, procedures, assign individual responsibilities, write questions, problems, sources and references, summaries, outlines, directions, practice individual drills or creative work, make graphic demonstrations, screen for still pictures, projections, symbolic representations and review the total lesson and announcements.
- It can be used to state questions, cite examples of work desired, pose problems and list sources for study.
- It helps in illustrating forms of charting and providing opportunity for nursing students to practice charting.
- It helps in clarifying abstract statements at the exposition stage and providing a summary containing the salient features at recapitulation stage.
- It provides a lot of scope for creative and decorative work.
- It helps in starting afresh by erasing writings and drawings.

C. Types of chalkboard

Blackboards can be fixed or portable and can be made of wood, slate, glass, magnetic materials or sun mica. The main types of boards are as follows:

- *Ordinary chalkboard held by an easel:* A portable and adjustable blackboard put on a wooden easel can be taken out of the classroom while taking the class in open, useful for teaching art subjects in a small class.
- *Roller type chalkboard with mat surface:* This type of chalkboard is very common in secondary, modern and infant schools. It is made of a thick canvas wrapped on a roller.
- *Magnetic board:* These boards are made up of PVC materials/sun mica. Small magnets are used to hold suitable objects fixed whenever they are put on this vertical surface. The teachers can make three-dimensional demonstrations with objects on a vertical surface.
- *Black ceramic unbreakable board:* These are framed with aluminium or wooden frames as per requirement and chalk is used as writing material.
- *Black or green glass chalkboard:* It is the same as the black ceramic unbreakable board but the boards are black/green in colour and made up of glass.
- *Lobby stand board:* A light weight board where the alphabets/figures are interchangeable and mainly used in lobbies. It is easy to carry and has a stand height of 6 feet.
- *Exhibition board:* It is easily foldable and expandable and both sides are useable. It is available in 2 panel, 3 panel and 4 panel where pamphlets and papers can be fixed with pushpins.
- *Double-side stand board:* In this type of board, one side is whiteboard that is used for marker writing. The other side is blackboard and is used for chalk-piece writing. It is easily moveable and fixed on a wheel stand.
- *Reception board:* It is generally used at the reception counters in the corporate sector, hotels, restaurants, etc. Golden letters are fixed and usually framed by golden coloured aluminium material.
- *Tariff board:* It is used at reception counters as a welcome to delegates, at weddings or at hotels to show price lists.

- *Paging board:* These are widely used as welcome boards for contacting people at airports and railway stations.
- *Pressing graph perforated board:* These perforated boards are commonly used in schools, colleges, corporate offices, hospitals and hotels to display essential information. The boards have either a vertical or horizontal display and have perforations where plastic or metallic alphabets and/or numbers are deployed. The usual size of these letters or numbers used for display on these boards range between ¾ and 1½ inches.
- *Write and wipe off whiteboard:* A whiteboard (also known by the terms marker board, dry-erase board, dry-wipe board, pen-board and the misnomer grease board) is a name for any glossy, usually white surface for nonpermanent markings. Whiteboards are analogous to chalkboards, allowing rapid marking and erasing of markings on their surface.
- *Information notice board:* Notice boards and pin boards fit nicely into any office environment where they are suitable and are used for posting notices, timetables and other information relating to company news and events. Notices are attached to the boards by pins so that they can be easily posted and removed. Notice boards and pin boards are also ideal for meetings and conferences for the same reason that it is quick and easy to display information and images. Notice boards can be used, for instance, for qualitative research purposes such as focus groups and workshops where images can be arranged quickly for brainstorming and image testing.

D. Guidelines for preparing and using a chalkboard

- A blackboard is generally prepared with a piece of plywood about 30 × 40 inch size and painted with blackboard paint.
- To carry from one place to another, it is made in two pieces and hinged in the middle.
- When writing on a blackboard, the teacher should stand on the side and not in front.
- The teacher should not turn his back to the audience for a long time.
- The teacher should write the letters and drawings in a large size.
- The teacher should avoid spelling mistakes.
- Writing should be in straight rows.
- The extreme lower corner of the blackboard should not be used as all members cannot see it.
- The teacher should avoid filling the board with words or figures.
- If the teacher has to write many things or make complicated drawings, he/she should write or draw in advance to save time.
- Abbreviations should not be used.
- Coloured chalks should be used to enhance attraction and clarity in understanding.
- The board should not be cleaned with hands; proper eraser should be used in an up and down motion.
- Before leaving the class, the teacher should make sure the blackboard is clean.

Advantages of a chalkboard

- It is simple to use with little practice.
- It is economical and reusable.
- It is easily available and can be used any time.
- It can be used in a wide variety of ways, for simple outlines, drawings, summary of main points, etc.

- It encourages active doing and seeing on the part of the audience.
- It is a natural supplement to all aids and mistakes can be quickly erased.
- It can be easily used for giving lesson notes to students.

Limitations of a chalkboard

- It cannot preserve written material.
- It cannot be used for a large audience.
- It requires imagination, initiation, practice and preparation.
- It interrupts communication.
- It becomes smooth and full of glare when used constantly.
- It makes students heavily dependent on the teacher.
- It makes the teacher paced.
- It makes the lesson a dull routine.
- It makes the chalk powder spread, which can be inhaled by the teacher and students.

II. CHART

A chart is a combination of pictorial, graphic and numerical materials, which presents a clear visual summary (Fig. 8.6). It is a diagnostic representation of facts and ideas. The main function of the chart is always to show relationships such as comparisons, relative amounts, developments, processes, classification and organization. Edgar Dale defines charts as, 'a visual symbol summarizing, comparing, contrasting or performing other helpful services in explaining subject-matter'.

A. Basic characteristics of a chart

- Size of the chart could vary based on the type and purpose. However, the standard size of a chart is considered 90 × 60 cm or 70 × 50 cm.
- Charts can be carefully stored and preserved for use in future.
- They have an educational value.
- Usually the charts are teacher made, but students can make it during their presentation as a visual aid.
- Charts display specific information.
- They are easy to carry and store.

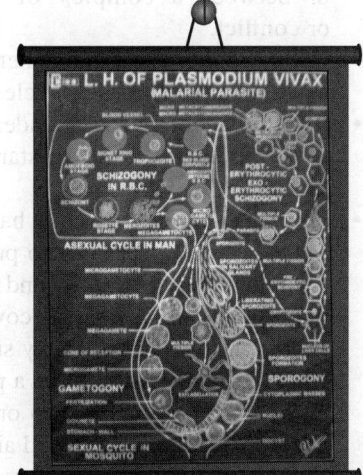

FIGURE 8.6
Chart.

B. Purposes of chart

Charts are essential educational aids generally used to:

- Present specific facts, figures and their relationships.
- Symbolically present the educational content.
- Illustrate continuity in a process of certain phenomenon.
- Present abstract ideas in visual forms.
- Present structural developments and organizational structures.

- Help in stimulating the thinking process through illustrative presentations.
- Provide students with motivation for learning.
- Show relationships between fazcts, figures and statistics.
- Summarize the large information so that comprehension of information may be obtained.

C. Types of charts

The main types of charts used for communication and educational purposes are as follows:

- *Flowchart:* Diagrams are used to show organizational elements/administrative/functional relationship boxes connected with lines to show the levels of lines of authority (Fig. 8.7). In this chart, lines, rectangles, circles or other graphic presentations are connected by lines showing the direction of flow.
- *Flip chart:* A set of charts related to specific topics that have been tagged together and hung on a supporting stand (Fig. 8.8). The individual charts carry a series of related materials or messages in a sequence. The salient features of specific topics are generally presented through these charts.
- *Timetable chart:* These are used to show the schedule of an activity or schedule of an individual. For example, timetable of a class, tour chart. It provides a chronological framework within which events and developments may be recorded. They develop a time sense in students and help them comprehend and visualize the pageant of time and relationships.
- *Cause and effect chart:* This kind of chart shows the arrangement of facts and ideas for expressing the relationship between rights and responsibilities, or between a complex of conditions and change or conflict.
- *Chain chart:* The arrangement of facts and ideas for expressing transitions or cycles.
- *Evolution chart:* Facts and ideas for expressing changes in specific items from the starting data and its projections in the future.
- *Striptease chart:* Strip chart has some peculiar characteristics such as (1) it enables speakers to present the information step by step; (2) it increases the interest and imagination of the audience; (3) the information on the chart is covered with thin paper strips applied either by wax, tape or sticky substance or pins; (4) as the speaker wishes to visually reinforce a point with words or symbols, he removes the appropriate strip or paper and (5) it produces interest and it increases learning and aids recall.
- *Pull chart:* It consists of written messages hidden by strips of thick paper. The message can be shown to the viewer, one after another by pulling out the concealing strips.

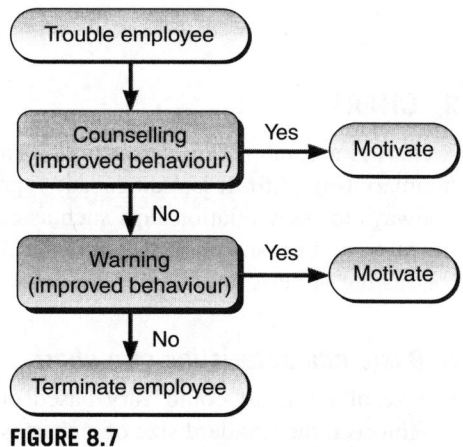

FIGURE 8.7
Flowchart.

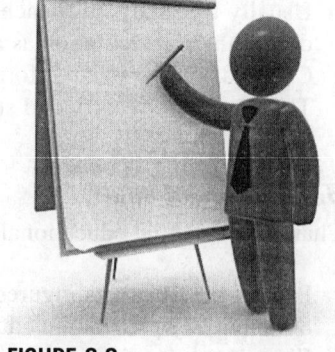

FIGURE 8.8
Flip chart.

- *Tabulation chart:* It shows the schedule of an activity or of an individual, for example, the timetable of a class. These are very valuable aids in the teaching situation where the breakdown of a fact or a statement is to be listed. Also, it is a useful aid for showing points of comparison, distinction and contrasts between two or more things. While making tabulation charts, a few points must be kept in mind. The chart should be 50 $\times$ 75 cm or more in size and captioned in bold letters. The vertical columns should be filled with short phrases rather than complete sentences.
- *Job chart:* A job chart includes the major responsibilities of the category of personnel for ready reference.
- *Tree chart:* Tree charts include the growth and development of specific phenomenons or organizations in a continuous growing process depicted in the form of a tree.
- *Overlay chart:* These charts consist of illustrated sheets that can be placed one over another conveniently and in succession. The drawing or illustration on each sheet forms a part of the whole picture. It enables the viewers to see not only the different parts but also see them against the total perspective when one is placed over the other. When the final overlay is placed the ultimate product is exposed to view.

D. Guidelines for preparing and using charts
- The chart should be of standard size (90 $\times$ 60 cm or 70 $\times$ 50 cm).
- The size of letters for captions and labels should be 2–3 cm and the line thickness should be 2–3 mm.
- Every detail depicted should be visible to everyone in the class.
- Display material should be contrasted with a background.
- Flat pictures and other material should be enlarged before placing on the chart.
- One chart should display information about one specific area in a subject.
- It should not contain too many details.
- It should be neat and tidy.
- The chart should be strong enough to stand for other rough use.

Advantages of a chart
- Charts are helpful in summarizing large information on a single paper so that comprehension and understanding of content can be prompted.
- Illustrative properties of charts catch the attention of students and motivate them for learning.
- The symbolic presentation of information increases quick learning in the learners.

Limitations of a chart
- If the selection of material for preparing charts is not good, they will not last long.
- It takes up a teacher's time if she has to prepare the chart.
- Charts only emphasize on the key points. This leaves the students in doubt if the clarification is not clear.
- Charts lose their charm if they contain too much written matter.
- Poor use of colour combination, improper spacing and margins create confusion in the minds of the students.

III. GRAPHS

Graphs are illustrations to present numerical and statistical data using dots, lines, shapes, colours and pictures. Graphical presentation is a visual art based on the use of visual symbolic and visual-abstract forms. They depict numerical, quantitative relationship or statistical data represented in the form of visual symbols. The common types of graphs are bar graph, line graph, pictorial graphs, histograms, pie graph and cumulative frequency graph.

A. Basic characteristics of graphs

The following basic characteristics must be kept in mind while constructing a diagram or graph.

- They must have a title and index.
- The proportion between width and height should be balanced.
- The selection of scale must be appropriate.
- Footnotes may be included wherever needed.
- Principle of simplicity must be kept in mind.
- Neatness and cleanliness in the construction of graphs must be ensured.

B. Purposes of graphs

The main purposes of using graphs in the teaching–learning process are as follows:

- Graphs are one of the most convincing and appealing ways in which statistical results may be presented.
- They give a bird's eye view of the entire information.
- The are attractive to the eye.
- They have a great memorizing effect on the learners.
- They facilitate comparison of data relating to different periods of time.

C. Types of graphs

The most commonly used graphs in the teaching–learning process are bar graphs, pie graphs, histograms, frequency polygons, line graphs, cumulative frequency curves and pictorial graphs.

- *Bar graphs:* It is a convenient graphical device that is particularly useful for displaying nominal or ordinal data. It is an easy method adopted for visual comparison of the magnitude of different frequencies. The length of the bars drawn vertically or horizontally indicates the frequency of a character. The bar charts are called *vertical bar charts* (or column charts) if the bars are placed vertically. When the bars are placed horizontally, they are called *horizontal bar charts*. There are three types of bar diagrams: simple, multiple and proportional bar diagrams (Fig. 8.9). The following points to be kept in mind while making a bar diagram:
  - The width of bars should be uniform throughout the diagram.
  - The gap between one bar and another should be uniform throughout.
  - Bars may be vertical or horizontal.
- *Line graphs:* It shows the relationships and trends of an event occurring over a period of time. A single line shows the relation and variation in the quantity (Fig. 8.10). The concepts are represented with the help of lines drawn either horizontally or vertically.

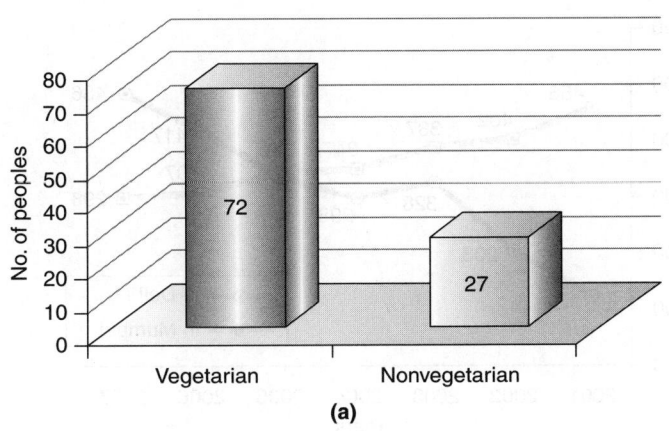

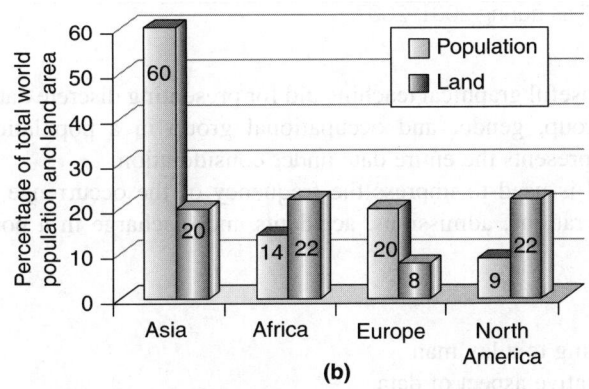

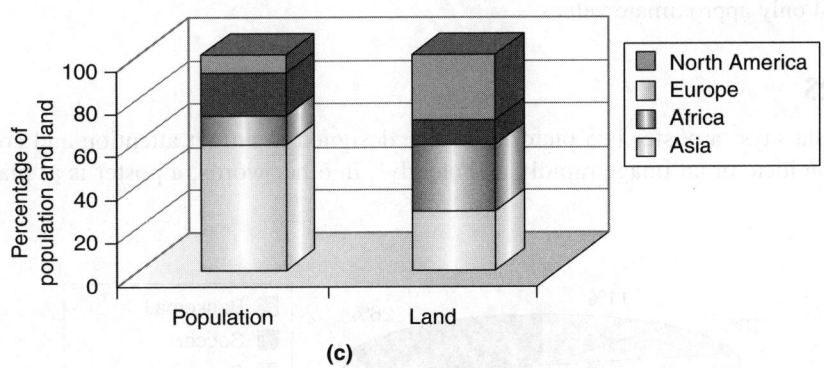

FIGURE 8.9

Different types of bar graphs: (a) simple bar graph, (b) multiple bar graph and (c) proportional bar graph.

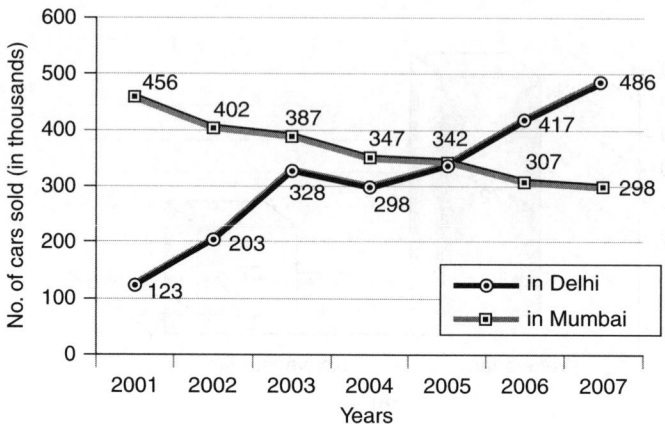

FIGURE 8.10

Line graph showing car sale in two cities during 2001–2007.

- *Pie/sector graph:* It is another useful graphical teaching aid for presenting discrete data of qualitative characteristics such as age group, gender and occupational group in a population (Fig. 8.11). The whole area of the circle represents the entire data under consideration.
- *Pictorial graphs:* This method is used to impress the frequency of the occurrence of events such as attacks, deaths, number operations, admissions, accidents and discharge in a population to the common man (Fig. 8.12).

Limitations of graphs

- Sometime may be quite confusing to a lay man.
- Generally presents only quantitative aspect of data.
- Can be used for presenting only one thing or smaller information at one time.
- Can present only approximate values.

IV. POSTERS

S.L. Ahulawalia says 'a poster is a pictorial device designed to attract attention and communicate a story, a fact, an idea, or an image rapidly and clearly'. In other words, a poster is a 'placard, usually

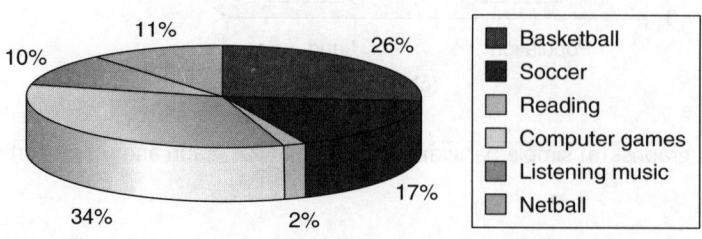

FIGURE 8.11

Pie diagram showing leisure activities in urban children.

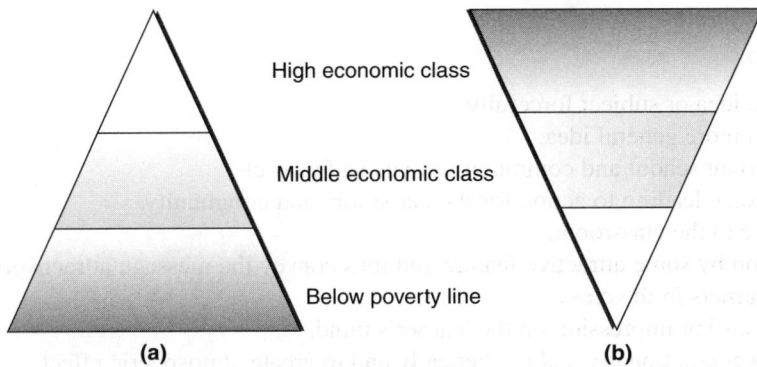

High economic class

Middle economic class

Below poverty line

(a)   (b)

FIGURE 8.12

Pictorial graph showing proportion of people with economic class: (a) developing countries and (b) developed countries.

pictorial or decorative, utilizing an emotional appeal to convey a message aimed at reinforcing an attitude or urging a course of action'. Posters are generally used for conveying a specific message, teaching a particular thing, giving a general idea, etc. Posters exert great influence on the observer (Fig. 8.13).

The poster can be further defined as a graphic representation of some strong emotional appeal that is carried through a combination of graphic aids like pictures, cartoons lettering and other visual arts on a placard.

Posters are the graphic aids with short quick and typical messages with attention capturing paintings.

A. Characteristics of a good poster

- A poster is any piece of printed paper designed to be attached to a wall or a vertical surface, and is typically good substitute for a first-hand experience.
- The ideal size of a poster must be 28 × 22 inches; however the size may vary based on the purpose of poster. For example, conference posters are generally large in size.
- Very effective visual aids vary from a simple printed card to a complicated and artistic design.
- There must be minimal use of words, i.e. only four to five words.
- The idea or feeling being presented must be original and clearly understandable.
- The layout of the poster must be simple so that it does not distract the student from the main content of learning.
- There must appropriate use of colours and fonts:
  - Use bold illustrations
  - Avoid fancy lettering style
  - Proper use of colour
- The poster must be as attractive as possible so that students can be motivated for learning.

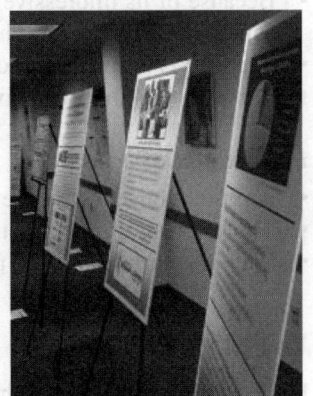

FIGURE 8.13

Posters.

B. Purposes of a poster

Posters are used to:

- Present a single idea or subject forcefully.
- Communicate a more general idea.
- Publicize important school and community events and projects.
- Thrust the message leading to action for the classroom and community.
- Add atmosphere to the classroom.
- Capture attention by some attractive feature and thus convey the message attractively and quickly.
- Motivate the learners in the class.
- Leave a strong lasting impression on the learner's mind.
- Satisfy the viewer emotionally and aesthetically and to create atmospheric effect.

C. Guidelines for preparing and using a poster

- Promote one point at a time.
- Support local demonstrations and exhibits.
- It should be planned for specified people on a specified topic and a theme should be provided.
- It should have instant appeal.
- It should tell the message in a single glance.
- It should be attractive enough and pleasing colours should be used.
- For headings, bold letters (20 × 30 inch) should be used.
- The language should be easy and simple.
- The most suitable words should be decided upon to provide a title or a slogan.
- A few layouts should be sketched and the best one should be decided on.
- All needed material should be gathered to prepare the poster.
- Smudge marks should be erased and finishing touches added.
- The poster must be displayed at a place with good provision of light and where a large number of people can see it.

Advantages of a poster

- Because of its impressive presentation, a poster captivates the eye, regardless of the message and is capable of being comprehended.
- A poster is a simple and dynamic medium of presenting a message in a compact form.
- A poster tells the story vividly with the desired effect.

Limitations of a poster

- A poster conveys a single theme and does not always give enough information.
- The lettering if not attractive and accurate makes the poster illegible.
- Smudge marks make the posters unattractive and futile.

V. FLASH CARDS

Flash cards are used for the presentation of an idea in the form of posters, pictures, words and sentences (Fig. 8.14). A single card or a whole series may be flashed in front of the class. In other words, flash cards are a set of pictured paper cards of varying sizes that are flashed one by one in a logical sequence. Flash cards can be self-made or commercially prepared and are made up of a chart or drawing paper or plain paper using colours or ink on them for drawings.

They aim to develop the power of observation, identification, quick comprehension and retention. Flash cards are small, compact cards, approximately 10×12 inches that are flashed before a group. Each card contains important highlights of the topic in the form of words, diagram, photograph and illustrations.

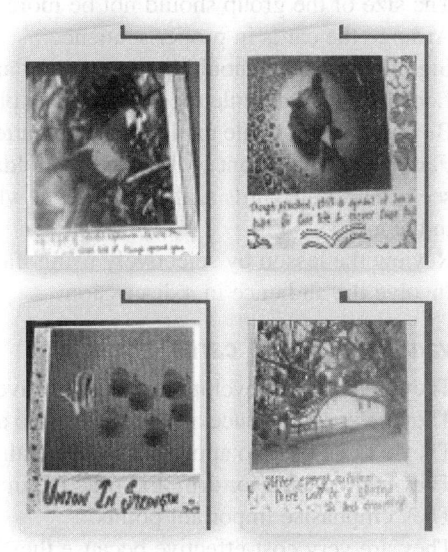

FIGURE 8.14

Flash cards.

A. Basic characteristics of flash cards

- Flash cards are small, compact cards of varying size approximately 10×12 inches in size.
- They are made out of cardboards or any other thick material.
- They are the simplest of all aids to present topic highlights in the form of words, diagrams, photographs and illustration.

B. Purposes of flash cards

Flash cards are generally used for the following purposes:

- The pictorial contents presented in a series are easily recognized by the group.
- They are flashed before the class one by one to bring home an idea.
- Communication of new ideas requires repetitive study methods, drill-work and review of the discussion that can be achieved through flash cards.
- They provide students with a systematic approach to drill.
- They are helpful to teach recognition by sight.
- They are easy to carry.

C. Guidelines for preparing and using flash cards

- The messages can be brief, simple line drawings or photographs, cartoons and the content is written in a few lines at the back of each card.
- They are commonly 10×12 inches in size.
- Ideally 10–12 cards can be used for one talk. The number of cards should not be less than 3 and more than 20.
- Preparing a picture for each idea which will give visual impact to the idea.
- The height of writing on the flash card is to be approximately 5 cm for better visualization.
- Selection of a topic and the content to be displayed should be planned.
- Illustrations and words should be simple and should give a brief introduction about the lesson to students.

- The size of the group should not be more than 30 students.
- Arrange the cards in proper sequence.
- Significant points should be pointed out and care should be taken not to cover them with hands.
- Look at the card while the concept is explained from the card.
- Be enthusiastic while explaining the matter.
- Flash the card in front of the class by holding it high with both your hands so that all the students can see it. Hold the cards at the chest level where people can see clearly; hold against the body and not in the air.
- Review the lesson by selectively using flash cards.
- Involve the audience in a discussion.

Advantages of flash cards
- They help in the development of cognitive abilities and recognition and recall of students.
- They help to introduce and present topic as well as review the topic.
- They can be used to apply information already gained by students to new situations.
- They can be used for drill and practice in the elementary class.
- They emphasise important points.
- They are very cost-effective because they can be prepared on simple papers.
- They are easy to make, require only hard papers and pens.
- They can work as a useful supplementary aid and can be effectively used with other materials.

Limitations of flash cards
- If used for a prolonged period, they become boring for students.
- The students cannot get a complete view of the concept, as the points are flashed one by one.
- They need to be carefully stored and prevented from bending.
- They are ineffective for large groups.
- They are time-consuming and cannot include the whole topic of presentation. Only a part of a topic can be presented through flash cards.

VI. FLANNEL BOARD

The flannel board or felt board is a piece of rigid material covered with cotton flannel, wool, suede cloth or paper (Fig. 8.15). A piece of rough flannel or khadi fixed over a wooden board provides an excellent background for displaying cut-out pictures, graphs, drawing and other illustrations. The cut-out pictures and other illustrations are provided with a rough surface at the back by pasting pieces of sand paper, felt or rough cloth. They adhere at once when put on the flannel. It is a very cheap medium, easy to transport and promotes thought and criticism.

A. Preparing flannel board
The following articles and steps are required for preparing the flannel board:
   Articles required:

- A piece of plywood, cardboard or poster board
- A piece of flannel large enough to cover the board
- A pair of scissors

- Duct tape (or a staple gun or upholstery tacks if using a plywood)
- Felt squares to make shapes and other cut-outs

Preparation procedure:

- Wrap the piece of flannel around the board you have chosen.
- Secure all edges around the back side with the duct tape, staples or tacks.
- The items to be displayed should also be pasted with the same flannel on back side which keeps it adherent to the board without visible support.

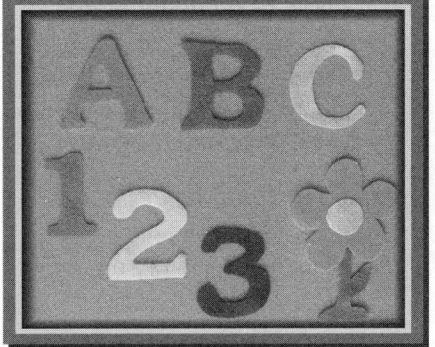

FIGURE 8.15

Flannel boards.

B. Purposes of a flannel board

The purposes of using flannel boards are given below:

- They can be used throughout the discussion whenever the needed item can be placed and explained on (if the purpose is served the item has to be removed).
- They help improve the visual artefact of the written content or illustrations to a large group of learners.
- They also facilitate the illustrative presentation of written content for easy understanding.
- Their use facilitate the auditory, visual and kinaesthetic learning.
  - *Auditory:* The learners can hear the content displayed on the board read by someone.
  - *Visual:* The learners can visualize the displayed content on the flannel board.
  - *Kinaesthetic:* They also can display pieces of information on the board.
- They are generally used as a bridge between the books and in story time programmes.
- They add variety to the storyline.
- They help communicate the idea in an effective manner.
- They describe the way of doing a particular item.
- They motivate the learner.
- They add variety to classroom activity.
- They intensify the impressions and vitalize the instructions.
- They provide information.
- They supplement and correlate information, so saves time.

C. Guidelines for using a flannel board

- The contents of the board should be organized around the central theme.
- Appearance must be neat and orderly.
- The material should be displayed in an attractive manner.
- Avoid overcrowding on the board.
- It should be clearly seen by the group members.
- The displayed pictures should be sufficiently large in size.
- Remove the picture as soon as their purpose is over.

Advantages of a flannel board

- Makes concepts easy to understand.
- Effectively used for small groups.
- Saves time during the presentation.
- Keeps students well motivated.

Limitations of a flannel board

- Cannot be used for large groups.
- Needs more preparatory time.

VII. BULLETIN BOARD

A bulletin board is a display board that shows the visual learning material on a specific subject. It is a soft board that holds pins or tags. It is a simple device placed either indoors or outdoors. Items like photographs, publications, posters, newspaper cut-outs are generally displayed (Fig. 8.16).

A bulletin board also known as a *pin board* or a *notice board* is a place where people can display public messages, for example, to advertise things, to buy or sell, announce events or provide information. Dormitory corridors, well-trafficked hallways, lobbies and freestanding kiosks often have cork boards attached to facilitate the posting of notices. At some universities, lamp posts, bollards, trees and walls often become impromptu posting sites in areas where official boards are sparse in number.

The items that can be displayed on the bulletin boards are photographs, CD covers, book jackets, news stories, sketches, newspaper and magazine clippings, drawings, cartoons, specimens, real objects, posters, poems, greeting cards, thoughts and even jokes.

A. Basic characteristics of bulletin boards

- They can be framed soft boards or straw boards or cork boards.
- Their size depends on the purpose.
- Dark blazer cloth works as a back drop.
- The height should be one meter above the ground.

B. Purposes of bulletin boards

Bulletin boards are used for the following purposes:

- Communication of ideas
- Giving correct initial impression
- Broaden the sensory experience
- Intensify impressions
- Vitalize instructions
- Add variety to classroom activity
- Provide information

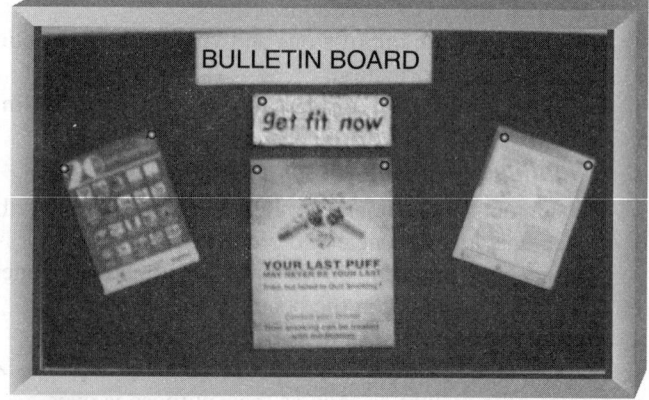

FIGURE 8.16

Bulletin board.

- Supplement and correlate instructions
- Save time
- Help students learn how to communicate ideas visually
- Facilitate class study of single copy material
- Encourage participation
- Provide a review

C. Types of bulletin boards

- Felt board
- Magnetic board
- Fixed type
- Movable type
- Folded type

D. Guidelines for preparing and using bulletin boards

- *Thumbnail sketches:* Make several and then select one.
- Procurement of material on a given subject.
- Sorting out relevant material.
- *Decide on a theme:* Words should catch attention of viewers.
- Use of attention-directing devices.
- Should be displayed in an aesthetic manner and the area should be well lighted.
- Should be kept a little above eye level.
- Place the bulletin board near the doorway.
- The content of a bulletin board should be organized around a central theme.
- Title of the topic must be fixed at the top and the material placed should be appropriately dated and revised from time to time.
- The material should be organized properly by dividing the board, overcrowding of content must be avoided.
- The board must have a neat, ordered and attractive appearance.
- Give due thoughts to eye catching leads.
- Make special reference during course of study.
- Students can be asked to collect display material.
- The content on the board should be changed regularly.
- There should be a separate board for posting routine notices of the institution.
- A bulletin board committee is responsible for editing the board from time to time.
- Do not leave the board for long after the teaching purpose is over.
- Take down displays from the board, return the borrowed items and file useful material.

Advantages of bulletin boards

- Display can be effectively used as a follow-up of chalkboard work.
- Adds colour and liveliness in communicating the message to the audience.
- Good supplement for other teaching aids.
- Introduces a new topic to a large number of people.
- Explains important events, reports and special activities.

Limitations of bulletin boards

- Not effective for illiterate groups.
- Takes a lot of time for preplanning and preparation.
- Cannot be used for an all inclusive teaching.
- Has to be used as a supplementary aid to other teaching aids.
- Collection of relevant materials for certain topics may sometimes be difficult.

VIII. CARTOONS

A cartoon is a humorous caricature which gives a subtle message. In a cartoon, the features of objects and people are exaggerated along with their general symbols. In short, a cartoon is a figurative and subtle graphic aid. It is a metaphoric representation of reality and makes learning more interesting and effective, as it creates a strong appeal to the emotions. A cartoon is an interpretative illustration which uses symbols to portray an opinion, a scene or a situation (Fig. 8.17).

Cartoons are a novel way of using pictures or symbols for presenting a message or a point of view concerning a personality, news, situation or an event. They are more attention drawing and providing a lot of imagination, particularly on current happenings, in a small space. They are blended with humour and satire.

A. Basic characteristics of cartoons

- Cartoons should be of appropriate size so that everyone can see them and understand the message appropriately.
- Cartoons must be drawn according to the age and educational level of the learners to ensure their appropriateness for the target group.
- The symbols used in cartoons must be clear and understandable.
- Use of text must be minimal and should be meaningful.
- Cartoons should be self-explanatory and instructive.
- Cartoons should be funny, interesting and humorous.

B. Purposes of cartoons

The main purposes of cartoons in the teaching–learning process are as follows:

- They are primarily designed for capturing the attention of the targeted group.
- They are successful tools for student motivation and the promotion of learning.
- They create humour and fantasy among the learners so educational stress can be minimized.
- A single cartoon can easily present multiple ideas and concepts.
- They trigger innovative thinking in the learners.
- They can present educational content in an interesting manner.

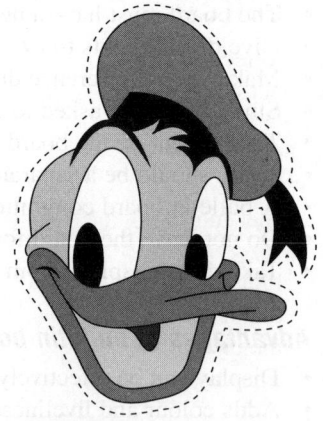

FIGURE 8.17

Cartoon.

Advantages of cartoons

- Cartoons are humorous caricatures so they capture the attention of the learners and prevent boredom among them.
- They are quite successful in motivating the learning and messages can be easily understood by the learners.
- They can easily present multiple ideas and concepts to the learners.

Limitations of cartoons

- A skilled specialist is required to prepare educational cartoons.
- Many educational topics can be presented only through cartoons.
- Cartoons as educational aids may sometimes distract the students from the main learning purpose and objectives.

THREE-DIMENSIONAL AUDIOVISUAL AIDS

Three-dimensional aids are considered good substitutes of real objectives. A variety of three-dimensional audiovisual aids are also known as *realia*. They are used to substitute the real objectives so that students can get the experience of real objectives in their natural setting. Sometimes it is not possible to provide a real object experience. In these cases the three-dimensional aids could be the best option to be used as a teaching tool. For example, a teacher can use a model of the heart to teach about the heart's anatomy, when real body dissection is not possible. On the other hand, sometimes real-life objectives could be too large or expensive to bring into the classroom, then the three-dimensional audiovisual objectives may be a good alternative. Three-dimensional objects stimulate the imagination, thinking and abstraction in the students by offering first-hand experiences about real-life situations. Some of the main three-dimensional audiovisual aids, i.e. objects and specimens, models, puppets, exhibitions, museums and dioramas, are discussed below.

I. OBJECTS AND SPECIMENS

A collection of real things for instructional use refers to objects. A specimen is a sample of the real object or material. Objects and specimens should be mounted in shallow boxes in an artistic way and the boxes should be covered with cellophane paper (Fig. 8.18). Also each object or specimen should be labelled using self-adhesive paper.

While using the specimen and objects as teaching aids, a teacher must keep the following points in mind:

- Planning of the object or specimen display should be such that a simple and direct visualization of the object or specimen is possible by all the learners with a great level of ease.
- The display of object or specimen must be supplemented with an active question–answer session, so that the teacher can be sure that students have clearly understood the object or specimen under observation.

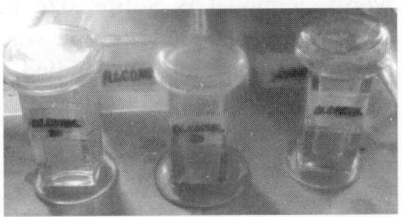

FIGURE 8.18

Specimen.

- The teacher must provide details of the structure of an object or specimen under display and offer clarification when and where needed.
- The teacher must ensure feedback and further practice so that students can learn the object or specimen thoroughly under observation.

A. Sources of objects and specimens

- Local markets.
- Manufacturers and factories.
- Discarded material from houses.
- Specimens found in nature can be collected by students from field trips and nature hunts.
- Plaster casts can be purchased.
- Wild flowers, leaves, shells, stones, butterflies, moths and insects can also be procured.

Advantages of objects and specimens

- Collection of objects and specimens by students requires interaction with others leading to the development of social skills and values.
- When students collect and display objects and specimens, they derive satisfaction of contributing something worthwhile to the school and the teacher.
- The student's power of observation and first-hand experience is enhanced by the collection of objects and specimens.
- Student's personal collection of objects and specimens can be a good source of doing investigatory projects.
- Collection of objects and specimens becomes an interesting educational pursuit of the teacher and the students alike.
- They arouse some interest in students for learning.
- They involve all the five senses in the process of learning.
- They heighten the reality in the classroom.

II. MODELS

A model is a recognizable representation of a real thing three dimensionally, that is height, width, and depth is felt as reality. In other words, a model is a life size miniature or over size or original size whether workable or not, whether it differs or not from original size of an object to be studied, which is very useful in teaching (Fig. 8.19).

Further, a model means imitation, replica and copy of the real-life object. However, if the model is larger or smaller than the real thing, the students should be given a clear idea of its actual size. In some cases, models are oversimplified, such models should be used with great caution.

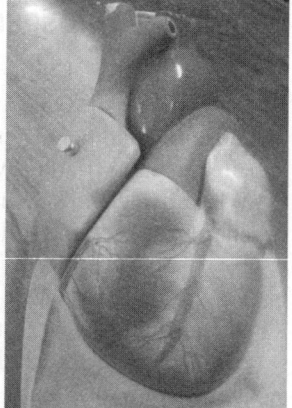

FIGURE 8.19

Model.

A. Purposes of models

Models are useful and necessary because

- The real thing may not be available in that season or may be far away from the institute.
- The real thing may be too big to be brought to the institute.
- The real thing may be too dangerous to be felt or handled by the students.
- The real thing may be too expensive.
- The real thing may be too small to be seen at all or seen properly.

Other core purposes of models used as teaching aids are as follows:

- Models simplify reality.
- Models help in clarifying the abstract concept of knowledge.
- They also facilitate visualization and learning of the large objects. It is generally not possible to visualize at one snapshot.
- Models also offer a clear and correct concept of invariably large real objects such as a dam, bridge and mountain, etc.
- Furthermore, functional models also help in understanding the real working of various objects, instruments and machines.
- Promotes creative interest in students.

B. Types of models

- *Solid models:* They are a replica of an original thing made with suitable material such as clay, plaster of Paris, wood and iron, to show the external parts of thing. For example, a globe, clay model of a human or animal.
- *Cutaway and x-ray models:* They are the replicas of the original things to show their internal parts. They show how something looks from inside. There are many situations particularly in technical subjects and in the study of hygiene where it is necessary to see the interior of an organ or a machine to understand how it works. Cross-sectional models are difficult to make in the classroom or institutions as they require expertise to construct them. For example, a cross-sectional model of the human body.
- *Working models:* These models are either actual working things or miniature replicas for illustration of an operation. In some lessons, working models that show how things function or operate in a simple way are very helpful. In many cases, they are used in place of real articles because they are easier to understand. For example, a motor, a generator or a model showing blood flow in the body.
- *Sand models:* Sand models are made by using sand, clay and saw dust. For example, a tribal village or a forest area.
- *Scale models:* In some study situations, we need a correct representation of things through exactness of a scale. Small-scale models of the Damodar valley and other projects help students as well as others form a good idea of big enterprises. Further, a scale is one measurement that represents another value of measurement. For example, architects may use a scale of ¼-inch = 1 foot for construction drawings. At this scale, a building of 100 feet on each side could be represented as a 25-inch square.

- *Simplified models:* There are, however, many learning situations in which models that show the external form of an object roughly are required. The animals, birds and fish which children of primary schools make out of clay, sand or straw have great educational value.

C. Essential qualities of a model

A model must have the following qualities:

- Usefulness
- Accuracy
- Simplicity
- Utility
- Solidity
- Ingenuity

Advantages of models

- Models heighten the reality of things and make learning direct and meaningful as they are three-dimensional.
- Models illustrate the application side of certain principles and laws.
- Models explain complex and intricate operations in a simplified way and thus make comprehension easier.
- Models are long lasting and ultimately work out to be cheaper teaching aids.
- Still models are easy to make with the help of discarded materials like empty boxes, pins, clips, nails and clay.
- Models should be reasonable in size and convenient to handle.
- Models involve the use of all the five senses and make learning effective.

Limitations of models

- They require expertise to make.
- They are time-consuming.
- Some models may be very expensive.

III. PUPPETS

One of the old and popular arts in Indian villages is puppetry. Puppetry is an education cum entertaining aid where puppets are manipulated by the performer (Fig. 8.20). In writing or selecting a puppet play, the age, background and tastes of students should be taken into consideration. A short puppet play is always preferable.

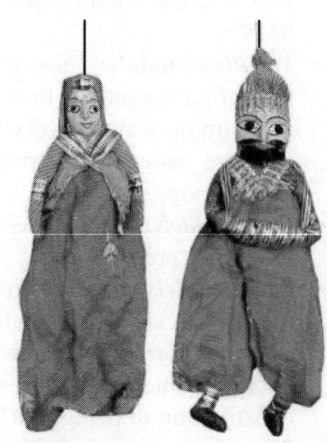

FIGURE 8.20

Puppets.

A puppet is a manipulative doll dressed as a character and the performer is a person termed as a puppeteer. A good puppeteer has to blend his art with dramatization to produce the desired effect. It is used as an effective teaching aid for languages and social sciences.

D. Types of puppets

- *String or marionette puppets:* Marionettes consist of puppets with hinged body parts which are controlled by nine strings producing the required movements in the puppet. These puppets are mainly manipulated by professional puppeteers.
- *Stick puppets:* Stick puppets are painted cut-outs attached by sticks. The actions of these puppets are manipulated by the teacher and students by hiding behind a screen so that only the puppets are visible to the audience or the class.
- *Shadow puppets:* Shadow puppets are silhouettes of cardboard that produce shadows on a white screen. The motion of these silhouettes is manipulated by the teacher and students.
- *Finger of hand puppets:* Hand puppets are round balls painted as heads with overflowing, colourful costumes. They are worn on fingers which operate their movements. They are operated from below the stage.

Advantages of puppets

- They create interest.
- They give knowledge in a brief period.
- They are an effective method in teaching.
- They motivate students.
- They are easy to carry and operate.

Limitations of puppets

- They need group cooperation and coordination.
- They require skills in preparation and supply.
- Skills are needed for presentation.

IV. EXHIBITIONS

Many times in the school, a department of the school or class puts up their work for showing it to the people outside the school, such a show is called an *exhibition* (Fig. 8.21). The pieces of work done by the students for an exhibition are called *exhibits*.

A. Basic characteristics of an exhibition

- The exhibition should have a central theme with a few sub-themes to focus attention to a particular concept.
- The exhibits should be clean and labelled properly.
- The concepts of contrast in colour and size should be used for laying out the exhibitions.
- The exhibits should be so placed so most visitors can see them.
- The place and exhibits should be well lighted.
- Both motion and sound should be utilized to capture the attention and interest of the visitors.

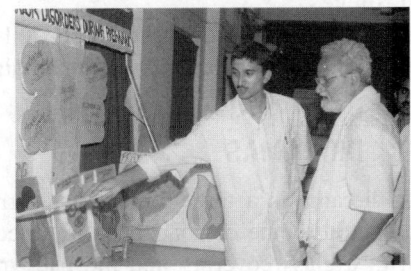

FIGURE 8.21

Exhibition.

- The exhibition should have some exhibits with operative mechanism such as switches and handles to be operated by the visitors to observe some happenings.
- The exhibition should include a lot of demonstrations as they involve the students and the visitors deeply.
- The exhibition should be able to relate various subject areas to provide integrated learning.

Advantages of an exhibitions

- Exhibitions inspire students to learn by doing things themselves and get a sense of involvement.
- Exhibitions give students a sense of accomplishment and achievement.
- Exhibitions develop social skills of communication, cooperation and coordination.
- Exhibitions foster better school community relations and make community members conscious about the school.
- Exhibitions couple information with pleasure.
- Exhibitions foster creativity in students.

Limitations of an exhibitions

- Exhibitions require thorough preparation.
- They are time-consuming.
- They require a large amount of funds or budget.

V. MUSEUMS

A museum is a building that displays a collection of historical relics, antiques, curiosities, works of arts, works of science, literature and other artefacts of general interest. Museums can be useful both for public education and specific classroom instructions.

A. Setting up a school museum

- Schools should have enough space.
- Take the help of students, collect old and new objects and articles.
- Accept donations from various organizations who donate articles.
- Students can be guided to prepare exhibits for museum.
- All the collected and prepared articles should be displayed and labelled.
- A detailed report book should be maintained giving a brief description of each museum pieces.
- The museum rooms should be well lighted.
- It should be clean and well maintained for use.

VI. DIORAMAS

A diorama is a three-dimensional arrangement of related objects, models and cut-outs to illustrate a central theme or concept. The objects and models are generally placed in a big box or showcased with a glass covering and the background is printed with a shade or a scene, e.g. a harvest scene, a planting scene.

Advantages of dioramas

- They provide a good opportunity to learn.
- They give the appearance of actual things which cannot be brought to the classroom.
- They are interesting and enhance creativity.
- Live things can also be shown in dioramas, for example, an aquarium.
- They provide an opportunity for the students to carry out a creative activity.

Limitations of dioramas

- Sometimes they are not a cost-effective method.
- They need expatriation for preparation.
- They may require a large budget.
- They may sometimes misguide the student if is not a replica of the actual thing.

PRINTED EDUCATIONAL AIDS

Printed educational aids have been used since a long time and are found essentially important in the classroom as well as mass education. However, rapid development in science and technology has revolutionized the use of educational aids in the teaching–learning process. Today, we have so many advanced educational aids which are far advanced in technology and usefulness than conventional educational aids. However, conventional educational aids still have their importance in the teaching–learning process. Some important printed educational aids are pamphlets, handouts, handbills and leaflets. However, this chapter presents the most commonly used printed eductional aids, i.e. pamphlets and leaflets.

I. PAMPHLETS

Pamphlets are a type of nonprojected audiovisual aids. A pamphlet is a paper that can be folded into two or three or five, and the matter can be printed either on a single or on both sides. In other words, a pamphlet is an unbounded booklet without a hard cover or binding. It may consist of a single sheet of paper that is printed on both sides and folded in half, in thirds, or in fourth, or it may consist of a few pages that are folded in half or stapled at the crease to make a single book. A pamphlet gives a chance to explain to the people who do not have time to stay and discuss the content of information. A pamphlet must be self-explanatory (Fig. 8.22).

A. Purposes of pamphlets

Pamphlets are used for the following purposes:

- To mobilize people to support a cause.
- To advertise a meeting or a specific event.
- To popularize a slogan or a message.

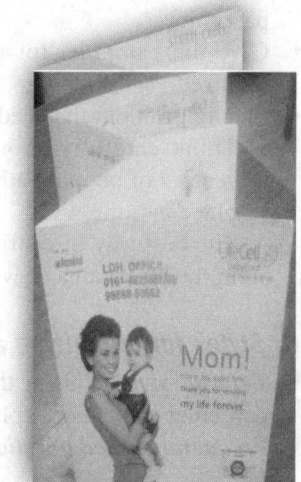

FIGURE 8.22

Pamphlet.

- Furthermore, pamphlets are used for the following purposes:
  - Explain an issue to the community.
  - Inform people of their rights.
  - Win support for a campaign you are running.
  - Win support for any organization's point of view.

B. Preparing pamphlets

To prepare a good pamphlet, the following things must be followed:

- Discuss the purpose, the message, the target people and content.
- Discuss the quantity and quality of pamphlets.
- If printing is done on both sides of a pamphlet, each side should have an interesting *bold* headline to get peoples' attention.
- Each side should also carry the organization's logo or name.
- Keep the language simple by avoiding long and complicated sentences.
- The best pamphlets are short and simple.
- All facts should be correct.

Steps for preparing pamphlets

- Initially, the purpose and nature of the pamphlets and the target group must be determined. The target group may be a general person, professionals such as doctors and nurses.
- The second priority should be to define the dimensions of the pamphlet. The best and most used size is with the dimensions of 8.5×11 inches^2.
- Some people, however, choose a larger, smaller and more expensive pamphlet sizes if the budget can handle it.
- Design the pamphlet by writing the content and identifying the images to be included in the pamphlet.
- Give the pamphlet for proof printing and then check for any mistake, ensure modification, if required.
- Finally print out the needed pamphlets and distribute them according to the best method.
  - Think carefully about the target group before you plan for distribution because different sectors of people gather in different places, e.g. outside the school gates, factory gates, public places.
  - The best way of distributing is door to door where a team drops the pamphlets off at each house in the target area or with newspapers.

C. Styles for organizing a pamphlet

- *Tutorial style:* This is the first and the most basic style of pamphlets. It gives information on a particular subject or explains how something is done.
- *Frequently asked question style:* This is a very effective technique to get an answer to any question fast.
- *Testimonial style:* This is a storytelling mode. A story is narrated about the pamphlet issue. The concepts are introduced one by one historically. This makes the learning process easier for most learners.

Advantages of pamphlets

- They are the best method of dissemination of information or a message to larger group of people.
- They save time and recourses in dissemination of information to a large group of people.

Limitations of pamphlets

- The main disadvantage of pamphlets is that they can waste a lot of money and time if printed pamphlets are not distributed properly.
- Only literate and educated people can be benefited with this educational aid. Furthermore, because of more written content, they capture less attention.
- They do not ensure that the targeted group has surely paid attention and time to read the pamphlet.

II. LEAFLETS

Leaflets are printed educational aids of a single sheet paper folded to make a full page of printed matter on a single side. A leaflet is commonly referred to as any piece of printed information, which includes fact sheets, guides, small booklets, brochures and usually distributed for a campaign to disseminate the information or message to a large population (Fig. 8.23). Leaflets are printed educational media used to propagate a message to a mass population in a short time.

A. Types of leaflets

- *Persuasive leaflets:* Persuasive leaflets are used to spread a message and convince people through the reason and logic printed in the leaflets.
- *Informative leaflets:* These leaflets are used to present the facts that are already known to the people in a target group, and therefore attract and satisfy their curiosity.
- *Directive leaflets:* As the name suggests, these leaflets are used to offer special instructions and directions to the people in a target group which is useful for directing and controlling their activities.

B. Guidelines for preparing leaflets

- A leaflet must be organized under the following headings:
  - *Heading:* Leaflet heading is the part which is most prominently responsible for catching the attention of people and is therefore considered as the most important part of the leaflet. The heading must be precise, focused on the main theme and written in eye catching words and colours.
  - *Subheadings:* Leaflet subheadings are essential when the main heading is not successful in covering the theme of the main text. Further, subheadings may be required if stress is required on a specific point or used to introduce a new paragraph in text so that a gap between the main heading and text can be obtained.

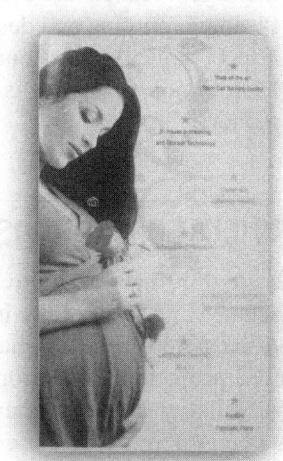

FIGURE 8.23

Leaflets.

- *Text:* The text in leaflets must be as brief as possible and should begin with impressive and interesting sentences to capture the attention of readers. Creditable and verifiable facts must be presented so that readers can believe in the content and can make use of those facts.
- *Pictures:* To make the leaflet more eye catching, the pictures are mixed in the text so that it becomes more easily understandable, interesting and meaningful.
- Good colour combinations and background must be used in organizing the leaflet so that leaflet could be more attractive and amazing.
- The size of leaflet must be customized so that it is easy to carry and read.
- The written words must be large enough so that everyone including the elderly people with diminished eyesight may read the content.
- Leaflets must be a good mixture of text, illustrations and pictures so that they become more interesting for the readers.

Advantages of leaflets

- Leaflets are a good combination of written words, illustrations and pictures so they are more widely accepted.
- They should have facts to enjoy a high level of credibility and prestige in readers.
- They are considered a permanent source of message which cannot be alerted until and unless the leaflet is tampered with.
- A wide range of people may be targeted to spread the message through leaflets.
- A very personal question can also be answered through leaflets which can be read in private, e.g. questions and answers related to safe sexual practices.

Limitations of leaflets

- Illiterate people can be targeted through leaflets to spread a message. They remain deprived of the message if leaflets are used as an education aid for them.
- Planning, printing and designing the leaflets requires a lot of time, effort, men and money.
- Expert, skilled professional manpower is required for planning and designing leaflets.
- Distribution of leaflet is not an easy task, it requires a strong coordination, efforts, time and money.

PROJECTED AUDIOVISUAL AIDS

The use of projected audiovisual aids is not a very recent phenomenon; however, rapid contribution of science and technology in the development of newer projecting audiovisual aids has revolutionized the field of audiovisual aids. Today, there is an availability of the most technologically advanced projecting educational aids such as liquid crystal display (LCD) projectors, which are the most widely media nowadays in educational purposes. The other projected audiovisual media that have been popular in the educational fraternity are overhead projectors, slide projectors, opaque projectors (epidiascope), television, VCR/VCD, cameras and microscopes. Some valuable projected audiovisual aids are discussed below, namely slide projector, overhead projector, opaque projector, filmstrip, television, video cassette recorder (VCR)/DVD player, camera, microscope and LCD player.

I. SLIDE PROJECTOR

A slide projector is a projecting audiovisual device, where small sized (about 2 × 2 inches) transparent pictorial or diagrammatic slides are arranged in a proper sequence for presentation on a large screen. Slide projectors were the most popularly used audiovisual aids in health sciences where teachers used them during lectures to show still pictures using slides prepared from photographs, pictures or a special diagram (Fig. 8.24).

A slide is a small piece of transparent material on which a single pictorial image or scene or graphic image has been photographed or reproduced. Slides are a form of projected media that are easy to prepare. They are still pictures on a positive film which you can process and mount individually yourself or send to a film laboratory. The standard size of the slides is 2 × 2 inches and any 35 mm camera will make satisfactory slides.

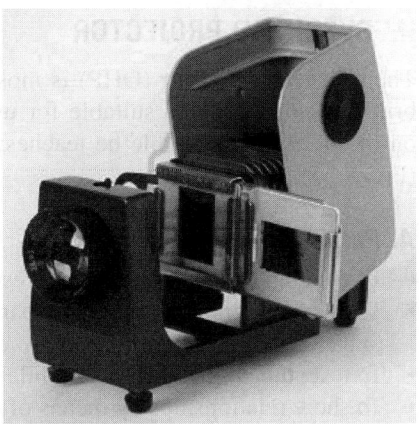

FIGURE 8.24

Slide projector.

The preparation of slides requires imagination and creative ability and they may be prepared from diagrams, pictures and photographs generally captured during life experiences or certain learning experiences such as a picture of a patient with a rare clinical presentation, a specific finding of a pathological laboratory test and so on. At the time of presentation, slides must be presented in a sequence of topics so that they may be used appropriately and efficiently during presentation.

A. Types of slides

- *Photographic slides:* The ideal size is 2 × 2 inches to 3 × 4 inches. Photographic slides could be black and white or coloured.
- *Handmade slides:* Slides used in slide projectors may be handmade using an acetate sheet, cellophane, etched glass, plain glass or a lumarith.

Advantages of a slide projector

- Requires only filming, processing and mounting by self or laboratory.
- Results in colourful and realistic reproduction of original subject.
- Preparation with any 35 mm camera for most uses.
- Easy to revise and update.
- Easily handled, stored and rearranged for various uses.
- Can be combined with taped narration or can be controlled for time during a discussion.
- May be adapted to group or individual use.

Limitations of a slide projector

- Only diagrams, pictures, photographs and abbreviated text can be presented. It can be used to present the written descriptive text.
- Slide preparation requires a lot of predevelopmental work such as collecting or taking a snapshot of the pictures or photographs.
- This method requires a significant amount of imaginative and creative skills.

II. OVERHEAD PROJECTOR

The overhead projector (OHP) is mostly used in all audiovisual aids. It projects transparencies with brilliant screen images suitable for use in a lighted room. The teacher can write or draw diagrams on the transparency while he teaches; these are projected simultaneously on the screen by the OHP (Fig. 8.25).

A. Purposes of an OHP

- To develop concepts and sequences in a subject matter area.
- To make marginal notes on transparencies for the teacher's use that can carry without exposing them to the class.
- To test student performances while other classmates observe.
- To show relationships by means of transparent overlays in contrasting colours.
- To give the illusion of motion in the transparency.

B. OHP transparencies

- Transparencies are a popular instructional medium. They are simple and easy to prepare and easy to operate with the OHP which is lightweight.
- A 10 × 10 inch sheet with printed, written or drawn material is placed on the platform of the projector and a large image is projected on the screen.
- The projector is used from rear to the front of the room with the teacher standing or sitting beside the projector, facing the student.

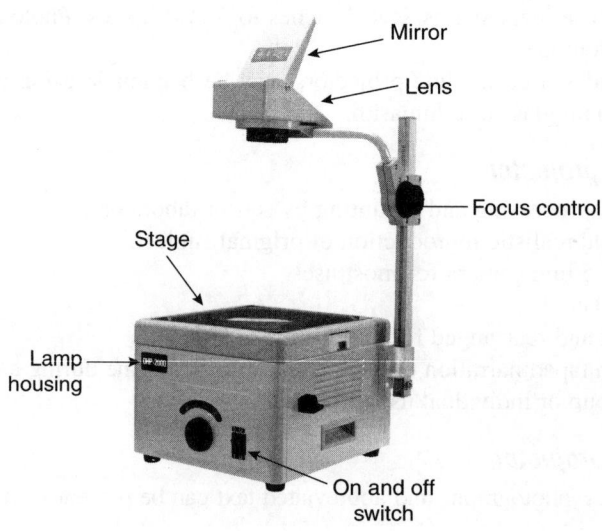

FIGURE 8.25

Overhead projector.

Source: www.uniconinstruments.com

Guidelines for making effective transparencies

- Have one main idea on each transparency.
- Include only related figures and diagrams.
- Ensure that all transparencies are as simple as possible and as easy to read.
- Avoid too much information on any single transparency.
- Use a simple letter style in writing.
- Do not use all capital letters.
- Do not overcrowd the transparency with written content.
- Use diagrams in proportion to its lettering.
- Keep the message clear and simple.
- Emphasize the key messages.
- Use colour and words with discretion.
- Colour can enhance a visual, but can also reduce the effectiveness of the message. Do not overuse the colours in texts of a transparency.
- Be sure what the transparency says is immediately evident in the transparency in the form of an illustration to enhance understanding.

C. Points to remember during an OHP presentation

- Keep the screen above the participants heads (Fig. 8.26).
- Keep the screen in full view of the participants.
- The presenter must make sure that he is not blocking anyone's view when presenting.
- Darken the room appropriately by blocking out sunshine and dimming nearby light.
- Turn the screen off between slides if you are going to talk for more than two minutes.
- Talk to the audience, not to the screen.
- Switch off the bulb of the OHP when not in use to save electricity but the fan must keep running to keep the OHP cool.
- Do not move the OHP when it is in use; it may increase the chances of losing the lamp of the OHP.

Advantages of an OHP

- Permits the teacher to stand in front of the class while using the projector, thus enabling her to point out features appearing on the screen by pointing to the materials at the projector itself and at the same time, to observe the students' reactions to her discussion.
- Gains the students' attention.
- Permits face-to-face interaction with the students.
- Can be used in daylight with a slight darkening of the room.
- Can present information in systemic developmental sequences.
- Requires limited planning and can be prepared in a variety of inexpensive methods.
- Use of an OHP can be quite cheap and transparencies can be used repeatedly.
- Easily available.
- Easy to operate and handle.

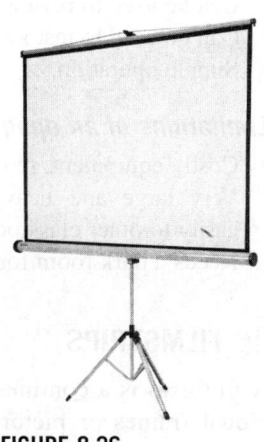

FIGURE 8.26

Projector screen.

Limitations of an OHP

- Cannot be used in situations of power supply interruptions.
- Requires careful handling as OHP bulbs are very sensitive to power fluctuations and jerky movements.
- Preparing transparencies is a time-consuming process and requires good handwriting abilities.

iii. OPAQUE PROJECTOR

Opaque projector is also commonly known as *epidiascope*. It can present images or printed matter or small opaque objects on a screen. Opaque projector is the only projector on which you can project a variety of materials like book pages, objects, coins, postcards or any other similar flat material that is nontransparent. The opaque projector will project and simultaneously enlarge all kinds of written or pictorial matter directly from the originals in any sequence derived by the teacher (Fig. 8.27).

It works on the principle of horizontal straight line projection with a lamp; plane mirror placed at a 45 degree angle over the projector reflects the light so that it passes through the projection lens forming a magnified image on the screen. This large size projector requires a dark room with a fixed place because it is not easily movable due to its heavy weight and size.

Advantages of an opaque projector

- Stimulates attention and arouses interest.
- Can project a wide range of materials like stamps, coins and specimens when one copy is available.
- Can be used for enlarging drawings, pictures and maps.
- Does not require any written or typed materials, handwritten material can be used.
- Helps students retain knowledge for a longer period of time.
- Can be used to review instructional problems.
- Can be used to test knowledge and ability.
- Simple operation.

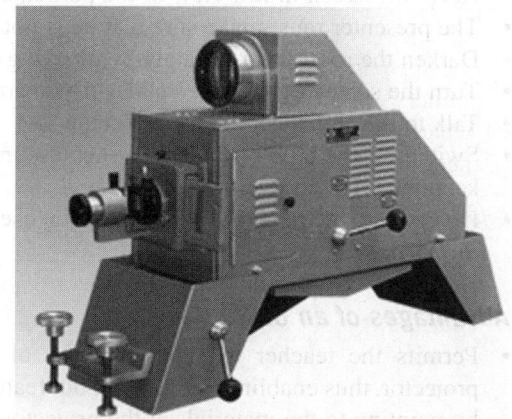

FIGURE 8.27

Opaque projector.

Source: www.uniconinstruments.com

Limitations of an opaque projector

- Costly equipment, requires careful handling.
- Very large and heavy object, cannot be moved easily to other classrooms or place.
- Needs a dark room for projection.

IV. FILMSTRIPS

A filmstrip is a continuous strip of film consisting of individual frames or pictures arranged in a sequence usually with a specific title (Fig. 8.28). In other words, filmstrips are a sequence of transparent still pictures with individual

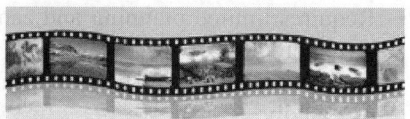

FIGURE 8.28

Filmstrip.

frames on a 35 mm film. A tape-recorded narration can be synchronized with a film strip. Each strip contains between 12 and 18 or more pictures. It is a fixed sequence of related stills on a roll of a 35 mm or an 8 mm film.

Filmstrips are basically used to present a process in a logical consistency and continuity with still pictures so that the whole filmstrip makes a complete presentation. Filmstrips are used to stimulate emotions, build attitudes and point out problems. Filmstrips have been very commonly used for presenting the still pictures in a sequence and continuity along with verbal or audiotape explanation to demonstrate common nursing procedures such as bed bath, back care, crutch walking, intravenous cannulation and nasogastric tube insertion.

A. Types of filmstrips

- *Discussion filmstrip:* It is a continuous strip of film consisting of individual frames arranged in a sequence usually with explanatory titles.
- *Sound slide film:* It is similar to a filmstrip but instead of explanatory titles or spoken discussion, the recorded explanation is audible and is synchronized with the pictures.

B. Guidelines for using filmstrips

- Select the filmstrips carefully to meet the needs of the topic to be taught and preview them before actual presentation.
- An appropriate and efficient congruence must be established between the filmstrip and the topic of study. Before starting the presentation of the filmstrip, it must be appropriately introduced so that the audience is adequately charged to receive the important message.
- The specific details and important points on the filmstrip must be focused by the presenter using a pointer.
- A part of the filmstrip may be shown again if the content needs to be stressed on or needs more specific study.

Advantages of filmstrips

- Filmstrips are compact, easy to handle and always in proper sequence.
- They can be supplemented with a recorded audiotape or verbal explanation.
- They are inexpensive when quantity reproduction is required.
- They are useful for group or individual study as the projection rate is controlled by the instructor or user.
- They are projected with a simple, lightweight equipment.

Limitations of filmstrips

- Preparing the slides is a cumbersome job and requires a lot of effort.
- If the filmstrip is not supplemented with an audiotape, the verbal explanation becomes difficult to understand, especially to the new learners.

V. TELEVISION

Television (TV) is a telecommunication medium for transmitting and receiving moving images that can be monochrome (black and white) or coloured with accompanying sound. Television is a very commonly and widely used medium for sharing and disseminating information between large groups. It is also very popular and widely viewed by different strata of the society because of its specific feature, the combination of audio and visual technology. Televisions have wide variety of uses such as entertainment, sharing information and may also be very effective for educational purposes because of their easy and wide accessibility (Fig. 8.29).

The educational use of television was first reported at the State University of Iowa, USA, in 1932. Later, the popularity of television steeply grew and by 1972 it had become a popular medium for educational instructions. India reportedly started the use of TV in 1959 and in the 1990s the popularity and use of TV grew steeply. Today, TV in India covers more than 70 million homes giving a viewing population more than 400 million individuals through more than 100 channels.

A. Educational uses of television

The instructional television may have the following principal educational uses:

- Television could be *interactive* (allowing the viewers to interact with the instructor or other students live) or *passive* (airing prerecorded programmes) to share educational material for general students that are broadcasted at a particular time so that everyone who is interested may view them.
- Television can be used in a classroom setting where either a telecasted or prerecorded programme may be displayed for students to supplement traditional learning.
- Television may be used for teaching students social, cultural, political and religious affairs of the country by exposing them with the general basic television programmes.
- Television may be used for behaviour modification through showing specific therapeutic programmes.
- Television may also be used for educational entertainment so that students can feel fresh to carry out the next traditional educational activity.

Advantages of television

Television is a visually stimulating medium and is of interest to children. Therefore, it can be used to assist reluctant learners by creating interest and removing pressure that can accompany traditional learning techniques. The main advantages of using television in education are as follows:

- A cost-effective educational media, which is easily available everywhere and large proportion of students may be covered by a single teacher in interactive television programmes.

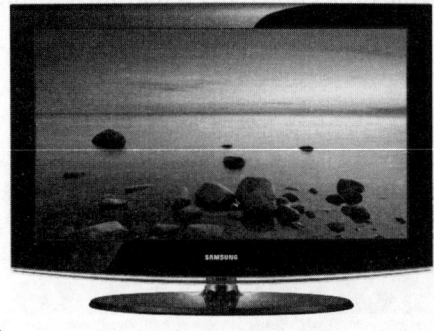 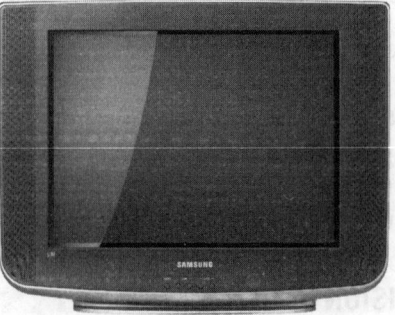

FIGURE 8.29

Television.

Source: www.samsung.com

- A multiple sensory stimulating educational media (sight and sound), which makes learning a recreational and leisure activity by providing real experiences in a stimulating way to learn faster and quicker.
- Television ensures uniformity in learning experience because it offers same basic ideas, information techniques to everyone viewing the educational programme.
- Television provides quicker and long-lasting visual and sound impression because it improves concentration by eliminating the possibilities of environmental distraction.
- Television stimulates and reinforces learning by repetitive presentation of ideas, information and beliefs to the learner that brings permanent change in the behaviour of an individual.
- Revision and repetition of the same educational programme is possible to telecast, which may be used to reinforce knowledge to achieve long-lasting learning.
- Real-life impossible experiences are achieved in the classroom through television because the naturally impossible things such as forests, wild animals and snakes may be brought to the classroom electronically through television.
- Media for mass education: Television is considered as a good education aid for teaching a large group because of television's universal availability.

Limitations of television

- Television educational instructions are generally a one-way process; therefore doubts of the students cannot be clarified.
- It is not a student-centric approach, where instructions are prepared and are not flexible to be moulded according to the situation of a particular group of students in a classroom.
- Underprivileged group of students in schools where television is not available remain deprived of these educational programmes.
- School schedules have to be customized according to the telecast schedule of television educational programmes.

VI. VIDEO CASSETTE RECORDER (VCR)/ VCD PLAYER

The video cassette recorder is an electromechanical educational medium which constitutes an electronic machine, prerecorded video cassettes and the television screen for display (Fig. 8.30). This educational medium is considered as a useful teaching aid because preplanned tailor-made teaching programmes may be prepared and used as and when required for multiple times with audio as well video stimulation for the learners. Gradually with the development of science and technology, the conventional VCR has been replaced by more sophisticated electronic advanced VCD players because of their handiness and cost factors.

A. Educational uses of VCR / VCD player

The VCR and the VCD player are considered as potential educational media for learning a wide range of motor, intellectual, cognitive, and interpersonal and affective skills. These audiovisual educational media have certain specific qualities to bring visual and auditory stimulus, which finally leads to a permanent memory impact and learning. They are used for a

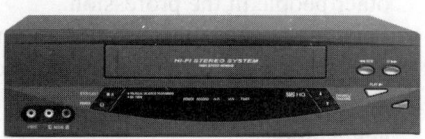

FIGURE 8.30

Video cassette recorder.

wide range of educational purposes ranging from simple classroom content delivery to facilitating distance education.

Advantages of VCR / VCD player

- Easy to access and use for educational purposes.
- Multiple use and repetition of the same content several times is possible.
- They can be used in daylight in the classroom without any special preparation.
- Recording and playing content does not require any special skills and techniques.
- Combines the advantages of both the motion pictures and a tape recorder.

Limitations of VCR / VCD player

- Older playback equipments are bulky and large to transport to different situations.
- Power supply is mandatory to run these equipments; without power supply they do not have any use.
- Recorded content cannot be edited in basic equipments.
- Good quality video recording is a time-consuming and cumbersome task.

VII. CAMERA

Camera is an electromechanical device capable of recording and storing still or movable images (Fig. 8.31). The camera is the most commonly used device in medical and nursing education. The use of camera has further increased with the availability of more advanced assistive education media such as slide projectors, film projectors and LCD projectors, where images taken from real clinical practice are used to educate students using the abovementioned assistive educational devices. The emergence of the digital camera has significantly influenced the use of camera in medical and nursing education because the user may obtain any image and can instantly use the image for teaching.

A. Educational uses of camera

The camera is very widely and significantly used in education; some of the most essential uses of a camera in education are as follows:

- Cameras can improve the teaching presentation by making it more illustrative by adding the images obtained through the camera.
- Some of the images of the patients' rarer clinical issues may be obtained and published to educate other people in the profession.
- Pursuing regular photography and making use of relevant images for teaching purpose.
- Assisting students in special education and autistic applications.
- Providing close-up, macro or micro views of objects, plants or animals.

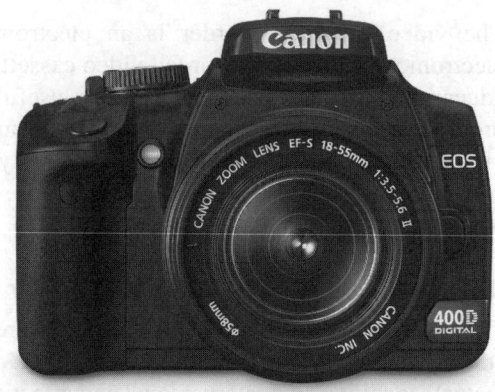

FIGURE 8.31

Camera.

Source: www.canon.co.in

- Enhancing slideshows or presentations by incorporating current relevant pictures from own scenario.
- Encouraging effort through immediate recognition of achievement.
- Recording student progress (including difficult-to-record evidence for process outcomes).
- Analysing physical education activities through photography.
- Recording sequences of events in science experiments (e.g. lifecycles, motion).

B. Some real-world examples of camera use in education

- Using camera for obtaining images of an advanced nursing procedure to disseminate knowledge to people sitting at remote places through telenursing.
- A nurse may monitor the progress of bedsore heeling in a diabetic patient by taking images at different intervals and the same may also be used for teaching the nursing students about the process of bedsore wound healing in a diabetic patient.
- A surgeon may take a few images of a rarer surgical procedure and may use these for publication, presentation in a conference and teaching students.

VIII. MICROSCOPE

The word *microscope* is derived from the Greek word *mikrós* meaning 'small' and 'to look' or 'see'. It is an instrument used to see objects that are too small for the naked eye (Fig. 8.32). The microscope is a device used for visualization of objects or living things such as tissue samples, microorganisms and micro-objects, which cannot be seen by naked eyes. In health sciences, a microscope is the most commonly used teaching device for preclinical and paraclinical subjects such as anatomy, physiology, biochemistry, microbiology, pathology and genetics. The initial microscope used for diagnostic and teaching purposes was the optical microscope where light was used to image the sample. Other advanced microscopes used for medical diagnostic tests and teaching are transmission electron microscope, scanning electron microscope and scanning probe microscope.

A. Uses of microscope in nursing and medical education

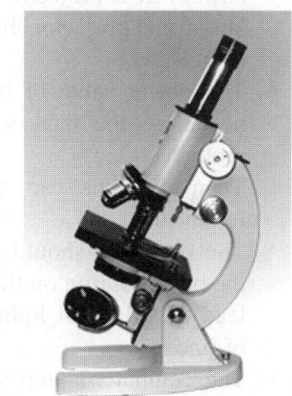

FIGURE 8.32

Microscope.

Source: www.uniconinstruments.com

- The microscope has played a significant role in nursing and medical education; microscope is used for teaching anatomy, physiology, microbiology and pathology to medical and nursing students.
- Microscopes are used in diagnostic laboratories to carry out tests, ranging from the simple blood test to the complex histo-pathological or genetic test, where students can be practically taught through showing live slides of the disease diagnostic tests. This live practical experience helps them comprehend the theory more conveniently and easily.
- Today, microscopes are used to produce and develop pictures of diagnostic findings, which could be used for teaching in classrooms.

IX. LCD PROJECTOR

An LCD projector is a type of video projector for displaying video, images or computer data on a screen or other flat surfaces (Fig. 8.33). The LCD projector was invented by the New York inventor, Gene Dolgoff, in 1984. LCD projectors are increasingly being used in meetings, training sessions, classroom education and visual entertainment. They appeal to all the sensory organs and the impact is always greater than simple speech.

B. Types of LCD projectors

According to their size and portability, LCD projectors are classified in the following three categories:

- Ultralight portable projectors
- Conference room projectors
- Fixed installation projectors

C. Guidelines for using LCD projectors

The following guidelines must be followed while using the LCD projector for educational purposes:

- ***Projection surface:*** White projecting, the surface should be a neutral colour and best suited for natural colour tones.
- ***Setting up the system:*** The following steps must be followed to set up the LCD projection system:
  - The LCD projector must be placed 5–15 feet away from the projection screen, either with a permanently fixed ceiling or placed on a stable surface.
  - Computer/laptop cable should be connected at the back of LCD projector on a video pot and computer/laptop and projector should be effectively connected (Fig. 8.34).
  - The power cable of the projector should be connected to the three-way electrical port which is grounded.
  - Then the lens cap of the projector should be removed.
  - The projector should be switched on by pressing the power button on the top of projector which will lead to a flash of light followed by the projection of image.
  - The computer/laptop should then be started. Then the teacher should right click on the desktop screen and proceed to the graphical properties and graphical output. There, the teacher should click on the Notebook + Monitor option to have content display

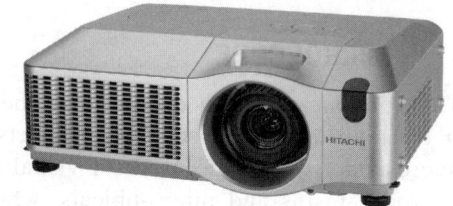

FIGURE 8.33

LCD projector.

Source: www.hitachiconsumer.com

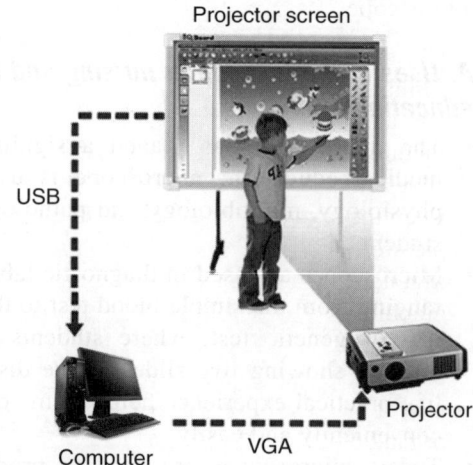

FIGURE 8.34

Connecting LCD projector with computer.

on the projection screen and computer/laptop screen both or the same may be done through the keyboard function key and F3 key.
- The content to be projected should be clearly projected on the projection screen. If projection is not clear then the focus of projection should be fixed using the rings on the lens.
- Further, projection may be adjusted by manipulating the foot of the projector on bottom at front and back.
- *Shutting down the LCD projector:*
  - To shut off the LCD projector, the power button should be pressed; a message may appear to check if you actually want to turn off the projector, the power button should be pressed again and finally projector will turn off.
  - The teacher should wait for the projector fan to off before the projector is unplugged from the electrical port. Also, it must be ensured that the flashing light is off before the projector is unplugged.
- *Warning lights:* In addition to the power button light there are two additional warning light buttons, which are lamp warning light and temperature warning light.
  - The blinking of lamp warning light notifies the need of the lamp to be changed.
  - The blinking of orange colour temperature status light notifies the need to change the air filter, and the red colour temperature status light notifies the increased temperature of the projector and the need to turn off the lamp and allow the running fan to cool the warm lamp.
- *Additional audio and video devices:*
  - The projector has several other additional ports to connect VCR, DVD and cameras which can further improve the utility of the LCD projector in education.

D. Guidelines for powerpoint presentations

PowerPoint presentations are the most popular audiovisual aid in the present educational community because they are believed to be more interesting and visually attractive. A PowerPoint presentation is preferred because of its flexibility in both preparation and presentation. The following guidelines must be followed for the preparation and presentation of PowerPoint presentations:

- Use the horizontal/landscape format for slides.
- Limit the information on each slide to a single topic or idea.
- Use action words and short phrases rather than sentences.
- Pictures, drawings and illustrations make the presentation interesting but as a general rule keep the slides simple and clear.
- Keep the slide simple and clear without overburdening the slides with special effects and irrelevant pictures. Irrelevant images and effects may distract the audience.
- Maintain consistency in use of colour throughout the slides and avoid overuse of multiple colours and graphics.
- Use dark-coloured text on a light background and vice versa, e.g. using white or yellow text on a black background slide.
- Use of bullets instead of numbers is always considered good; only use the numbers to show sequence or rank of presented content.
- Do not overboard the slide with text; try to keep enough open space around the written text on slide.
- Use the 6 × 6 rule that is 6 lines of text and 6 words per line.

- Ensure the text on the slide is readable. It is recommended to use a minimum of 36 points for the slide title and 24 points for the body text.
- Ensure the use of standard styles of written text such Arial fonts, which are easily readable.
- Avoid using only uppercase text (CAPITAL), rather, use upper and lower case text, which is more legible.
- Use contrasting colours to present and highlight specific points but avoid small red text, which is generally not visible.
- Significant points in text may be presented using bold, italic and large size fonts to ensure emphasis.
- To make the presentation more interactive, limit the written content and use simple illustrations.
- Do not use multiple animations and transition effects on a single slide. Limit to one or two animations or transition effects per slide.
- Try developing visual aids that are visually pleasing as well as clear.
- It is generally considered good to limit the number of slides to the number of minutes the presenter has in hand.

Advantages of LCD projectors

- It is a technologically advanced audiovisual aid that can be used for presentation of still slides as well as videos. Slide show and video can be clubbed together and customized in a single presentation.
- It is considered very interesting and visually attractive for the audience.
- Back and forth movement of presenting content can be easily carried out for reinforcing or recapitalizing the whole presentation.

Limitations of LCD projectors

- It is quite an expensive electronic gadget that is not easy to afford.
- Teachers and faculty require technical skills of computer and PowerPoint presentation while using LCD projector.
- In case of power failure or technological failure, it may cause a lot of problems, which are very difficult to manage at the last minute.

AUDIO EDUCATIONAL AIDS

Audio educational aids are popularly known as *auditory aids* and are considered significantly important educational aids because of their access, cost-effectiveness and easy operability. Audio educational aids are very popular in language-learning strategies. The common educational aids that come under this category are radios, taperecorders and gramophones, and most commonly used is tape recorder, which is discussed below.

I. TAPE RECORDER

A tape recorder is a portable electronic gadget used to record, reproduce, erase and rerecord sound on a magnetic tape. This device can be used without any problem by anybody by operating the press buttons attached to the recorder, namely stop, play, wind, rewind, record, pause and eject (Fig. 8.35).

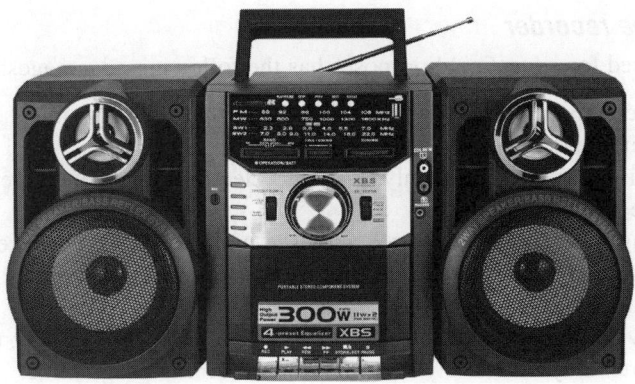

FIGURE 8.35

Tape recorder.

A. Using of a tape recorder in teaching

A record player can be used in the following ways in the actual classroom situation:

- Supplementing a lesson with tape recorder to provide additional information or content.
- Can be used as an appreciation lesson in music or literature class.
- Can be used for students to acquire singing ability, deliver a speech properly and recite a poem in the right way.
- Can be used for reviewing a lesson already presented.
- A tape recorder can be used for physical exercises, yoga or meditation accompanied with relevant music.
- It could be used for recording interviews, talks, discussions of various experts, which could be later used for teaching purposes.

B. Guidelines for using a tape recorder in teaching

The following guidelines must be followed for using the tape recorder for educational purposes:

- The teacher must be familiar or practice the basic functioning of the tape recorder before using it in the classroom setting.
- Proper functioning of the tape and recorded cassette must be ensured by the teacher before final use in the classroom.
- The teacher must prepare, customize and practice the tape-recorded lesson before use in the actual classroom.
- The teacher must prepare tape-recorded material and catalogue it properly.
- The teacher may use prerecorded programmes in a tape recorder from previously recorded actual lessons, radio educational programmes, television programmes, etc.
- The teacher must maintain a tape recorder cassette library on particular subjects which could be used later by the teacher or other faculty members.

Advantages of a tape recorder

Tape recorder when used for educational purposes has the following advantages:

- Tape recorders are commonly available educational aids that are economical as recording tapes can be used multiple times and erasing and rerecording is also possible.
- The tape recorder is the most commonly available electronic gadget; therefore, most people are familiar with its use and functioning.
- A valuable recording can be recoded, stored and used multiple times whenever required.
- In language learning, a tape recorder is very useful because spoken conversation can be recorded and replayed for correcting the individual.
- Hearing of one's own recorded voice provides a positive psychic stimulation; therefore, by using the tape recorder, children may be actively involved in the learning programme.
- Recorded cassettes of interviews or discussion can become an evidence of facts having high legal value and may be used in case of disputes.

PUBLIC ADDRESS SYSTEMS

A public address system is an electronic amplification system made up of the tape recorder, amplifier and loudspeaker to distribute the sound to a large group of people. For example, loudspeakers used for speeches for a large group of people, DJ playing prerecorded music (Fig. 8.36). Small public address systems are commonly used in schools and colleges in the auditorium and examination halls. They may also be used in playgrounds for making announcements and address a large group of students.

I. TYPES OF PUBLIC ADDRESS SYSTEMS

- *Small public address systems:* The simplest public address system consists of a microphone, a modestly powered mixer amplifier and one or more loudspeakers. Simple public address systems of this type, often provide 50–200 watts of power, are often used in small venues such as school auditoriums, churches and small bars. A sound source such as a CD player or a radio may be connected to a public address system so that music or sound can be played through the system.
- *Large public address systems:* Some public address systems have speakers that cover an entire campus of a college or an industrial site, or an entire outdoor complex (e.g. an athletic stadium). More often than not, this public address system is used as a voice alarm system that makes announcements during emergencies to evacuate the occupants in a building.

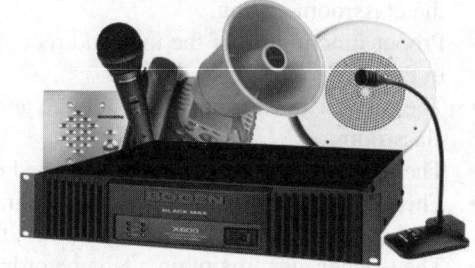

FIGURE 8.36

Public address systems.

COMPUTER

A computer is a programmable machine designed to sequentially and automatically carry out a sequence of arithmetic or logical operations. The particular sequence of operations can be changed readily, allowing the computer to solve more than one kind of problem. A computer is an electronic machine that can work under the control of stored programmes, automatically accepting data to produce the desired results (Fig. 8.37). Conventionally, a computer comprises two basic components, i.e. hardware and software.

Computers are extremely fast, information processing machines. They take a given input, process it and deliver a certain output. The developments in microelectronics and transistors have gone so far that computers are classified in terms of different generations. The first computer ENIAC (Electronics Numerical Integrator and Calculator) was invented in 1946. From that point, we have moved into the age of the fifth generation of supercomputer (based on artificial intelligence). In our lives today, however, fourth generation personal computers are predominantly used. At present, we have the most sophisticated, handy and modern cost-effective computers that have become an essential part of the education system. Computers have become an integral part of each discipline of human operation including the education system because of its specific qualities and characteristics like speed, accuracy, diligence, versatility, vast memory for storage and automation. Unfortunately, the computer has no brain.

I. IMPORTANCE OF A COMPUTER IN EDUCATION

Educational uses of the computer are concerned with more effective learning with the help of the computer. In fact, the computer should be regarded as an add-on rather than a replacing device. It is a technological tool that deserves to be used at the right time, to the right extent and in the right way to improve what has been learnt using other media and source material. The decision of when, how and how much computers should be used for learning should ideally be left to the teacher. The educational applicability of the computer covers almost all subjects ranging from mathematics (the most structured) to music (one of the least structured). The essential uses of computers in education as an educational aid are as follows:

- Computers facilitate active learning in students as they learn through working with computers.
- Computers help in improving the recall ability of learners because of visual impressions.
- They also offer fresh innovative instructional stimuli so that undivided attention of the learner may be ensured.
- They also enhance interactive learning through constant, systematic and desired feedback.
- The interactive computer system can make the learners more autonomous and help them assume greater responsibility for their learning by providing individual adaptive instructions supported by graphics, synthesized speech and modelling software.
- The educational uses of the computer have special significance in distance education because of economic reasons. The computer enables a large number of students in distance education to develop

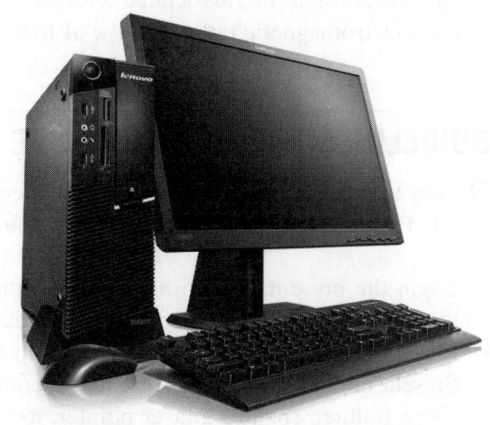

FIGURE 8.37

Computer.

Source: www.lenovo.com

new skills at a much lower cost than is possible through the formal learning system. In distance education, the computer can function as a surrogate for the human tutor even though it lacks the latter's intelligence and flexibility.

Advantages of a computer

Certain essential capabilities and qualities that make computers highly suitable for use in education and training are as follows:

- Computers help to work in a fast and accurate way.
- They are reliable.
- They save time because they perform operations at a high speed.
- They help in doing repetitive work.
- Ideas can be understood quickly and easily through a presentation.
- Photographs or images can be transferred to computers with the help of a scanner or a digital camera.
- They are used as a voice recognition system.
- They store huge amounts of information in formats such as text, sound, picture and film.
- They take up very little space, usually that of one table; you can also have just a *notebook*-type computer on your palm.
- They are portable. One can work on a *notebook* or *laptop* computer even while making a trip.
- They are highly interactive and also enable communication from one place to another.
- They are user-friendly and easy to operate.

Disadvantages of a computer

- Computer is not a very cost-effective tool to be used in all educational settings. Everyone cannot afford the computer for educational purposes.
- Health and safety is crucial to the effective operation of a computer. Stress is widely accepted as a common and possibly the most dangerous aspect of using a computer.
- Computer use is also associated with physical problems such as musculoskeletal problems, eye strain and electromagnetic radiation risk of foetus in pregnant women.

GUIDELINES FOR EFFECTIVE USE OF AUDIOVISUAL AIDS

The key to using graphics and visual aids effectively requires using them so that they make the maximum impact (Table 8.1). The principles of using audiovisual aids are as follows:

- Begin the presentation with no aids, as presenters want their audience to be listening to them, not looking at props, specimens or other visual aids.
- Present the aid at the appropriate point in the presentation and then remove it immediately.
- Present the aid, give audience a few seconds to comprehend it and then comment on the aid.
- Use a pointer, such as a laser pointer, to focus the audience on the part of the graphic that is being discussed by the presenter.
- Be sure to speak slowly and deliberately as the presenter; explain or use a graphic to avoid confusing the audience.

Table 8.1 Comprehensive Description of Selected Types of Audiovisual Aids

Types of Audiovisual Aids	Standard Size	Essential Characteristics	Basic Guidelines for Preparation and Use
Graphic Audiovisual Aids			
1. Charts	90 × 60 cm or 70 × 50 cm	One chart should display information about one area Should display specific information Can be carefully stored and preserved for use in future	Size of letters for caption, labels should be 2–3 cm Every detail depicted should be visible Display material should be contrasted Should not contain too many details Should be neat and tidy
2. Graphs	Various sizes based on purpose	Principle of simplicity must be kept in mind Give bird's eye view of entire information Attractive to the eye Facilitate comparison of data relating to different periods of time	Must have a title and index Proportion between width and height must be balanced Selection of scale must be appropriate Footnotes should be included wherever needed Neatness and cleanliness must be ensured
3. Flash cards	10″ × 12″	Made out of cardboard Simple and understandable 10–12 cards can be used for one talk Message written should be brief	Height of writing should be 5 cm Size of group should not be more than 30 students Arrange in proper sequence Do not cover content with hands while displaying Should be held at chest level against body, not in air
4. Posters	22″ × 28″	Minimal use of words (4–5) Presented idea must be simple and understandable Must be attractive Language should be easy and simple	Use bold illustrations Avoid fancy lettering Attractive and pleasing colours should be used
Display Audiovisual Aids			
1. Chalk-board	5 m × 6 m	Surface should be rough and dull Mounted on appropriate height	Write letters and drawings in large size Writing should be in straight rows Extreme lower corners should not be used Do not use abbreviations Coloured chalks can be used to enhance attraction Avoid spelling mistakes
2. Bulletin board	Size depends on purpose	Framed soft board, straw board or cork board Dark blazer cloth to work as a back drop Height should be 1 m above the ground	Words should catch attention Sort out relevant material Title of the topic must be fixed at the top Should be kept little above the eye level Place bulletin board near the door Board must have neat, ordered and attractive appearance Change the content on the board regularly Overcrowding of the contents must be avoided

Continued

Table 8.1 Comprehensive Description of Selected Types of Audiovisual Aids—cont'd

Types of Audiovisual Aids	Standard Size	Essential Characteristics	Basic Guidelines for Preparation and Use
3. Flannel board	1.5 m × 1.5 m	A piece of rigid material covered with cotton flannel, wool, suede cloth and paper The cut-outs are provided with rough surface at the back by pasting pieces of sandpaper	Content should be organized around the central theme. Material should be displayed attractively Must be neat and orderly Avoid overcrowding on the board Displayed material should be of sufficient size Remove the material as soon as its purpose is over
Three-Dimensional Aids			
1. Specimen	–	Boxes should be covered with cellophane paper Should be mounted in shallow boxes in an artistic way Label each object or specimen	Plan teaching with certain simple and direct observation of objects and specimen Clarify and emphasize important structural details Provide review and practice to make learning permanent
2. Model	–	Three-dimensional Simplifies reality Explains the various processes of objects and machine	Must be of adequate size Relevant appearance closely resembling the actual organ/object Material and colours must be of good quality and appropriate in appearance to illustrate originality Must be used for a small group of students so that presentation and visibility can be enhanced Ideal models may have written labels for promotion of self-explanation
3. Puppets	–	Educational cum entertaining aid Easy to carry and operate Material used should be cost-effective and easily available	Age, background and taste of the audience should be considered while writing the puppet play Puppet plays should be short to maintain the interest of audience Size of the puppets should be appropriate Puppeteer should blend his art with dramatization to produce the desired effect Local language should be used while narration of story

- In addition, remember to talk to the audience maintaining eye contact with them, not only to the visual aid.
- When using slides, tell the audience what they will see, show them the slide, give them time to digest what they are seeing, then comment on the slide.
- Turn off the projector lamp between slides.
- Do not begin talking about another topic while a slide, depicting a past topic, is still showing.
- Remember people cannot see and listen at the same time.

- Use colour to influence mood and emotion.
- The colours for type, illustrations and backgrounds influence the way they are perceived. Here is a basic guide to using colour in presentations:

Red: excitement, alert	**Purple:** dignity, sophistication
Green: growth	**Yellow:** confidence, warmth, wisdom
Blue: truth, trust, justice	**White:** professionalism, new, innocence
Black: authority, strength	**Orange:** action, optimism
Brown: friendliness, warmth	**Grey:** integrity, maturity

- **Text size:** Projected text should be large enough to be read by all viewers (even the people at the end of the room). Ideally, the following text size must be followed:
  - *Headline text:* 36–44 points
  - *Subtext:* 34–36 points
  - *Second-level text:* 24–28 points
  - 28–24 points is a minimum for most situations.
- **Font style:** Regarding the font style, the following guidelines must be followed:
  - Use simple bold running styles of written text content.
  - Use only standardized font styles, such as Arial font, which are easily readable.
  - Do not use only capital text, they are difficult to read; use both upper and lower case text.
- **Images**
  - Use images to supplement text content, which improves understanding.
  - Use images for emphasizing the specific points of the presentation.
  - Do not use an image or illustration to fill the space.
  - Do not use irrelevant pictures or images with text. Those will rather distract the learner.
- **Animation:** It is good to use animation in presentations but keep the animations simple and effective.
- **Other miscellaneous principles**
  - The instructional programme should be organized and administered such that the audiovisual material functions as an integral part of the educational programme.
  - The audiovisual education programme should be organized and administered in such a way that the programme is centralized with a specialized direction and leadership.
  - The audiovisual education programme should be flexible. In addition to those education communication media which are available through purchase, rental or loan, opportunities should be provided which encourage the teacher to personalize their instruction through the preparation of their own instructional materials where feasible.
  - An advisory committee should be appointed to assist in the selection and coordination of audiovisual materials.
  - Audiovisual materials should be available as and when they are needed if they are to be utilized effectively as an integral part of the curriculum.
    - They eliminate frequent duplication of materials.
    - Pooling of equipment makes for more frequent and better use of equipment.
    - They are readily available and accessible to the entire instructional staff.
    - They provide for space for adequate preparation or production of audiovisual materials.

- Provision should be made for helping the instructors to acquire skills in the use of audiovisual materials.
- Budget appropriation should be made regularly for the audiovisual education programme.
- Evaluation of the audiovisual education programme should be made at regular intervals. Evaluation of the function and the use of each audiovisual aid should be done continuously.
- Legal aspects should be considered in the production and the utilization of educational communication media.

- **Additional presenter tips:** A presenter may follow the following tips to make presentation more successful:
  - Arrive early for the presentation so that the presenter can feel psychologically comfortable and ready.
  - Check out the equipment, lights and set-up so that the presentation may proceed smoothly later.
  - Get oriented to rooms, lighting and audiovisual aid for effective operation during needs.
  - Brush up on giving your presentation to feel comfortable.
  - Give yourself time to feel prepared and confident before the presentation.

REVIEW QUESTIONS

Long-Answer Questions

1. Discuss audiovisual aids.
2. Explain the importance of audiovisual aids in teaching nursing and describe the principles in use for any two educational aids.
3. Discuss audiovisual aids and their use in teaching. Explain with suitable examples.
4. Discuss audiovisual aids in nursing education.
5. Discuss blackboard/chalkboard.
6. Define audiovisual aids and write the importance of using audiovisual aids in nursing education.
7. Discuss bulletin board and its principles.
8. List the various audiovisual aids and discuss how a blackboard is a simple and effective visual aid used for teaching.
9. Differentiate between blackboard and bulletin board.
10. Discuss educational communication media.
11. Discuss effective use of overhead projector.
12. Discuss the role of a teacher in using teaching aids effectively.
13. Enumerate the criteria for the selection of audiovisual aids.
14. Discuss flash cards.
15. Discuss the importance of a blackboard.
16. List the purposes of audiovisual aids in nursing education and elaborate the advantages of computer as a teaching aid.
17. List the types of audiovisual aids and write about three-dimensional aids used in nursing education.

18. Discuss posters.
19. Write about projected teaching aids.
20. Discuss puppets.
21. Discuss slide projectors.
22. Write about tape recorders.
23. Explain the uses of a flannel board.
24. Discuss the types and advantages and disadvantages of blackboards.
25. Discuss the principles in use in audiovisual aids.
26. Discuss the role of audiovisual aids in teaching.
27. Discuss the various types of audiovisual aids.
28. Discuss graphic audiovisual aids.
29. Enumerate sources of audiovisual aids.
30. Explain the principles to be followed for the effective use of audiovisual aids.
31. Explain different types of chart.

Short-Answer Questions

1. Discuss briefly four characteristics of good audiovisual aids.
2. Mention four types of blackboard.
3. List down the projected audiovisual aids.
4. Classify instructional aids.

Multiple-Choice Questions (MCQs)

1. Leaflet is made up of
   (a) Full page
   (b) Two pages
   (c) Half page
   (d) Five pages
2. How many folds do pamphlets contain?
   (a) 2 to 5
   (b) 2 to 6
   (c) 2 to 7
   (d) 2 to 8
3. Full page, single side printed material is called
   (a) Leaflet
   (b) Handout
   (c) Pamphlet
   (d) Flash card
4. A paper that is both sides printed with three-fold is known as
   (a) Leaflet
   (b) Pamphlet
   (c) Handout
   (d) Flash card

5. What is the appropriate size of flash card?
   (a) 10″ × 10″
   (b) 10″ × 12″
   (c) 12″ × 14″
   (d) 12″ × 12″
6. Flash card can be used for group of
   (a) 40
   (b) 20
   (c) 35
   (d) 45
7. Ideally how many flash cards can be used for one health talk/one session?
   (a) 01 to 02
   (b) 10 to 12
   (c) 20 to 25
   (d) 25 to 30
8. Appropriate size of letter for making posters
   (a) 10″ × 20″
   (b) 15″ × 25″
   (c) 22″ × 28″
   (d) 5″ × 15″
9. Percentile, quartile deviation can be drawn on
   (a) Cumulative frequency
   (b) Ogive
   (c) Histogram
   (d) Frequency polygon
10. Angle of pie graph is
    (a) 90°
    (b) 180°
    (c) 360°
    (d) None of these
11. Graphical presentation of data can be drawn for
    (a) Qualitative data
    (b) Quantitative data
    (c) Raw data
    (d) Abstract data
12. Which one of the following is not a type of a map?
    (a) Relief maps
    (b) Historical maps
    (c) Distribution map
    (d) Overlay maps
13. To show the complication of disease you will use
    (a) Job chart
    (b) Flow chart
    (c) Tree chart
    (d) Pie chart

14. To show family history of patient, you will use
  (a) Tabulation
  (b) Genealogy chart
  (c) Flow chart
  (d) Tree chart
15. Which one of the following is one-way communication aid?
  (a) Television
  (b) Radio
  (c) Both (a) and (b)
  (d) None of these

Answer to the Mulitple-Choice Questions

1. (a), 2. (a), 3. (b), 4. (b), 5. (b), 6. (b), 7. (b), 8. (a), 9. (c), 10. (c), 11. (b), 12. (c), 13. (b), 14. (d), 15. (c).

FURTHER READING

Alexander, M., Lenahan, P., & Pavlov, A. (2005). *The future of cinemeducation*. Abingdon, UK: Radcliffe Publishing.

Amory, A. (2001). Building an educational adventure game: Theory, design, and lessons. *Journal of Interactive Learning Research*, 12(2–3), 249–263.

Anglin, G. J., Vaez, H., & Cunningham, K. L. (2004). *Visual representations and learning: The role of static and animated graphics*. Mahwah, NJ: Lawrence Erlbaum Associates Publishers.

Atkinson, R. K. (2005). *Multimedia learning of mathematics*. New York: Cambridge University Press.

Barron, A. E. (2004). *Auditory instruction*. Mahwah, NJ: Lawrence Erlbaum Associates Publishers.

Belliveau, P. P., & Perla, R. J. (2007). Antibiogram-derived radial decision trees: Innovative visual educational tools for discussing empirical antibiotic selections. *Pharmacy Education*, 7(1), 43–51.

Betrancourt, M. (2005). *The animation and interactivity principles in multimedia learning*. New York: Cambridge University Press.

Block, G., Miller, M., Harnack, L., Kayman, S., Mandel, S., & Cristofar, S. (2000). An interactive CD-ROM for nutrition screening and counselling. *American Journal of Public Health*, 90(5), 781–785.

Bouman, M. (2004). *Entertainment-education television drama in the Netherlands*. Mahwah, NJ: Lawrence Erlbaum Associates Publishers.

Brett, R. P. (2003). Allocation of support levels to hearing-impaired children: Moving away from using audiometric descriptors. *Deafness & Education International*, 5(3), 167–181.

Burn, A., & Durran, J. (2006). *Digital anatomies: Analysis as production in media education*. Mahwah, NJ: Lawrence Erlbaum Associates Publishers.

Carey, M., Schofield, P., Jefford, M., Krishnasamy, M., & Aranda, S. (2007). The development of audio-visual materials to prepare patients for medical procedures: An oncology application. *European Journal of Cancer Care*, 16(5), 417–423.

Casarotti, M., Filipponi, L., Pieti, L., & Sartori, R. (2002). Educational interaction in distance learning: Analysis of a one-way video and two-way audio system. *PsychNology Journal*, 1(1), 28–38.

Chang, C. K. (2004). Constructing a streaming video-based learning forum for collaborative learning. *Journal of Educational Multimedia and Hypermedia*, 13(3), 245–263.

Clark, R. C. (2005). *Multimedia learning in e-courses*. New York: Cambridge University Press.

Clark, R. E., & Feldon, D. F. (2005). *Five common but questionable principles of multimedia learning*. New York: Cambridge University Press.

Clarke, J. O. (1975). Improving teaching techniques through the use of A-V materials. *Journal Pendidikan*, U.K.M., No. 14, 7–59.

Claudet, J. (2002). Integrating school leadership knowledge and practice using multimedia technology: Linking national standards, assessment, and professional development. *Journal of Personnel Evaluation in Education*, 16(1), 29–43.

Claudet, J. (2002). Issues and directions in technology-integrated personnel assessment and professional development. *Journal of Personnel Evaluation in Education*, 16(1), 7–10.

Cobb, S., & Fraser, D. S. (2005). *Multimedia learning in virtual reality*. New York: Cambridge University Press.

Copley, J. (2007). Audio and video podcasts of lectures for campus-based students: Production and evaluation of student use. *Innovations in Education and Teaching International*, 44(4), 387–399.

Creighton-Zollar, A. (2006). *Communicating across preferences: A comparative family systems example*. New York: Haworth Press.

Croker, S. (2003). Review of secrets of the mind CD ROMs. *Psychology Learning & Teaching*, 3(1), 69–70.

Damore-Petingola, S., Lightfoot, N., Vaillancourt, C., Mayer, C., Steggles, S., & Gauthier-Frohlick, D. (2002). Hear how I feel: Evaluation of a video depicting the experiences of adolescents and young adults with a parent diagnosed with cancer. *Journal of Psychosocial Oncology*, 20(4), 57–69.

Davies, D. K., Stock, S. E., & Wehmeyer, M. L. (2002). Enhancing independent task performance for individuals with mental retardation through use of a handheld self-directed visual and audio prompting system. *Education & Training in Mental Retardation & Developmental Disabilities*, 37(2), 209–218.

Dewald, B. W. A. (2000). Turning part-time students' feedback into video programs. *Education & Training*, 42(1), 33–39.

Dillon, A., & Jobst, J. (2005). *Multimedia learning with hypermedia*. New York: Cambridge University Press.

Douglas, G. (2001). ICT, education, and visual impairment. *British Journal of Educational Technology*, 32(3), 353–364.

Dowaliby, F., & Lang, H. G. (1999). Adjunct aids in instructional prose: A multimedia study with deaf college students. *Journal of Deaf Studies and Deaf Education*, 4(4), 270–282.

Elbon, S., Nsubuga, P., Knowles, J., Bobrow, E., Parvanta, I., Timmer, A., et al. (2006). Micronutrient action plan instructional tool (MAPit): A training tool to support public health professionals' efforts to eliminate micronutrient malnutrition. *Innovations in Education and Teaching International*, 43(4), 353–368.

Finlayson, R., Schneider, J., Wan, M., Irons, R., & Sealy, J. (1999). Sexual addiction portrayed in cinema. *Sexual Addiction & Compulsivity*, 6(2), 151–159.

Fleming, M. (1982). Changing conceptions in research on pictures. *Communication & Cognition*, 15(1), 53–60.

Fletcher, J. D., & Tobias, S. (2005). *The multimedia principle*. New York: Cambridge University Press.

Franks, F. L., & Glass, R. (1985). Microslide Cassette Programs for low vision students. *Education of the Visually Handicapped*, 17(1), 11–16.

Galvez Diaz, V., & Waldegg, G. (2004). Science and scientific knowledge in educational television. *Ensenanza de las Ciencias Revista de investigacion y experiencias didacticas*, 2(1), 147–158.

Goodman, S. (2005). *The practice and principles of teaching critical literacy at the educational video center*. Malden, MA: Blackwell Publishing.

Gouzouasis, P. (1994). Multimedia constructions of children: An exploratory study. *Journal of Computing in Childhood Education*, 5(3–4), 273–284.

Graff, M. (2003). Assessing learning from hypertext: An individual differences perspective. *Journal of Interactive Learning Research*, 14(4), 425–438.

Graves, D., Ray, R., & Thompson, D. (1986). Audiovisual training materials to support mainstreaming. *Pointer*, 31(1), 29–33.

Hayes, M. T., & Petrie, G. M. (2006). We're from the generation that was raised on television: A qualitative exploration of media imagery in elementary preservice teachers video production. *International Journal of Qualitative Studies in Education*, 19(4), 499–517.

Hegarty, M. (2005). *Multimedia learning about physical systems*. New York: Cambridge University Press.

Hernandez-Ramos, P. (2007). Aim, shoot, ready! Future teachers learn to 'do' video. *British Journal of Educational Technology*, 38(1), 33–41.

Higgins, J. A., & Dermer, S. (2001). The use of film in marriage and family counselor education. *Counselor Education and Supervision*, 40(3), 182–192.

Hizal, A. (1983). *Uzaktan Ogretim Surecleri ve Yazili Gerecler (Distance Teaching Process and Print Materials)*. Ankara, Turkey: Ankara Universitesi Egitim Fakultesi Yayinlari.

Jeste, D. V., Dunn, L. B., Folsom, D. P., & Zisook, D. (2008). Multimedia educational aids for improving consumer knowledge about illness management and treatment decisions: A review of randomized controlled trials. *Journal of Psychiatric Research*, 42(1), 1–21.

Jewell, J., Hupp, S., & Luttrell, G. (2004). The effectiveness of fatal vision goggles: Disentangling experiential versus onlooker effects. *Journal of Alcohol and Drug Education*, 48(3), 63–84.

Johnson, L. (2006). Lights…camera…educate: A tool to engage and enthuse students in medical education. *PsycCRITIQUES*, 51(9), 2006.

Jonassen, D. H., Lee, C. B., Yang, C. C., & Laffey, J. (2005). *The collaboration principle in multimedia learning*. New York: Cambridge University Press.

Jones, L., & McNamara, O. (2004). The possibilities and constraints of multimedia as a basis for critical reflection. *Cambridge Journal of Education*, 34(3), 279–296.

King, J. (2002). Using DVD feature films in the EFL classroom. *Computer Assisted Language Learning*, 15(5), 509–523.

Kirkpatrick, H. A. (2005). *Technological considerations*. Abingdon, UK: Radcliffe Publishing.

Kompolt, P. (1984). Function and tasks of film in education. *Jednotna Skola*, 36(3), 243–253.

Konrad, J. L., & Yoder, J. D. (2000). Adding feminist therapy to videotape demonstrations. *Teaching of Psychology*, 27(1), 57–58.

Kozma, R., & Russell, J. (2005). *Multimedia learning of chemistry*. New York: Cambridge University Press.

Krupinski, E. A., Lopez, A. M., Lyman, T., Barker, G., & Weinstein, R. S. (2004). Continuing education via telemedicine: Analysis of reasons for attending or not attending. *Telemedicine Journal and e-Health*, 10(3), 403–409.

Lajoie, S. P., & Nakamura, C. (2005). *Multimedia learning of cognitive skills*. New York: Cambridge University Press.

Lan, W. Y., & Morgan, J. (2003). Videotaping as a means of self-monitoring to improve theater students' performance. *Journal of Experimental Education*, 71(4), 371–381.

Lancioni, G. E., O'Reilly, M. F., Singh, N. N., Sigafoos, J., Oliva, D., Baccani, S., et al. (2004). Technological aids to promote basic developmental achievements by children with multiple disabilities: Evaluation of two cases. *Cognitive Processing*, 5(4), 232–238.

Lemaire, E. D., & Greene, G. (2003). A comparison between three electronic media and in-person learning for continuing education in physical rehabilitation. *Journal of Telemedicine and Telecare*, 9(1), 17–22.

Lepard, D. H. (2002). Using peers and technology to strengthen leadership. *Journal of Personnel Evaluation in Education*, 16(1), 11–28.

Lowe, R. K. (2005). *Multimedia learning of meteorology*. New York: Cambridge University Press.

Mayer, R. E. (2005). *Introduction to multimedia learning*. New York: Cambridge University Press.

Mayer, R. E. (2005). *Principles for managing essential processing in multimedia learning: Segmenting, pretraining, and modality principles*. New York: Cambridge University Press.

Mayer, R. E. (2005). *Principles of multimedia learning based on social cues: Personalization, voice, and image principles*. New York: Cambridge University Press.

Metha, A. A. (2003). *Learning in high dimensional spaces: Applications, theory, and algorithms. Dissertation Abstracts International: Section B: The Sciences and Engineering*. Washington DC: University of Washington.

Moreno, R. (2005). *Multimedia learning with animated pedagogical agents*. New York: Cambridge University Press.

Moss, J., Deppeler, J., Astley, L., & Pattison, K. (2007). Student researchers in the middle: Using visual images to make sense of inclusive education. *Journal of Research in Special Educational Needs*, 7(1), 46–54.

Ofiesh, N. S., Rice, C. J., Long, E. M., Merchant, D. C., & Gajar, A. H. (2002). Service delivery for postsecondary students with disabilities: A survey of assistive technology use across disabilities. *College Student Journal,* 36(1), 94–108.

Olivero, F., John, P., & Sutherland, R. (2004). Seeing is believing: Using videopapers to transform teachers' professional knowledge and practice. *Cambridge Journal of Education,* 34(2), 179–191.

Parish, S. J., Weber, C. M., Steiner-Grossman, P., Milan, F. B., Burton, W. B., & Marantz, P. R. (2006). Teaching clinical skills through videotape review: A randomized trial of group versus individual reviews. *Teaching and Learning in Medicine,* 18(2), 92–98.

Parra-Medina, D., Wilcox, S., Thompson-Robinson, M., Sargent, R., & Will, J. C. (2004). A replicable process for redesigning ethnically relevant educational materials. *Journal of Women's Health,* 13(5), 579–588.

Pearson, S., & Ralph, S. (2007). The identity of SENCos: Insights through images. *Journal of Research in Special Educational Needs,* 7(1), 36–45.

Peraya, D. (1984). Audiovisual pedagogy: Myths and actual trends. *Revue Belge de Psychologie et de Pedagogie,* 46(185–186), 19–32.

Plass, J. L., & Jones, L. C. (2005). *Multimedia learning in second language acquisition.* New York: Cambridge University Press.

Prosser, J., & Loxley, A. (2007). Enhancing the contribution of visual methods to inclusive education. *Journal of Research in Special Educational Needs,* 7(1), 55–68.

Puzanov, B. P. (1983). Use of graph-projector at the history lessons in the school for mentally retarded children. *Defektologiya,* 2, 44–47.

Ramirez, A. (2000). *Assessing the cognitive fit of hypertext-based learning aids for advanced learning in complex and ill-structured domains. Dissertation Abstracts International Section A: Humanities and Social Sciences.* Washington DC: University of Washington.

Reinking, D. (2005). *Multimedia learning of reading.* New York: Cambridge University Press.

Rieber, L. P. (2005). *Multimedia learning in games, simulations, and microworlds.* New York: Cambridge University Press.

Robertson, M., & Collins, A. (2003). The video role model as an enterprise teaching aid. *Education & Training,* 45(6), 331–340.

Rouet, J.-F., & Potelle, H. (2005). *Navigational principles in multimedia learning.* New York: Cambridge University Press.

Roy, M., & Chi, M. T. H. (2005). *The self-explanation principle in multimedia learning.* New York: Cambridge University Press.

Schnotz, W., & Rasch, T. (2005). Enabling, facilitating, and inhibiting effects of animations in multimedia learning: Why reduction of cognitive load can have negative results on learning. *Educational Technology Research and Development,* 53(3), 47–58.

Shapiro, A. M. (2005). *The site map principle in multimedia learning.* New York: Cambridge University Press.

Sharma, V. (1988). Educational technology and multi-media language learning: A psychological consideration. *Psycho-Lingua,* 18(1), 1–10.

Shephard, K. (2003). Questioning, promoting and evaluating the use off streaming video to support student learning. *British Journal of Educational Technology,* 34(3), 295–308.

Skouge, J. R., Rao, K., & Boisvert, P. C. (2007). Promoting early literacy for diverse learners using audio and video technology. *Early Childhood Education Journal,* 35(1), 5–11.

Slavenas, R. D. (1981). *The effect of audiovisual presentation on interest in books of preschool children.* Dissertation Abstracts International.

Sloan, D., Stratford, J., & Gregor, P. (2006). Using multimedia to enhance the accessibility of the learning environment for disabled students: Reflections from the skills for access project. *ALT-J Research in Learning Technology,* 14(1), 39–54.

Sweller, J. (2005). *Implications of cognitive load theory for multimedia learning.* New York: Cambridge University Press.

Sweller, J. (2005). *The redundancy principle in multimedia learning.* New York: Cambridge University Press.

Thierry, K. L., Goh, C. L., Pipe, M.-E., & Murray, J. (2005). Source recall enhances children's discrimination of seen and heard events. *Journal of Experimental Psychology: Applied,* 11(1), 33–44.

Thompson, D. E., Brooks, K., & Lizarraga, E. S. (2003). Perceived transfer of learning: From the distance education classroom to the workplace. *Assessment & Evaluation in Higher Education,* 28(5), 539–547.

Wiley, J., & Ash, I. K. (2005). *Multimedia learning of history.* New York: Cambridge University Press.

Wilksch, S. M., Tiggemann, M., & Wade, T. D. (2006). Impact of interactive school-based media literacy lessons for reducing internalization of media ideals in young adolescent girls and boys. *International Journal of Eating Disorders,* 39(5), 385–393.

Williams, C., Griffin, K. W., Macaulay, A. P., West, T. L., & Gronewold, E. (2005). Efficacy of a drug prevention CD-ROM intervention for adolescents. *Substance Use & Misuse,* 40(6), 869–878.

Zabel, B. (2007). *Using technology and music to motivate science students.* Thousand Oaks, CA: Corwin Press.

Zahn, D. K. (1973). *A study to evaluate the effectiveness of audio-tutorial, slide/tape instruction versus the flowcharted method of self-instruction in machine calculation.* Dissertation Abstracts International.

Zeedyk, M. S., & Wallace, L. (2003). Tackling children's road safety through edutainment: An evaluation of effectiveness. *Health Education Research,* 18(4), 493–505.

9

Assessment

Assessment efforts should not be concerned about valuing what can be measured but, instead, about measuring that which is valued.
—B.N. Sharma

LEARNING OBJECTIVES

This chapter is designed to enable the reader to

- Understand the concept of measurement, assessment and evaluation
- Describe the meaning, purposes, scope and types of assessment
- Appraise the criteria for selection of assessment techniques and methods
- Classify the assessment tools and techniques
- Discuss the concept, purposes, features, principles, advantages and disadvantages of different assessment techniques, such as essay type questions, short answer questions, multiple-choice questions, observation checklist, rating scale, practical examination and viva voce
- Demonstrate the skills in conducting the objective structured clinical examination
- Explain the concept, purposes, features, principles, advantages and disadvantages of different attitude measurement scales such as Likert scale and semantic differential scale

KEY TERMS

INTRODUCTION

Assessment is part of the everyday activities of nursing professionals. People also regularly check out our life progress by evaluating our achievements in life. Assessment is the most important but often neglected part of nursing education as well as nursing care provided by nurses through the nursing process approach. Assessment is the only way by which a teacher can know how successful his teaching was and what areas in teaching need improvement. Similarly, a student can know his learning difficulties and also at what position he stands in the crowd of students. Assessment is also necessary to determine to what extent the curriculum objectives have been achieved and the need for improvement.

CONCEPTS OF MEASUREMENT, ASSESSMENT AND EVALUATION

Evaluation, measurement and assessment are three different terms that are certainly connected and interchangeably used. However, it is essential to consider them distinct as well as interconnected ideas and processes.

Measurement refers to the process by which the physical specifications (length, height, weight) of an object are determined. Measurement is the process of assigning a number to an attribute (or phenomenon) according to a rule or set of rules. The term can also be used to refer to the result obtained after performing the process. Measurement is a collection of quantitative data. Measurement is made by comparing a quantity with a standard unit. As this comparison cannot be perfect, measurements are subjected to error.

Educational settings may involve the measurement of attitude, IQ, etc. For measurement, we require standardized tools and a person who is skilled in administering those tools. For example, we require a thermometer to measure temperature, a BP instrument to measure blood pressure, a pulseoxymeter to measure oxygen saturation and so on. We will also require a physician or nurse to administer these tools to gather data. The end result of measurement is the collection of data. Measurement is the application of a standard scale or measuring device to an object, event or condition, according to practices accepted by those who are skilled in the use of the device or scale.

Now let us see what *assessment* means. Students frequently hear from a teacher that they will have an assessment test on so and so date. The idea of assessment should now be clear in your mind; it is simply a test that is conducted to test the progress of the student against some predetermined learning objectives. Remember, all tests are assessments but all assessments are not tests. Sometimes, a teacher may require some tools for the assessment, for example, basic life support skill assessment checklist to assess the BLS skills of undergraduate nursing students. Assessment is the specified condition by which the behaviour laid down in an objective may be ascertained. Such specifications are usually in the form of written descriptions. So, assessment is the process of documenting, usually in measurable terms, knowledge, skills, attitude and beliefs.

Evaluation is perhaps the most frequently used and the least attended term. It is not simply administering the test, checking answer sheets and announcing marks to the students. What remains in the heart of evaluation is the 'value or quality judgement'. Without using these two core words, evaluation cannot be explained. Evaluation is the most powerful tool in the hands of the teacher to enhance learning. Evaluation is a process that starts with the specification of the criteria or objectives for evaluation; preparing and administering the test (reliable and valid) based on the prespecified criteria; gathering data and facts, and making a judgement whether the objectives are achieved or not; making judgements about the quality, appropriateness, worthiness, validity and goodness of this achievement; and if the criteria or objectives are not achieved, searching for reasons behind this failure, generating solutions to overcome the barriers leading to failure. Evaluation is the process of systematically assessing the design, implementation and impact of programmes, policies or projects.

For example, I often tell my students if they wanted to determine the temperature of the classroom they would need to get a thermometer and take several readings at different spots, and perhaps average the readings. That is simple measuring. The average temperature tells us nothing about whether or not it is appropriate for learning. To do that, students would have to be polled in some reliable and valid way. That polling process is what evaluation is all about. An average classroom temperature of 75°F is simply information. It is the context of the temperature for a particular purpose that provides the criteria for evaluation. A temperature of 75°F may not be very good for some students, while for others, it is ideal for learning.

MEANING OF ASSESSMENT/EVALUATION

Evaluation is the process of determining to what extent the educational objectives are being realized.

—Ralph Tyler

Evaluation is the process of determining the extent to which objectives are being achieved, the effectiveness of the learning experiences provided in the classroom and how well the goals of education have been accomplished.

—NCERT

Evaluation is the assessment of merits and or worth.

—Scriven

Evaluation is a value judgment on an observation, 'performance test' or indeed any data whether directly measured or inferred.

—International Dictionary of Education

Evaluation is a systematic examination of educational and social progress.

—Conbach et al

Educational evaluation is a process of estimating and appraising the degree and dimensions of student's achievement. Further, it is also a process of estimating and appraising the proficiency level of the particular educational practice, which is being conducted. It is a way of appraising the application of educational theory in practice.

—K. Sudha Rao

Evaluation in education is a systematic process which enables the extent to which the student has attained the educational objectives to be measured. Evaluation always includes measurements (quantitative or qualitative) plus a value judgment.

—J.J. Gulbert

Evaluation involves assessing the strengths and weaknesses of programs, policies, personnel, products, and organizations to improve their effectiveness.

—American Evaluation Association

Continuous evaluation is evaluating patient needs and their progress and determining how well their health care needs are being met. Evaluation is a means of helping an individual or a group to become self-directing; it assists in the establishment of goals which, in turn, serve as a criterion for judging desirable changes. A complete evaluation programme for a teacher of nursing would encompass the evaluation of the following:

- Educational objectives
- Teaching and learning procedures
- Student's progress outcome

TYPES OF ASSESSMENT/EVALUATION

The description of the types of assessment or evaluation may be seen in Box 9.1.

PURPOSES OF ASSESSMENT/EVALUATION

Evaluation serves distinct purposes for students, teachers, curriculum and society. The teacher should have a complete programme of evaluation, which should be considered an integral, continuous part of teaching as it enables the teacher to accomplish essential purposes. Imagine what will happen if individuals are provided with nursing degrees without proper and objective evaluation? It will ultimately lead to a compromised and poor quality nursing care because incompetent candidates may obtain nursing degrees or licenses in the absence of an efficient evaluation system, which may be disastrous for

BOX 9.1 DESCRIPTION OF TYPES OF ASSESSMENT/EVALUATION

Parameters	Formative assessment	Summative assessment
Meaning	It is an ongoing assessment of the student's achievement while the instructional course/programme is in progress.	It is the final assessment of the student's achievement at the end of a unit/course/programme.
Purposes	To monitor the progress of students and provide feedback for improvement while instructions are in progress.	To finally assign the grades or pass/fail status in a particular educational module or programme.
Frequency	Carried out quite frequently ranging from daily to weekly while instructions are in progress.	Carried out monthly, biannually, annually or at the end of a semester course/progress.
Content focus	Detailed focus on content.	General and broad content scope.
Methods	Methods of formative assessment include classroom questioning, daily assignments, regular formal/informal observation, class tests and internal assessments.	Methods of summative assessment include project evaluation, term examination and final external examination.

the profession in long term. Evaluation serves the following distinct purposes for students, teachers, curriculum and society:

- To provide short-term goals to the students to work towards the achievement of educational objectives.
- To clarify the intended learning outcome.
- To determine the level of knowledge and understanding in students.
- To diagnose the strengths and weaknesses of students.
- To encourage student learning by measuring their achievement and informing them about their success.
- To provide information to students for overcoming learning difficulties and selecting future learning experiences.
- To estimate the effectiveness of the instructional media used and the usefulness of instructional materials.
- To help students acquire the attitude and skills of self-evaluation.
- To assess the nonscholastic domains of the student's personality (interests, attitudes and values).
- To provide feedback to the students about their strengths and weaknesses requiring their special attention.
- To assess the student's progress throughout the year.
- To determine whether a particular student is competent enough to be advanced to the next class.
- To ascertain if the teaching strategies are effective and if there is a need to change the teaching strategies.
- To improve curriculum in light of recent advances.
- To satisfy the university requirements for a curriculum.
- To recommend the names of students eligible for a degree to the university.
- To report the student's progress to parents.
- To prevent the society from quacks and incompetent professionals by blocking them from getting degrees/diplomas.
- Evaluation is carried out for general and educational research.

SCOPE OF ASSESSMENT/EVALUATION

There is a broad and wide scope of assessment and evaluation as discussed below (Fig. 9.1).

- **Selection of students:** Selection of students in the institute is the first and foremost scope of assessment because the right students in the right educational programmes are essential for the ultimate growth and development of a country. This can be ensured through the means of assessment for student selection.
- **Feedback to students:** Feedback is necessary for efficient remedial measures in time. Therefore, assessments have a wide scope to offer timely feedback to students so that they can improve and the educational objectives may be achieved.
- **Feedback to teachers:** Assessment does offer feedback to teachers about the student's progress so they can plan and implement corrective measures to support the students in achieving the educational objectives.
- **Incentive to learning:** Students feel an incentive to learning when they are assessed and feedback is given to them. They get a feeling of incentive that reduces boredom in the routine, monotonous teaching–learning process.

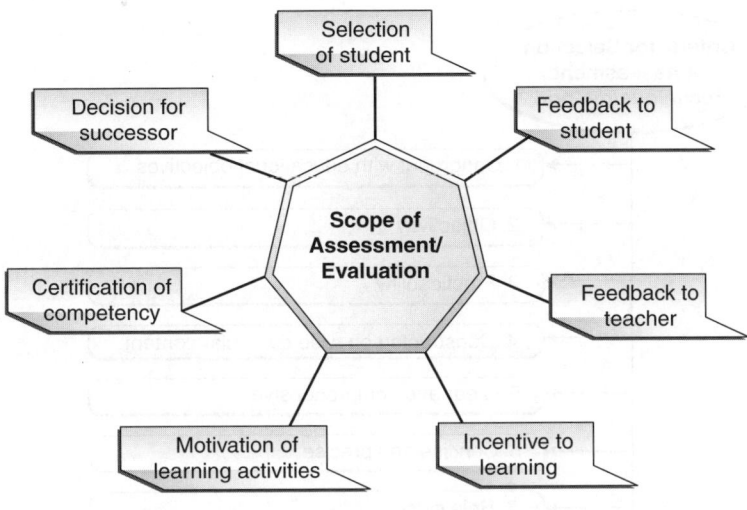

FIGURE 9.1

Scope of the assessment/evaluation.

- **Motivation of learning activities:** The teaching–learning activities do not remain interesting without timely assessment and evaluation. Therefore, scheduled assessment processes are required for motivating students.
- **Certification of competence:** Student assessment is one of the principle prerequisite to certify the competence or knowledge in a particulate aspect of curriculum.
- **Decision for success or failure:** Assessment offers the ability to decide about the ultimate success or failure of students in the achievement of preplanned educational objectives.

CRITERIA FOR SELECTION OF ASSESSMENT TECHNIQUES/METHODS

Each assessment technique and method has unique features; however, the selection of an assessment technique and method requires careful consideration of the criteria shown in Fig. 9.2 so that the assessment process can be efficient. Assessment is considered the most tedious task, therefore, the selection of an appropriate technique and method is an essential responsibility of an evaluator. These criteria are also known as *qualities of good assessment tools, techniques and methods.*

- **Congruent with educational objectives:** The assessment techniques and methods must be directly related to the educational objectives so that planned educational objectives can be met. Therefore, evaluators generally base their evaluation techniques and methods on the respective educational objective of a particular curriculum.
- **Objectivity of assessment techniques/methods:** Objectivity is the extent to which independent and competent examiners agree on what constitutes a good answer for each of the elements of a measuring instrument. A good tool used for assessment must be objective so that the evaluator's subjective bias may be avoided. For example, multiple-choice questions, short answer questions, objective

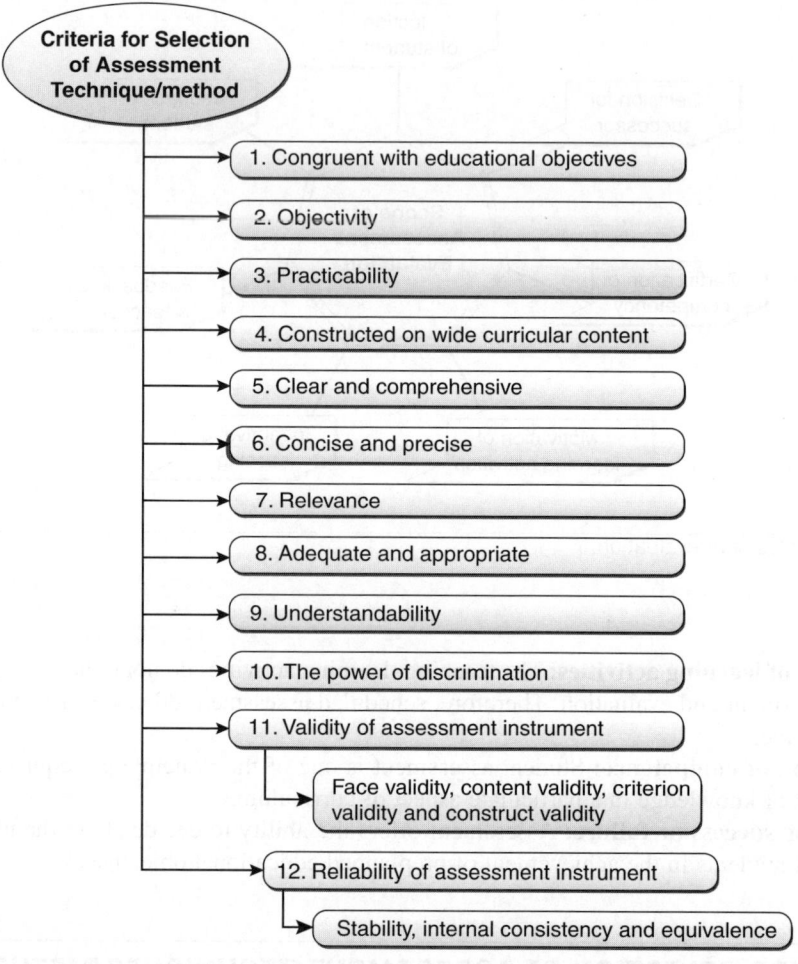

FIGURE 9.2

Criteria for the selection of assessment technique/method.

structured clinical examinations are more objective methods of evaluation where there is a minimal risk of subjective bias of the evaluator. However, essay type questions or informal observation in practical examinations may have a high risk of subjective bias and may not be considered an objective means of evaluation.

- **Practicability of measuring techniques/methods:** Evaluators sometimes develop complex methods and tools of evaluation in overenthusiasm. However, it is not practically possible to implement such complex tools and methods of evaluation. For example, a set of multiple-choice questions may not be practical to assess clinical skills of nursing students. An evaluator may require an observational rating scale or checklist to appropriately measure their clinical skills.
- **Evaluation tools constructed on wide curricular content:** A good evaluation tool must be constructed from the wide curricular content so that essential and vital areas may not be neglected and the evaluator is assured that the learner is competent in all the essential curricular areas and domains.

- **Clear and comprehensive:** The constructed evaluation tools must be clear to promote understanding in students and they should be comprehensive so that unnecessary time is not wasted in learning and comprehension is easy.
- **Concise and precise:** An evaluation instrument must be as concise as possible and precise so that the face and contract validity of the evaluation tools may be ensured. Furthermore, a concise and precise evaluation tool makes the evaluation process more easy and convenient.
- **Relevance:** The measuring tool must be relevant in reference to the curricular content to be evaluated, the domain of learning to be evaluated and the learner's age and ability to answer the constructed items.
- **Adequate and appropriate:** An evaluation tool must be adequate enough to cover all the essential aspects of the content to be evaluated and it must be appropriate for the evaluation of the domain of learning and the student's ability.
- **Understandability:** An evaluation tool must be easily understandable by the respondent; the understandability of an evaluation tool may be enhanced by using simple and familiar language, avoiding ambiguity in the written content of the items and clear presentation.
- **The power of discrimination:** The basic and essential function of each evaluation tool and technique is to efficiently discriminate in the particular domain of learning among students. Before the selection of an evaluation tool, it must be ensured that it has the ability and strength to discriminate between students with poor and good knowledge. The power of discrimination in an evaluation tool signifies that the students with good knowledge will be able to score more marks as compared to poor students.
- **Validity of assessment instrument:** Validity of an evaluation technique and method is the extent to which the particular evaluation tool and technique measures what it is intended to measure. The validity of an evaluation tool is the most primary and essential characteristic of evaluation tools and techniques because if a tool is not valid then it will not measure what it is supposed to measure. For example, a valid evaluation tool developed to assess the ECG interpretation skills of nursing students must include only the items related to the different clinical ECG situations rather than simple ECG knowledge-related questions. Generally, the validity of an evaluation tool is ensured by seeking the opinions and suggestions from experts of the respective fields. Furthermore, developing standardized evaluation tools may require the statistical measure to establish the validity of the respective evaluation tool. Validity of an evaluation tool may be affected by unclear directions to attempt the questions in a test or examination, difficult professional jargons used to construct the questions, ambiguous terms and sentences, use of unfamiliar language for respondents/students and inexperienced and unqualified persons preparing the questions. Basically, the validity of an assessment tool is classified into the following four categories:
  - *Face validity:* Face validity involves the overall look of an instrument regarding its appropriateness to measure a particular aspect of knowledge and skill or to affect the domain of learning. Though face validity is not considered a very important and essential type of validity for an instrument, it may be taken in consideration to assess the other aspects of validity of an evaluation instrument. In simple words, this aspect of validity refers to the face value or the outlook of an instrument. For example, for a questionnaire constructed to assess the knowledge of nursing regarding 'endotracheal suctioning', an expert of the respective field or evaluator may judge the face value of this instrument (whether it looks good or not), but it provides no guarantee about the appropriateness and completeness of an evaluation instrument with regard to its content, construction and measurement score.

- *Content validity:* It is concerned with the scope of coverage of the content area to be measured. It is often applied in tests of knowledge measurement. It is a case expert judgement about the adequacy, appropriateness and completeness of the content area included in the evaluation instrument to measure a particular phenomenon. Judgement of the content viability may be subjective and based on the previous researcher's and expert's opinion about the adequacy, appropriateness and completeness of the content of the instrument. Generally, this viability is ensured through the judgements of experts about the content.
- *Criterion validity:* This type of validity is a relationship between the measurements of the instrument with some other external criteria. The instrument is valid if its measurements strongly respond to the score of some other valid criterion. The problems with criterion-related validity is finding a reliable and valid external criterion. Mostly, we are to rely on a less than perfect criterion because the rating found by empirical and supervisory methods may be computed mathematically that can correlate the score of the instrument with the score of criterion variable. The range of coefficient ≥ 0.70 is desirable. Criterion-related validity may be differentiated by predictive validity and concurrent validity.
  - *Predictive validity:* It is the degree of forecasting judgement; for example, some personality tests and academic futures of students can be a predictive behaviour pattern. It is the differentiation between the performances on some future criterion and instruments ability. An instrument may have predictive validity when its score significantly correlates with some future criteria.
  - *Concurrent validity:* It is the degree of the measures in the present time. It relates to the present specific behaviour and characteristics, hence the difference between the predictive and concurrent validity refers to the timing pattern of obtaining the measurements of a criterion.
- *Construct validity:* Construct validity is a key criterion for assessing the quality of an evaluation instrument. It has most often been addressed in terms of measurement issues. The key construct validity questions with regard to measurements are as follows: What is this instrument really measuring? Does it adequately measure the abstract concept of interest? Construct validity gives more importance to testing the relationship predicted on theoretical measurements. The evaluator can make predictions in relation to other such type of constructs. One such method of construct validation is known as *group technique.*
- **Reliability of the assessment instrument:** Reliability is the degree of consistency and accuracy with which an instrument measures the attribute it is designed to measure. Further, reliability is defined as the ability of an instrument to create reproducible results. Therefore, reliability is concerned with consistency of the measurement tools. A tool can only be considered reliable if it measures an attribute with similar results on repeated use. There are several ways to measure the reliability of research tools, which depends on several factors such as nature of the instrument as well as aspects of reliability the evaluator wants to measure. The main aspects of reliability that are considered important in evaluation are stability, internal consistency and equivalence.
  - *Stability:* The stability aspect of reliability means that the research instrument provides the same results when it is administered consecutively two or more times. Stability is estimated to make sure that the research instrument is consistent in providing similar results with repeated administrations. It is also known as *test-retest reliability.* To assess test-retest reliability, the test is administered twice at two different points in time. It is used to assess the consistency of a test across different times. This type of reliability assumes that there will be no change in the quality or construct being measured. Test-retest reliability is best used for things that are stable over time, such

as intelligence. Generally, reliability will be higher when little time has passed between tests. The test-retest method is a relatively easy and straightforward approach to establish reliability. It is used for questionnaires, observation checklists and observation rating scales. It can be statistically calculated the Karl Person's correlation coefficient formula.

- *Internal consistency:* Internal consistency is also called *homogeneity*. It ensures that all the subparts of a research instrument are measuring the same characteristics. An evaluation tool can only be considered internally consistent if all the subparts of the tool are measuring the same characteristics. One of the most primitive approaches of assessing the internal consistency is the split half technique. However, to overcome its drawback as an estimation tool of different correlation coefficient results with different combination of split half (odd–even or first half–second half, etc.). This method is replaced by formulas that compensate this deficiency such as Cronbach's alpha and Kunder–Richardon formula-20.
- *Equivalence:* This aspect of reliability is estimated when an evaluator is testing the reliability of a tool, which is used by two different observers to observe a single task performed by the learner independently or two presumably parallel instruments are administered to the individual at about the same time. For example, a rating scale is developed to assess wound dressing skills among nursing students. This rating scale may be administered to observe the clinical skills of nursing students for wound dressing by two different observers simultaneously but independently. This is also known as *interrater reliability* or *interobserver reliability*, which is estimated by the administration of tools to observe single events simultaneously and independently by two or more trained observers.

CLASSIFICATION OF ASSESSMENT TOOLS AND TECHNIQUES

The basic classification of assessment tools and techniques is given in Box 9.2.

BOX 9.2 CLASSIFICATION OF ASSESSMENT TOOLS AND TECHNIQUES

Assessment of knowledge	Assessment of skills	Assessment of attitude

• Essay type questions
  • Extended response essay
  • Restricted response essay
	• Observation checklist
	• Rating scale
	• Anecdotal records
		• Likert attitude scale
		• Semantic differential scale

• *Short answer questions*
  • Fill in the blank type
  • Statement completion
  • Labelling a diagram
  • Short answer in 5–10 words
	• Cumulative records
	• Written clinical assignments
	• Critical incident record
	• Practical examination
	• Viva voce (Oral examination)	

• *Objective type of questions*
  • Multiple-choice questions
  • Multiple response questions
  • True and false questions
  • Matching type question
	• Objective Structured Clinical Examination (OSCE)
	• Objective Structured Practical Examination (OSPE)	

ESSAY TYPE QUESTIONS

Educators choose essay questions over other forms of assessment because essay items challenge students to create a response rather than to simply select a response. Some educators use them because essays have the potential to reveal students' abilities to reason, create, analyse, synthesize and evaluate. In short, essay items are used for the advantages they offer. Despite the advantages associated with essay questions there are numerous disadvantages also. However, essay type questions are the most frequently used method of evaluation in most Indian universities, colleges and schools.

Essay questions are defined as a test item which requires a response composed by the examinee, usually in the form of one or more sentences, of a nature that no single response or pattern of responses can be listed as correct, and the accuracy and quality of which can be judged subjectively only by one skilled or informed in the subject.

—John M. Stalnaker

An essay type test presents one or more questions or other tasks that require extended written responses from the persons being tested.

—Robert L.E. and David A.F.

Essay type questions are a test containing questions requiring the students to respond in writing. It emphasizes recall rather than recognition of the correct alternative.

—Gilert Sax

Based on Stalnaker's definition, an essay question should meet the following criteria:

- They should require examinees to *compose* rather than select their response.
- They should elicit student responses that must consist of many interlined sentences.
- They should allow different or original responses or a pattern of responses.
- They should require subjective judgement by a competent specialist to judge the accuracy and quality of responses.
- They should provide students with an indication of the types of thinking and content to use in responding to the essay question.

Essay questions are different from these other constructed response items because they require more systematic and in-depth thinking. An effective essay question will align with each of the four criteria given in Stalnaker's definition and provide students with an indication of the types of thinking and content to use in responding to the essay type question.

I. FEATURES OF ESSAY TYPE QUESTIONS

- Questions are used both as formative and summative assessments.
- They require a great deal of thought and planning.
- Students prepare their own answers.
- They evaluate knowledge areas alone.
- Student's handwriting, spelling, neatness, organization and way of expressing ideas may be considered while scoring the items.
- No single answer can be considered thorough or correct.
- The examinee is permitted freedom of response.
- Answers vary in their degree of equality or corrections.

II. PURPOSES OF ESSAY TYPE QUESTIONS

Essay type questions are subjected to criticism by educationists but are still used in university exams across the globe. One might wonder if there are so many loopholes, why they are consistently being used for evaluation in nursing. This is because essay type questions serve distinct purposes which cannot be accomplished by any other type of questions. These purposes are discussed below:

- *Students get a chance to express own views:* It provides students with an opportunity to express their views on particular phenomena.
- *To assess factual recall of knowledge:* Sometimes teachers might be interested in knowing how well students can recall the facts they have learned. This purpose can be fulfilled by having essay type questions in the test paper.
- *Analysis and explanation of relationships:* When the teacher is interested in knowing how well the students can explain the relationship between two or more concepts, essay type questions are used because no other form of question can serve this purpose.
- *Assessment of non-content-related attributes of students:* Creativity, writing style, organization, neatness and cleanliness are some other attributes that can be more appropriately assessed through essay type of questions.

III. PRINCIPLES FOR CONSTRUCTION OF ESSAY TYPE QUESTIONS

The following guidelines must be followed for the construction of essay type questions:

- The learning objective supposed to be evaluated by an essay type question should be clearly defined in simple words.
- If a learning objective can be evaluated by any other type of question, the use of essay type question should be avoided.
- It is always better to use several short essay type questions instead of a long one.
- The question and the task in a problem situation should be clearly defined by ensuring the following:
  - Clearly define the question so that students understand what to write.
  - Delimit the scope of the question so that students do not feel that they need to write infinite number of pages.
  - Clearly develop the problem or problem situation so that students can be focused.
- The approximate time and word limit for each essay type question should be specified.
- The distribution of marks for different segments of a particular question and organization, neatness, expressive language should be explained.
- The use of complex and ambiguous words should be avoided.
- Questions that are too broad in scope and allow for blunders should be avoided.
- Words like differentiate and compare should be used at the beginning of the question to restrict the scope of the question.
- Simple unambiguous language well understood by all students should be used.
- A reasonable question should be presented to students, so that they do not feel that it is outside their ability and scope to answer.
- Questions can be written in declarative as well as interrogative statements.
- The relative point value and the approximate time limit should be specified in clear directions.
- The criteria for grading should be stated so that students know what to include in answer.

- The use of optional questions which may confuse the students and make evaluation difficult should be avoided.
- The essay question should be improved through preview and review.

Preview: Before administration the evaluator must

- Predict student responses.
- Write a model answer.
- Ask a knowledgeable colleague to critically review the essay question, the model answer and the intended learning outcome for alignment.

Review: After the administration of essay type questions, the evaluator must

- Review student responses to the essay question.

Advantages of essay type questions

- Assess higher-order or critical-thinking skills in learners.
- Evaluate student thinking and reasoning.
- Provide an opportunity to assess the problem solving and decision making abilities in learners.
- Help evaluate thinking, recall, analysis and synthesis of facts.
- Provide an opportunity for creative expression and organization of facts.
- Are relatively easy to construct but require a good knowledge of essay type question contraction among evaluators.
- Provide very limited scope of guessing answers.

Disadvantages of essay type questions

- These questions lead to vague answers if wording of questions is ambiguous and difficult to understand.
- They assess a limited sample of the range of content from the entire curriculum.
- It is difficult and time consuming to grade the answers.
- Evaluation is subjective; different teachers may mark the same answer differently.
- There is a scope of a lot of subjective biasness.
- These questions provide practice in poor or unpolished writing.
- They have a limited range of application.

SHORT ANSWER QUESTIONS

Short answer questions (SAQs) are very similar to objective items as a clearly-defined answer is required in both. However, in short answer questions the answer has to be generated and supplied by the learner rather than chosen from a number of options provided. SAQs are sometimes called *objective questions*, because they can be marked with a very high degree of reliability, if suitably designed. Strictly speaking, however, they are not truly objective as the marker may sometimes have to exercise a certain amount of subjective judgement in deciding whether an answer is satisfactory. The evaluator may, for example, have to decide whether a wrongly-spelt word, a partly correct answer or a perfectly good answer that the question setter did not anticipate is acceptable, and may also have to decide whether an explanation or description is satisfactory. Obviously, the subjective judgement involved tends to increase with the length and complexity of the required answer, while the degree of 'objectivity' shows a corresponding fall.

I. PURPOSES OF SAQs

- Useful to assess the recall ability of students (lower cognitive domain).
- Used to assess students in a classroom while a lecture is in progress.
- Useful in formative assessment.
- May be used in summative evaluation to supplement other forms of questions.

II. PRINCIPLES FOR CONSTRUCTION OF SAQs

The following guidelines must be followed for the construction of essay type questions:

- The learning objective which is supposed to be evaluated by the short answer type question should be clearly defined in simple words.
- The overall purpose and content of the item should be determined.
- Short answer questions should be written using the following guidelines:
  - The item should be expressed in such a way that only a single, brief answer is possible.
  - The item should be expressed in a clear, simple language, making it as concise as possible while avoiding looseness or ambiguity.
  - The item should be expressed in a positive form wherever possible as it has been found that positively phrased test items tend to measure more important learning outcomes than negatively phrased items.
  - One should try to avoid providing clues to the required answer unwittingly.
  - Where a numerical answer has to be supplied, the degree of precision expected and (if appropriate) the units to express it should be indicated. For example, how many milligrams of Lasix a nurse will administer to a patient with renal failure in a day?
  - Precise, simple and unambiguous language should be used.
  - Action-oriented verbs should be used.
  - Each question should deal with important content area of a unit.
  - Long complex sentences should be avoided and the questions should be kept as simple as possible.
  - Phrases like 'write briefly on, short notes on' should be avoided.
  - Space should be provided for answers below each question per the requirement of the question being asked.
  - Specific problems for questions that will have distinct specific answers should be chosen.
  - Fill in the blank type questions should use statements that omit only one or two key words (answer) at the end of sentence.
- While finalizing the layout of questions, it must be ensured that:
  - The item is presented in such a way that the learners are in no doubt as to what they are expected to do and how they are required to indicate their response.
  - The wattage for each question and criteria for marking is mentioned clearly.

- Items to be evaluated by the subject experts panel: An expert must ensure the availability of the following information before finalizing the evaluation of each short answer item:
  - Is the item relevant to the course/module/syllabus to which it relates?
  - Is the item style appropriate to the topic being covered and the specific educational skills or outcomes being assessed?
  - Does the item present the learners with a clearly-defined task?
  - Is the item logically and structurally sound?
  - Is the item stated in a simple and clear language?
  - Is the item free from extraneous clues?
  - Is the stated difficulty of the item likely to prove accurate?
  - Is this stated difficulty appropriate?

III. TYPES OF SAQs

Fill in the blank type

Example: **Q.1:** A patient is diagnosed with brain tumour. The nurse's assessment reveals that the patient has difficulty in interpreting visual stimuli. Based on these findings, the nurse suspects injury in the.....................lobe of the brain.

Answer: Occipital

Statement completion

Example: **Q.1:** A 45-year-old patient is admitted with excruciating paroxysmal facial pain. He reports that the episodes occur most often after feeling cold draft and drinking cold beverages. Based on these findings, the nurse determines that the patient is most likely suffering from...

Answer: Trigeminal neuralgia

Labelling a diagram

Example: **Q.1:** An elderly patient fell and fractured the neck of his femur. Identify the area where the fracture occurred.

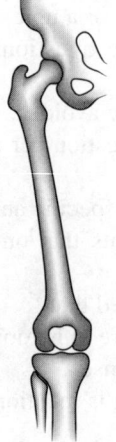 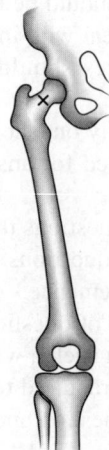

Short answer in 5–10 words

Example: **Q.1:** Mention the five commonly occurring signs and symptoms of hypothyroidism.

1. _____   2. _____
3. _____   4. _____
5. _____

Advantages of SAQs

- Provide the opportunity to cover a much wider content of the syllabus to evaluate the students.
- Can be administered to a large group of students for a short formative assessment.
- Useful to assess the recall of information without any assistance or cues or alternatives.
- Provide less scope for guesswork.
- Require less stationary as compared to essay type questions.
- Less scope of subjectivity as compared to essay type questions when judging answers.
- Easy to administer and mark the tests; ensure more objective scoring.

Disadvantages of SAQs

- They are not particularly well suited for testing some types of higher cognitive and noncognitive outcomes, especially if these are of a multifaceted or complex nature, or involve the assessment of 'life skills'.
- They can lead to cheating within a group of students if the examination hall is not spacious enough.
- They can lead to difficulties in scoring if not worded carefully.
- They provide no scope to assess the writing ability, expression, organization of answer, etc.

MULTIPLE-CHOICE QUESTIONS

Multiple-choice questions (MCQs) are the form of assessment where respondents are asked to select the best possible answer (or answers) out of choices from a list. Although E.L. Thorndike developed an early multiple choice test, Frederick J. Kelly was the first to use such items as part of a large-scale assessment. MCQs are a special type of questions that are widely used in various entrance exams where thousands of students attempt the exams. These are standardized tests with high reliability and validity. A typical MCQ begins with a *stem* which may be an incomplete statement, picture or a graph, which is followed by 4–5 *alternatives* or choices. All the wrong answers or alternatives are known as *distractors*. The correct answer/answers are known as the key (Fig. 9.3). Clear instructions are provided at the beginning of the questionnaire about the selection of the answer (e.g. choose one response that is correct; choose all responses that are correct) or instructions are provided within the questionnaire whenever necessary. Scoring in MCQs is easier as compared to essay type and short answer type questions but the other side of the coin is that it is equally difficult to construct good quality MCQs and there is a high chance of cheating and guesswork practices.

I. STRUCTURE AND CHARACTERISTICS OF MCQS

- Multiple-choice questions consist of a stem and a set of options. The *stem* is the beginning part of the item that presents the item as a problem to be solved, a question asked to the respondent or an incomplete statement to be completed and any other relevant information.

Q.1: Which artery is most commonly used to assess the pulse rate in a two-year-old child? } **Question Stem**

a) Radial artery
b) Femoral artery } Distracters
c) Pedal artery
d) Apical artery } Answer

(a–d) } Alternatives

FIGURE 9.3

Basic structure of multiple-choice questions.

- The stem follows by 4–5 options. The options are possible answers that the examiner can choose from with the correct answer called the *key* and the incorrect answers called *distractors.* Generally, only one answer can be keyed as correct. However, when more than one answer is keyed as correct, then these questions are named as *multiple response questions* (Box 9.3).
- Usually, a correct answer earns a set number of points towards the total marks and an incorrect answer earns nothing. However, tests may also award a partial credit for unanswered questions or penalize students for incorrect answers to discourage guessing.
- Markings of the answers made by the teacher are objective as there is no scope of subjectivity.
- Answers can be checked by computers or by any other person supplied with the answer key.

II. GUIDELINES TO CONSTRUCT GOOD MCQS

The following basic rules must be observed for writing good multiple-choice questions:

A. General tips

- Design each item to measure an important learning objective or learning outcome.
- Before writing a question, think about what it is that you want to test. Lecture notes, textbook readings, assigned problems and other course materials can be an inspiration to write items.

BOX 9.3 EXAMPLES OF MULTIPLE CHOICE AND MULTIPLE RESPONSE QUESTIONS

Multiple-choice question

Q: A patient is admitted to the hospital with a diagnosis of chronic bronchitis. He has a 10-year history of emphysema. The nurse should place him on which of the following positions?

A. Side-lying
B. Supine
C. High-Fowler's
D. Semi-Fowler's

Answer: C

Multiple response question

Q: The nurse is assessing a 2-year-old patient diagnosed with bacterial meningitis. Which of the following signs and symptoms of meningeal irritation is the nurse likely to observe?

Select all that apply:

A. Generalized seizures
B. Nuchal rigidity
C. Positive Budzinski's sign
D. Positive Kernig's sign
E. Babinski reflex
F. Photophobia

Answer: B, C, D, F

- Control the difficulty of the item either by varying the problem in the stem or by changing the alternatives.
- Make certain that each item is independent of the other items in the test.
- Make sure that each item is grammatically accurate to avoid ambiguity in understanding.
- Keep the question stem and alternatives as short as possible. Use few words. Avoid repeating words from the question stem in the alternatives.
- Make sure to have a sufficient number of easy and more challenging questions so that the poor, fair, good and excellent students are effectively judged and separated.
- Try to make the first few MCQs relatively quick and easy, to help calm students down so they can focus on the more challenging questions to come.
- Avoid the temptation to test many things in one question. If possible, try to write more than one MCQ rather than test multiple concepts in one question.
- Ask more than one questions when a fair amount of information must be provided as it takes time for students to carefully read and understand the information you provide in a test. For example, you could give them a table of results, a graph, or a scenario and then ask two or three different MCQs about it.
- Do not try to write the entire test in one day; it takes time, creativity and thought to write good MCQs.
  - After constructing the MCQ test, a try-out may be planned on nearly similar subjects and an item analysis must be carried out before preparation of a final draft of the test.

B. Construction of the stem

- Present a single, clearly formulated problem in the stem of the item/question.
- Phrase the question stem as clearly and concisely as possible, avoiding complex language.
- State the stem of the item in a positive form, wherever possible.
- Emphasize negative wording whenever it is used in the stem of an item; for example, which of the following is **NOT** an appropriate method of back massage?
- Avoid verbal clues, which might enable students to select the correct answer or to eliminate an incorrect alternative. Similarity of wording in both the stem and the correct answer is one of the more obvious clues.

C. Construction of alternatives

- Make certain that the intended answer is correct or clearly the best.
- Make all alternatives grammatically consistent with the stem of the item and parallel in form.
- Avoid the use of the alternative 'all of the above' and use 'none of the above' with great caution.
- Do not include alternatives such as 'both (A) and (D)' or 'all but (C)', as these complicate the structure of the question and tend to confuse students and/or slow them down.
- Vary the position of the correct answer in a random manner.
- Vary the relative length of the correct answer to eliminate length as a clue.
- There is no set rule about the number of options you should include in MCQs. The greater the number of options, the smaller the mathematical chance of correct guesswork. Therefore, generally 4–5 alternatives are used.
- Make the distracters plausible and attractive to the uninformed, by:
  - Using common misconceptions or common errors of students as distracters.
  - Using good sounding words (e.g. accurate, important, etc.) in the distracters, as well as in the correct answers.

- Making the distracters similar to the correct answer in both length and complexity of wording.
- Stating the alternatives in the language of the student.
- Construct the destructors as close as possible to the correct answer to make most effective destructors.

D. Advantages of MCQs
- Easy to use and administer.
- Can cover a large content area of syllabus.
- Easy to check answers.
- High reliability and validity.
- No scope of subjective biasness.
- Allow more adequate sampling of content.
- Tend to more effectively structure the problem to be addressed.
- Questions can be used more efficiently and reliably than just supplying items.
- Different response alternatives can provide diagnostic feedback about the planned questions (item analysis is possible).
- Questions can be constructed to address various levels of cognitive complexities.

E. Disadvantages of MCQs
- Not useful to test the highest level of cognitive domain.
- Difficult to construct good MCQs.
- Provide an opportunity to guess the answer if the question is not properly constructed.
- More suitable format for cheating in students if the invigilator is not highly keen in observing students.
- A time-consuming process to construct good questions.
- Can lead the instructor to favour simple recall of facts.
- High degree of dependence on student's readings and instructor's writing ability.
- Measuring synthesis and evaluation can be difficult.
- Inappropriate for measuring the outcomes that require skilled performance.

ITEM ANALYSIS

It is important that a newly constructed MCQ test must be valid and reliable, which depends on characteristics of each question item included in the test. The value and suitability of each constructed question item are evaluated through a specific method named as *'item analysis'* so that eventually the final draft of test is functional and useful. The item analysis is one of the important phases of test construction (see Box 9.4).

Item analysis is referred to as a specific method of systemically examining the effectiveness of each item created for the test that includes three main characteristics, which are evaluating the item difficulty, discrimination index and effectiveness of destructors.

> **BOX 9.4 PHASES OF AN MCQ TEST CONSTRUCTION**
>
> 1. Preparing a draft of items.
> 2. Tryout of test in similar setting.
> 3. Item analysis
> 4. Final draft of test

PURPOSES OF ITEM ANALYSIS

The item analysis serves the following main purposes:

- Item analysis provides information about (i) difficulty level of each item in test, (ii) discriminating power of each item in test and (iii) effectiveness of each destructor used in an item.
- It is helpful in construction of a functional, useful and a more effective test.
- It helps in accepting the good items and revises or rejects the poor items to construct the most suitable test for the target group.

COMPONENTS OF ITEM ANALYSIS

The main characteristics of the item analysis are the item difficulty, discrimination index and effectiveness of destructors.

(a) *Item difficulty:* It is a proportion of students who are with the correct answer for a particular test item.

$$\text{Item Difficulty} = \frac{\text{No. of students with correct answer}}{\text{Total No. of students}}$$

For example, MCQ No. 03 is answered correctly by 45 students out of 80 students. The item difficulty (*p*-value) for this MCQ item will be 45/80 = 0.56. The ideal range of item difficulty is 0.26–0.75; the items with *p*-value in this range should be considered with appropriate difficulty. However, an item with *p*-value above the 0.76 is considered very easy and a *p*-value below 0.25 is considered very difficult. Therefore, those items need to be revised or discarded.

(b) *Discrimination index:* It is a difference between the proportion of the upper group who are with the correct answer and the proportion of the lower group who are with the correct answer.
Discrimination Index = DU − DL

$$\text{DU} = \frac{\text{No. of students in the upper 25\% with correct answer}}{\text{Total no. of students in upper 25\%}}$$

$$\text{DL} = \frac{\text{No. of students in the lower 25\% with correct answer}}{\text{Total no. of students in lower 25\%}}$$

For example, in a question item, 15 students are with correct answer in upper 25% students (20 students) and the same question item is answered correctly by 5 students among lower 25% students (20 students). In this case, DU = 15/20 = 0.75 and DL = 5/20 = 0.25. Thus, the discrimination index will be 0.75 − 0.25 = 0.50. The discrimination index ranges between −1.0 and 1.0. The discrimination index score between −1.0 and −0.50 can discriminate but the item is questionable and this must be discarded. Furthermore, the discrimination index score between −0.55 and 0.45 is considered as non-discriminatory and thus it must be revised, while score of discrimination index between 0.45 and 1.0 is considered as discriminating score for the particular item and this item must be included in the test.

(c) *Effectiveness of destructors:* It is very important in the MCQ test that the destructors created are very effective. The effectiveness of a particular destructor can be evaluated by the total number of students who have chosen a destructor in a particular item in a tryout test. A destructor chosen by less then 5% student is considered as inappropriate and must be revised.

OBSERVATION CHECKLIST

An observation checklist is the most commonly used instrument for performance evaluation. A checklist enables the observer to note only whether a trait is present or not. It consists of a listing of steps, activities or behaviours the observer records when an incident occurs. The observer has to judge whether a certain behaviour has taken place.

Observation checklist is simply a list of the performer's behaviours associated with particular nursing interventions within a space for the assessor to check or tick off whether or not that particular behaviour occurred (Box 9.5).

DEFINITIONS OF CHECKLIST

A checklist is a simple instrument consisting prepared list of expected items of performance or attributes, which are checked by a evaluator for their presence or absence.

Checklists are constructed by breaking a performance and the quality of a product, which specifies the presence or absence of an attribute or trait which is then 'checked' by the rater/observer.

CHARACTERISTICS OF A CHECKLIST

- Observe one respondent at one time.
- Clearly specifies the characteristics of the behaviour to be observed.

BOX 9.5 CHECKLIST FOR EVALUATION OF STUDENT'S PERFORMANCE DURING INTRADERMAL INJECTION

Steps	Place for (✓) tick mark		Remarks
	Yes	No	
1. Wash hands			
2. Collect all articles			
3. Check the medication order with medication card			
4. Load the syringe with the required amount of medicine			
5. Identify the patient by name and other details			
6. Explain the procedure to the patient			
7. Select the site and clean the area with a sprit swab			
8. Stretch the patient's skin tightly with the thumb and finger			
9. Insert the needle at 5–15° angle, advance about 3 mm through the epidermic layer			
10. Inject contents watching for a bleb			
11. Do not massage the area			
12. Mark with a pen around the wheel and note the date, time sight and medication			
13. Wash hands and replace the articles			

*Each step carries one mark   Total marks obtained: ....
Signature of examiner: ....   Date: ....

- Use only carefully prepared checklists to avoid more complex traits.
- The observer should be trained how to observe, what to observe and how to record the observed behaviour.
- Use checklists only when you are interested in calculating a particular characteristic.

CONSTRUCTION OF A CHECKLIST

While constructing or preparing checklists, the following points should be kept in mind:

- Express each item in clear, simple language.
- An intensive survey of the literature should be made to determine the type of checklist to be used in a particular assessment/evaluation.
- The list of items in the checklist may be continuous or divided into groups of related items.
- These lists of the items are formulated on the basis of the judgement of experts and each item is evaluated with respect to the number of favourable and unfavourable responses.
- Avoid negative statements whenever possible.
- Avoid lifting statements verbatim from the text.
- Ensure that each item has a clear response: *yes* or *no*, or *true* or *false*.
- Review the items independently.
- Checklists must have the quality of completeness and comprehensiveness.

A. Advantages of checklists

- Checklists allow inter-individual comparisons.
- They provide a simple method to record observations.
- They are adaptable to subject matter areas.
- Checklists are useful in evaluating learning activities expected to be performed.
- They are helpful in evaluating procedure work.
- Properly prepared checklists allow the observer to constrain the direct attention.
- Checklists have objectivity to evaluate characteristics.
- Useful for evaluating the processes that can be subdivided into a series of actions.
- Decreases the chances of errors in observation.

B. Disadvantages of checklists

- Checklists do not indicate quality of performance so the usefulness of checklists is limited.
- Only a limited component of overall clinical performance can be evaluated.
- Only the presence or absence of an attribute, behaviour or performance parameter may be assessed. However, the degree of accuracy of performance can be assessed.
- It has limited use in qualitative observations.
- Checklists are not easy to prepare.

RATING SCALE

Rating is the term used to express opinion or judgement regarding some performance of a person, object, situation and character. The rating scale involves qualitative description of a limited number of aspects of a thing or traits of a person. When we use rating scales, we judge an object in absolute terms against some specified criteria, i.e. we judge properties of objects without reference to other similar objects.

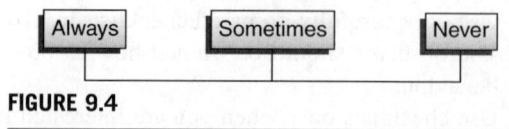

FIGURE 9.4

Three-point rating scale.

I. DEFINITIONS OF A RATING SCALE

Rating scale refers to a scale with a set of opinion, which describes varying degree of the dimensions of an attitude or a phenomenon being observed.

Rating scale is a device by which judgements may be qualified or a opinion concerning a trait can be systematized.

—**Suresh K. Sharma**

A rating scale is a tool in which one person simply checks off another person's level of performance. It could be a 3-point (Fig. 9.4), 5-point (Fig. 9.5) or 7-point rating scale. Rating scales measure how much or how well something happened, where generally quantitative and qualitative terms are used to judge the performance. A wide variety of attributes may be assessed by using rating scales; details may be perused from Box 9.6.

Q. How frequently do you discuss with your clinical instructor the difficulties encountered during clinical posting?

Q. The overall performance of the student in a mouth care procedure.

II. TYPES OF RATING SCALES

(a) *Graphic rating scale:* In this scale, the performance is printed horizontally at various points from lowest to highest. It includes the numerical points on the scale. It is anchored by two extremes presented to the respondents for the evaluation of a concept or object. For example: How satisfied are you with the lecture delivered by Professor X?

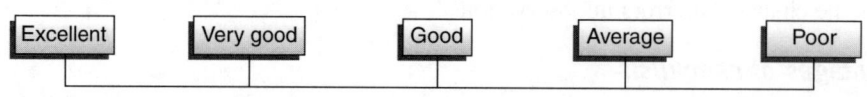

FIGURE 9.5

Five-point rating scale.

BOX 9.6 COMMON CONTENT OF APPRAISAL IN RATING SCALE			
Quantity of work	**Volume of work**	**Quality of work**	**Dependability**
Reliability	Initiative	Judgement	Neatness
Accuracy of work knowledge	Cooperative	Ability to work	Willingness

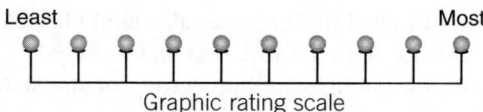

Graphic rating scale

(b) *Descriptive rating scale:* This type of rating scale does not use numbers but divides the assessment into a series of verbal phrases to indicate the level of performance.

For example: Q. Judge the level of performance of the nursing personnel in a medical ICU.

Nursing Personnel in a Ward	Level of Clinical Performance			
	Very Active	**Active**	**Moderately Active**	**Passive**
1. *Amandeep*				
2. *Jasveen*				
3. *Tara*				
4. *Kirandeep*				

(c) *Numerical rating scale:* It divides the evaluation criteria into a fixed number of points and defines only numbers except at the extremes. In these scales, each statement is generally assigned a numerical score ranging from 1 to 10 or even more. For example: Pain assessment numerical scale.

(d) *Comparative rating scale:* In this type of rating scale, the rater makes a judgement about a person's attributes by comparing with an other similar person(s). For example, Mr Ram's decision making abilities closely resemble that of Mr Shyam and Mr Gopal. In this type of rating scale, the rater must have prior knowledge about the selected attributes of the people with whom the subjects are supposed to be compared.

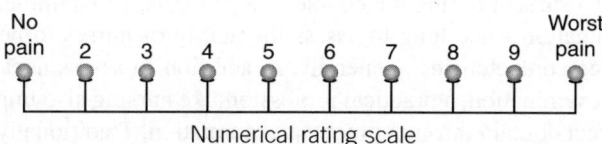

Numerical rating scale

III. CHARACTERISTICS OF A RATING SCALE

* Rating scales are value judgements of the attributes of one person by another person.
* These scales are most commonly used tools to carry out structured observations.
* They are generally developed to make quantitative judgements about qualitative attributes.
* They provide more flexibility to judge the level of performance or presence of attributes among subjects.
* Guiford (1954) identified that a rating scale must have the following basic characteristics that must be taken care of while constructing a rating scale.
    * *Clarity:* The rating scale must be constructed using short, concise statements in simple and unambiguous language.

- *Relevance:* The statement designed in a rating scale should be relevant to the phenomenon and should be exactly in accordance with the variables under study.
- *Variety:* While developing the rating scale, monotony of the statements must be avoided and variety in different statements must be ensured.
- *Objectivity:* The statement formed in a rating scale must be objective in nature so that it is convenient for the rater to judge the attributes or performances of the subjects under study.
- *Uniqueness:* Each statement constructed in a rating scale must be unique in itself so that the attributes can be judged appropriately.

A. Advantages of a rating scale

- Rating scales are easy to administer and score the measured attributes.
- They have a wide range of application in nursing educational evaluation.
- Graphic rating scale is more easy to make and less time-consuming.
- Rating scales can be easily used for a large group.
- They are also used for quantitative methods.
- They may also be used for the assessment of interests, attitudes and personal characteristics.
- They are used to evaluate performance, skills and product outcomes.
- Rating scales are adaptable and flexible assessment instruments.

B. Disadvantages of rating scales

- It is difficult or dangerous to fix up rating about many aspects of an individual.
- Misuse can result in a decrease in objectivity.
- There are chances of subjective evaluation thus the scales may become unscientific and unreliable.

PRACTICAL EXAMINATION

Practical examination is concerned with the assessment of practical performance skills and practice competency acquired by a student during the course of a particular programme. The nursing profession has used practical examination since long to assess the ability of nurses to perform specific expected practical tasks or practice competencies. Generally, in addition to assessment of cognitive domain of learning through theory examination, a practical profession like nursing also imposes a demand to assess the psychomotor and affect domain through practical examination. Traditionally, practical examinations are conducted in practice laboratories or real-life practice areas such as patients admitted in a hospital ward. The successful completion of a nursing programme requires a nursing student to pass the practical examination of a particular subject independently over and above the theoretical assessment. Practical examination is considered the most essential part of the overall assessment process in nursing because it is believed that merely theoretical knowledge of a nurse does not make them a qualified, competent nurse. Therefore, nurses must be assessed for their practical skills through practical examinations.

I. PURPOSES OF PRACTICAL EXAMINATIONS

Traditionally, practical examinations are used in nursing for the following purposes:

- To assess the practical skills and practice competencies of nursing students.
- To assess the development in practice domain of students by observing their reactions to real-life or simulated situations.

- To assess the student's problem solving skills.
- To assess the recording and reporting skills of nursing students.
- To assess how well the students are successful in transforming their theoretical knowledge in practice.
- To assess multiple performance tasks such as assessment, planning, implementation, communication and evaluation.

II. GUIDELINES FOR CONDUCTING PRACTICAL EXAMINATIONS

The following guidelines may be followed for conducting the practical examinations:

A. Planning phase of practical examination

- Consider the learning experience and learning objectives before planning the practical examination.
- Decide the appropriate place for the practical examination. Preliminary practical examinations must be conducted on simulators in a nursing laboratory. However, the final practical must be conducted on real-life situations. For example, patients admitted in the respective ward of a hospital or a field area for community health nursing.
- Preferably, plan to conduct the practical examination in a familiar place for students so that they can be psychologically comfortable.
- The selected area for practical examination must have an adequate supply to carry out the expected nursing procedures and the area should be well planned to accommodate the nursing students and examiners.
- The ward nurse managers or clinical area in-charges must be informed well in advance so that they are well prepared to support in the conduction of the practical examination.
- The overall evaluation criteria must be planned and students must be informed about the evaluation criteria so that they can prepare accordingly.

B. Conducting phase of practical examination

- Students and examiners must reach the place of examination as scheduled well in advance so that necessary changes may be adapted comfortably without any undue discomfort.
- Students must be called in a group and they must be conveyed with all the rules and regulations of the examination and examination stations or the patients may be randomly assigned through the lottery method to avoid subjective bias.
- Students must be assigned with routine nursing procedures performed by them regularly to make them psychologically comfortable with the practical situation.
- Generally, students feel nervous and anxious during practical examinations so a stress-free atmosphere must be offered to students so they can perform better without undue stress and pressure.
- Practical examinations must proceed using the steps of the nursing process such as assessment, planning, implementation and evaluation. For example, a student may initially assess the assigned patient, then plan and implement the care for priority needs and finally evaluate the effect of implemented care.
- Each student must be given sufficient time to perform the nursing procedure and accomplish the practical examination. Each examiner should not examine more than 20 students in a day (INC, 1986).
- Any sort of undue discomfort to the patients during practical examination must be avoided.

- On completion of the practical examination, the marks obtained by students must be compiled and sent to the examining body, i.e. university or nursing board in a sealed envelope under confidentiality.

C. Advantages of practical examinations

- Practical examination provides an opportunity to assess the skills and competency acquired by the students.
- Practical examination offers an opportunity to the examiners for assessing the use of compartmentalized knowledge in an integrated manner by a student while providing holistic nursing care to the assigned patient.
- An examiner also gets an opportunity to assess the communication and interpersonal skills of the students along with their clinical competence in performing the nursing procedures.

D. Disadvantages of practical examinations

- Practical examination is not considered a standardized assessment practice when students are assessed while working with patients.
- It is not considered an objective method of assessment because there are higher chances of subjectivity and personal bias.
- It is a time consuming process when an examiner assesses the complete practices and procedures of a student.
- It cannot be considered a feasible method for assessing a large group of students.
- Sometimes it is considered as unethical to expose patients for examining students.
- The emergencies and complex ward routines may be considered as disturbance factors to the smooth conduction of the practical examination.

VIVA VOCE

Viva voce is a Latin phrase literally meaning *with living voice*, but is most often translated as *by word of mouth*. Furthermore, viva voce is also termed as an *oral examination* which consists of a dialogue between the examiner and a student where the examiner asks question and the student replies. The examiner may ask short open questions, multiple-choice questions or a series of other type of questions not necessarily related to each other.

In nursing, viva voce is generally used to supplement the practical examination where two examiners, i.e. internal and external, ask several questions related to a particular subject matter. The viva voce might form a part of the validated assessment for a course, assessed by an oral examination. In these situations, the viva voce is a useful tool that assists in authenticating that the student has got enough knowledge in the subject matter.

I. PURPOSES OF VIVA VOCE

There are a variety of circumstances which might require the use of a viva voce and provision for these is contained in the academic and organizational regulations. There are several legitimate reasons for asking a student to attend a viva voce examination, all of which may have a different impact on the student. The main purposes of viva voce are mentioned below:

- To assess student's ability to communicate with another person.
- To supplement the information obtained through other evaluation techniques.

- To use stimulation methods like role play and telephone conversation.
- To identify and analyse the student's presence of mind.
- To evaluate the student's spontaneity and mannerism.
- To acquire soundness of knowledge through various forms of question.
- To diagnose the student's limitation and weakness and take remedial action.

II. PRINCIPLES TO CONDUCT VIVA VOCE

- The viva should not be limited to a single topic but should cover a range of different issues to avoid the results of the viva being skewed by selecting a topic which the candidate can answer exceptionally well or about which he/she knows nothing of. All questions should be strictly relevant to the purpose of the viva.
- Do not use long preambles to questions. Examiners should talk as little as possible during the viva.
- The chair of the examiners must remain in charge of the session and must deal appropriately with any problem candidate or difficult situation.
- When the last question is being asked, allow the student to complete his/her answer and end the session formally.
- Viva voce examinations should not normally exceed 30 minutes.
- Candidates should be examined individually.
- Candidates should be given adequate notice of the possibility of being called to attend a viva, and this should normally not be less than 24 hours.

A. Advantages of a viva voce

- Provides direct contact with the candidates to assess their communication, presentation skills and overall impression.
- Provides opportunity to mitigate circumstances into accounts.
- Provides flexibility in moving the candidates from strong to weak points.
- Makes students formulate replies without cues, and the reaction is observed for a specific stimulus.
- Facilitates simultaneous assessment by two or more examiners.
- Provides an opportunity for the examiner to get feedback on the performance of the students and the university.

B. Disadvantages of a viva voce

- Lacks standardization, objectivity and reproducibility of the result.
- Permits favouritism and cannot be used for future references.
- Suffers from undue influence of irrelevant factors.
- Costly in terms of professional time.

OBJECTIVE STRUCTURED CLINICAL EXAMINATION (OSCE)

Objective structured clinical examination (OSCE) is a modern type of examination often used in health sciences (e.g. medicine, dentistry nursing, pharmacy and physiotherapy) to assess clinical skill performance and competence in skills such as communication, clinical examination, medical and nursing procedures/ prescription, exercise prescription, joint mobilization/manipulation techniques and interpretation of results.

I. DEFINITIONS OF OSCE

Objective Structured Clinical Examination (OSCE) is a form of performance-based testing used to measure candidates' clinical competence. During an OSCE, candidates are observed and evaluated as they go through a series of stations in which they interview, examine and treat standardized patients who present with some type of medical problem.

The OSCE is an approach to the assessment of clinical competence in which the components of competence are assessed in a planned or structured way with attention being paid to the objectivity of the examination.

—Harden

OSCE is an assessment tool in which the components of clinical competence such as history taking, physical examination, simple procedures, interpretation of lab results, patient management problems, communication, attitude etc. are tested using agreed check lists and rotating the student round a number of stations some of which have observers with checklists.

—N. Ananthakrishnan

II. USES OF OSCE

OSCE can be used for undergraduate as well as postgraduate nursing students to assess their clinical competencies. Generally, ranges of basic and advanced clinical practice skills are assessed by using a 10-station OSCE session which comprises practice stations such as physical examination stations, history-taking stations, stations that cover communication skills and stations to perform nursing procedures followed by response stations to ask related multiple choice or short answer questions. Generally, the following range of practical skills are typically assessed in nursing using OSCE:

- Interpersonal and communication skills
- History-taking skills
- Physical examination of specific body systems
- Mental health assessment
- Clinical decision making, including the formation of differential diagnosis
- Clinical problem-solving skills
- Interpretation of clinical findings and investigations
- Management of a clinical situation, including treatment and referral
- Patient education
- Health promotion
- Acting safely and appropriately in an urgent clinical situation
- Basic and advanced nursing care procedure practices.

III. ORGANIZING THE OSCE

- The OSCE examination consists of about 10–15 stations, each of which requires about 4–5 minutes. The number of stations and time spent on each station may vary based on needs of evaluation.
- All stations should be capable of being completed in the same time.
- The students are rotated through all stations and have to move to the next station at the signal.

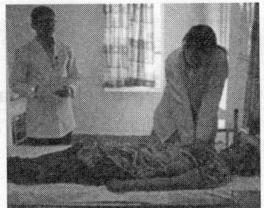
BLS skill station

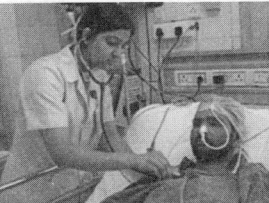
Chest examination station

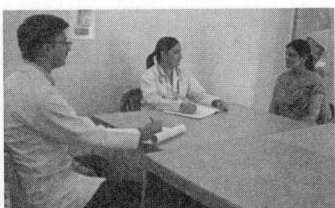
History taking station

FIGURE 9.6

Examples of a procedure station.

- As the stations are generally independent, students can start at any procedure stations and complete the cycle.
- Thus, using 15 stations of 4 minutes each, 15 students can complete the examination within 1 hour.
- Each station is designed to test a component of clinical competence.
- At some stations, called the *procedure stations*, (Fig. 9.6) students are given tasks to perform on patients or simulators (some of the essential examples of procedure stations that may be used for first year B.Sc. Nursing students are given in Box 9.7). At all such stations there are observers with agreed upon checklists or rating scales to score the student's performance (Box 9.8).
- At other stations called *response stations* (Fig. 9.7), students respond to questions of the objective type or interpret data or record their findings of the previous procedure stations. An example of a mode OSCE is depicted in Box 9.9.

IV. SIMULATED VS. REAL-LIFE OSCE STATIONS

This is one of the controversial issues; however, most of the clinicians support real-life OSCE station for procedures. A study conducted on the preference and efficacy of simulation vs. real-life OSCE station revealed that students preferred and felt comfortable in simulated stations. But candidates who performed better over simulators were not found to be confident real-life practitioners. However, simulators and real-life OSCE stations have their unique positive aspects as discussed below (Fig. 9.8):

The positive aspects of simulated OSCE stations are as follows:

- They are controlled and safe.
- Feedback from modern sophisticated simulators can be obtained.
- Simulators are readily available when required.
- Simulated stations can be tailored to the level of skill to be assessed.

BOX 9.7 EXAMPLES OF THE PROCEDURE STATION FOR FIRST YEAR B.SC. NURSING STUDENTS

- Brief history taking
- Chest assessment
- Identifying nursing needs
- Identification and uses of different gadgets

- Oral medication
- Back care
- Intramuscular injection and such nursing procedures

BOX 9.8 PROCEDURE STATION CHECKLIST

Procedure: Oral medications

Steps to be followed	Please tick (✓) mark	
	Yes	No
1. Wash hands		
2. Recall safety measures, locate the drug, read the label on the bottle and see that it is the right medicine and shake the bottle		
3. Collect medicine into the container		
4. Measure liquids accurately with a minim glass and read the lower level of the meniscus		
5. Pour liquid from the opposite side of the label, wipe the mouth of the bottle and recap the bottle		
6. Take the tablet/capsule in a spoon or medicine cup		
7. Identify the patient with the patient chart		
8. Explain the procedure		
9. Place patient's towel under the chin		
10. Position the patient comfortably in the upright sitting position		
11. Administer each drug separately followed by water		
12. Record the drug administering details of dose, route, date, time, signature and omissions		
13. Clean and replace the articles		

Each step carries one mark
Signature of examiner: …………………………………… Date: ……………………………

- Scenarios that are distressing to real patients can be simulated.
- In simulated stations, the patient variable in examination is uniform across trainees.

The positive aspects of real-life OSCE stations are as follows:

- Real-life stations provide actual competence of a person on performance because idealized 'textbook' scenarios may not mimic real-life situations.
- They allow assessment of complex skills which may not be possible at simulated stations.
- Real-life situations may be more cost-effective.

RESPONSE STATION-1

Interpret the following ABG report.

$pH = 7.27$

$PaCO_2 = 49$

$HCO_3 = 24$

$PaCO_2 = 92$

Name this condition: …………………

RESPONSE STATION-2

Patient-G had prescription of 1200 mL fluid for 12 hours. How many drops per minute nurse will administrator through macro drip set?

a) 27

b) 30

c) 32

d) 40

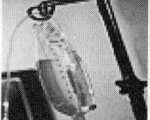

FIGURE 9.7

Examples of response stations for OSCE.I

BOX 9.9 EXAMPLE OF A MODEL OSCE FOR CRITICAL CARE NURSING STUDENTS

PROCEDURE STATION-1

Assess the patient X; identify the three priority nursing needs:

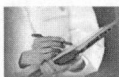

i ....

ii ....

iii ....

PROCEDURE STATION-2

Conduct chest assessment of patient A and identify two abnormal respiratory findings:

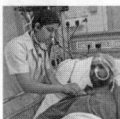

i ....

ii ....

PROCEDURE STATION-3

Carryout ET suctioning of patient Y and record the procedure:

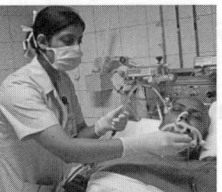

PROCEDURE STATION-4

Change 'PEEP' from 10 to 5 of patient Z, who is on ventilator:

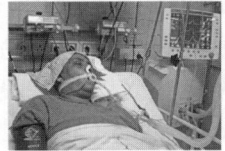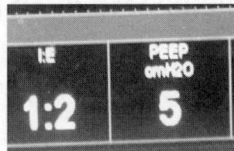

RESPONSE STATION-5

Interpret this ABG report:

$pH = 7.27$
$PaCO_2 = 49$
$HCO_3 = 24$
$PaCO_2 = 92$

Name this condition: ....

RESPONSE STATION-6

Patient G had a prescription of 1200 mL fluid for 12 hours. How many drops per min nurse will the administrator through macro drip set?

a) 27

b) 30

c) 32

d) 40

PROCEDURE STATION-7

Mention indications, dose and any four nursing consideration of this medicine:

i. Indication: ....

ii. Dose: ....

iii. Three essential nursing considerations:

....

....

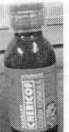

RESPONSE STATION-8

Interpret the following ECG strip:

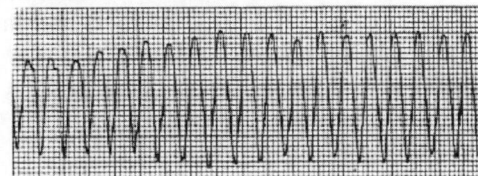

Name the condition: ....

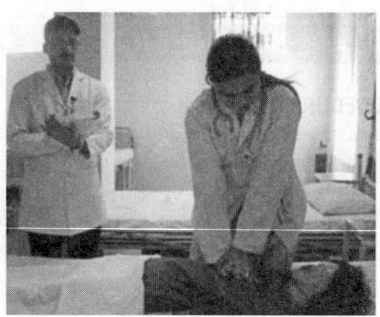 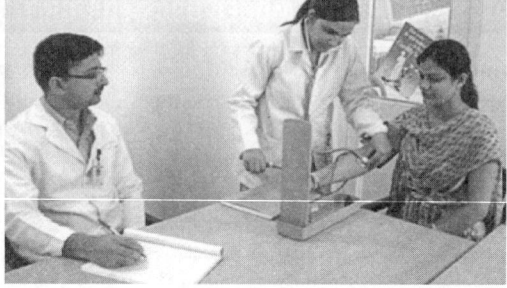

Simulated OSCE station   Real life OSCE station

FIGURE 9.8

Simulated vs. real-life situation for an OSCE station.

V. PROBLEMS OF USING OSCE IN THE INDIAN SCENARIO

The main reasons OSCE has not become a routine assessment method for clinical examination of nursing students either for formative or summative evaluation in India are as follows:

- Lack of feasibility due to time constrains.
- Shortage of training for use of OSCE.
- Shortage of observers/examiners.
- Lack of interest in examiners.
- Lack of enforced guidelines for practical examination by universities (number of students examined and format of evaluation used).

A. Advantages of OSCE

- More valid than the traditional approach to clinical examinations.
- Examiners can decide in advance what is to be tested and can then design the examination to test these competencies.
- Examiners can have better control on the content and complexities.
- Emphasis can be moved away from testing factual knowledge to testing a wide range of skills including advanced clinical skills.
- More reliable because variables of the examiner and the patient are removed to a large extent.
- The use of checklists by examiners and the use of multiple-choice questions results in a more objective examination.
- More practical because it can be used with a large numbers of students.

B. Disadvantages of OSCE

- Students' knowledge and skills are tested in compartments and they are not tested on their ability to look at the patient as a whole.
- Demanding for both examiners and patients.
- Examiners are required to pay close attention to students repeating the same task on a number of occasions.

- The time involved in setting up the examination is greater than for the traditional examination.
- Maintaining uniform difficulty levels is not always possible.

ATTITUDE SCALES

An attitude is a dispositional readiness to respond to certain situations, persons or objects in a consistent manner, which has been learned and has become one's typical mode of response. An attitude has a well-defined object of reference. For example, one's views regarding a class of food or drink, sports and maths are attitudes.

A scale is a device designed to assign a numeric score to people to place them on a continuum with respect to attributes being measured, like a scale for measuring attitudes or weight. These rating scales are used to assess the attitudes and feelings of self-concept. The expressions in view of any point are accounted as measurements towards any item, object or concept. It shows a person's positive or negative attitude towards any concept. Measuring the score between two opposite words tells us the attitude, feeling and perception of a person or study subject towards the directions of positive or negative attitude in a scale. Visual scales illustrate visual depiction of any culture; photographs are given to get feelings, belief, opinions about contrast, texture, colour and elements.

I. TYPES OF ATTITUDE SCALES

There are two attitude scales commonly used to assess the attitude of individuals: Likert scale and semantic differential scale.

LIKERT SCALE

Likert scale was named after a psychologist Rensis Likert, who developed it in 1932 as a psychological concept measurement scale. Likert scale is the most commonly used scaling technique. It was developed to measure the attitudes, values and feelings of people. Primarily, the original version of this scale was developed with a five-point scale (strongly agree, agree, uncertain, disagree and strongly disagree) containing a mixture of positive and negative declarative statements regarding measuring variables (Box 9.10). However, one can even observe the Likert scale now with four point (strongly agree, moderately agree, disagree and uncertain) to seven point (very strongly agree, strongly agree, agree, uncertain, disagree, strongly disagree and very strongly disagree) scaling categories.

I. DEFINITIONS OF A LIKERT SCALE

Likert scale is a composite measurement scale used to measure attitude, values and feelings of the people that involve summation of scores on the set of positive and negative declarative statements regarding measuring variables to which respondents are asked to indicate their degree of agreement or disagreement.

Likert scale is a composite measure of attitudes that involve summation of scores on set of items (statements) to which respondents are asked to indicate their degree of agreement or disagreement.

BOX 9.10 EXAMPLE OF THE FIVE-POINT LIKERT SCALE TO ASSESS THE ATTITUDE WITH HIV/AIDS

Statement	Please tick (✓) in appropriate column for each statement				
	Strongly agree	Agree	Uncertain	Disagree	Strongly disagree
1. Person with multiple sex partners are at high risk of AIDS					
2. You can get AIDS by sharing utensils					
3. You may have HIV by sharing needles with others					
4. Only gay men can get AIDS					
5. One way of getting AIDS is infected blood transfusion					
6. AIDS is a curable disease					

II. USES OF A LIKERT SCALE

- It is basically used to measure the attitudes, values and feelings of the people about a specific concept such as a situation, people, place, object, programme, practice and policy.
- This scale is used to have quantified measurement of the qualitative attributes of people such as feelings, values and attitude.
- It may also be used to assess the opinion of people about a particular abstract concept.
- It spreads out people with various attitudes, emotions and feelings towards a particular concept.

III. CHARACTERISTICS OF A LIKERT SCALE

The main characteristics of a Likert scale are are as follows:

- *Psychological measurement tool:* Likert scale is basically a psychological measurement tool to assess the attitudes, values and feelings of the people about a specific concept.
- *Illustrative in nature:* This scale is generally illustrative in nature, where each statement in the scale is stated in an explicitly graphical way so that a person can make a clear judgement about the degree of agreement or disagreement with the particular item of scale.
- *Neutral statements:* The scale must contain neutral statements without incorporation of any bias of the evaluator.
- *Bipolar scaling method:* This is composed with an alternative mixture of positive and negative declarative statements, so that the respondent's casual response bias can be eliminated. Positive statements get a high score with agreement and negative statements get a high score with disagreement with the statement.
- *Measurement of the specific number of scaling categories:* This scale is originally developed with five scaling categories and later the scales even developed with four, six and seven scaling categories.

IV. SCORING OF THE LIKERT SCALE

Scoring of the Likert scale is done on the basis of the type of statement and the level of the respondents' agreement with the statement.

- For a positive statement, respondents get a higher score if there is agreement with a statement. However, in case of negative statements, respondents get a higher score, if there is disagreement with a statement or vice versa as depicted in Box 9.11.

V. GUIDELINES FOR THE CONSTRUCTION OF LIKERT SCALE

- A five-point or seven-point Likert scale may be designed with appropriate degrees of agreement and disagreement phrases.
- The statements should be brief, concise and precise.
- Each statement should convey only one complete thought. More than one idea should not be included in a single statement; it is better to construct more statements.
- The statement should belong to the attitude variable that is to be measured.
- Care should be taken about language:
  - use simple sentences
  - avoid double negatives
  - avoid: all, always, none or never
  - use with care: only, just, merely
  - avoid words with more than one meaning.
- The statements should cover the entire range of the affective scale of interest.
- Statements should be such that they can be endorsed or rejected (agreed/disagreed)
- Acceptance and rejection should indicate something about the attitude measured.

A. Advantages of a Likert scale

- It is relatively easy to construct this scale.
- Likert scale is considered more reliable and valid tool to measure psychosocial variables.
- It is easy to administer as the respondents only have to place a tick in the provided spaces against each statement.
- It is less time consuming during construction and administration.

BOX 9.11 SCORING OF STATEMENTS IN LIKERT SCALE

Statement	Strongly agree	Agree	Uncertain	Disagree	Strongly disagree
(Positive statement)	5	4	3	2	1
1. Person with multiple sex partners are at high risk of AIDS					
(Negative statement)	1	2	3	4	5
2. You can get AIDS by sharing utensils					

B. Disadvantages of a Likert scale

- In a Likert scale, the respondents may feel forced to answer the question against each preplanned item and its categories.
- Feelings of the respondents may not be fully assessed due to researcher's preplanned statements and categories.
- Difficulty in justifying the selection of the number of categories and numerical assignment to these categories.
- Casual approach of respondents in these scales may provide misleading data.

SEMANTIC DIFFERENTIAL SCALE

Semantic differential scale is the most effective and most widely used technique these days. In 1967, Osgood, Suci and Tannenbaum introduced this method for the first time in their book, *The Measurement of Meaning*. Although the original purpose of the scale was not necessarily to measure the assessment of attitude, the procedure was well adopted for attitude assessment.

Semantic differential questions measure people's attitude towards stimulus, words, objects and concepts. This question type consists of a series of contrasting adjective pairs (e.g. good–bad, beneficial–harmful) listed on opposite ends of a bipolar scale. Many studies have shown that semantic differential questions can work effectively with different age groups, cultures and languages. This scale is popular because it is extremely easy to construct and administer, and provides reasonably valid and reliable quantitative data. An example of a semantic differential scale to assess the attitude of student nurses towards patients is illustrated in Fig. 9.9.

I. DEFINITION OF A SEMANTIC DIFFERENTIAL SCALE

Semantic differential scale is a type of rating scale designed to measure the connotative meaning of objects, events and concepts. These connotations are used to derive the attitude of the objects, events and concepts.

Experience Working with Patients

	1	2	3	4	5	6	7	
Unpleasant	1	2	3	4	5	6	7	Pleasant
Rude	1	2	3	4	5	6	7	Polite
Cold	1	2	3	4	5	6	7	Warm
Callous	1	2	3	4	5	6	7	Considerate
Inhuman	1	2	3	4	5	6	7	Human
Noncommunicative	1	2	3	4	5	6	7	Communicative
Disrespecting	1	2	3	4	5	6	7	Respectful
Insincere	1	2	3	4	5	6	7	Friendly
Unconcern	1	2	3	4	5	6	7	Empathy

FIGURE 9.9

Example of a semantic differential scale to assess the attitude of student nurses towards patients.

BOX 9.12 ADJECTIVE PAIRS USED FOR CONSTRUCTION OF SEMANTIC DIFFERENTIAL SCALE		
Evaluation	**Potency**	**Activity**
Good — Bad	Hard — Soft	Active — Passive
Kind — Cruel	Strong — Weak	Fast — Slow
Wise — Foolish	Heavy — Light	Hot — Cold
Beautiful — Ugly	Deep — Shallow	Motivated — Aimless
Happy — Sad	Potent — Impotent	Moving — Still
Sociable — Unsociable	Large — Small	Excitable — Calm
Friendly — Unfriendly	Simple — Complex	Alive — Dead
Willing — Unwilling	Difficult — Easy	Emotional — Unemotional
Honest — Dishonest	Submissive — Assertive	Bright — Dim

II. CONSTRUCTING A SEMANTIC DIFFERENTIAL SCALE

For the preparation of semantic differential scale, the following adjective pairs are used (Box 9.12):

- The bipolar adjective pairs can be used for a wide variety of subjects.
- The adjective pairs are selected according to the objectives of the survey.
- The adjective pairs can be grouped into three large categories and each survey question usually includes a few points from each category. These categories are evaluation, potency and activity.
- Often, the attitude scale needs to be constructed for a particular aspect that one wishes to measure and the following steps are used in construction of an attitude scale:
  - Specify the attitude variable that is to be measured.
  - Collect a wide variety of statements.
  - Edit the statements.
  - Sort out the statements into (an imaginary) scale.
  - Calculate the scale value.

A. Advantages of a semantic differential scale

- A convenient method to assess beliefs, attitudes and values in quantitative form.
- Easy to administer.
- Provides reasonable, valid and reliable quantitative data.

B. Disadvantages of a semantic differential scale

- It is difficult to select the relevant concepts that are appropriate for any given investigations.
- It is time consuming, if anyone is not able to find the appropriate adjective pairs.

REVIEW QUESTIONS

Long-Answer Questions

1. Describe the advantages and disadvantages of essay type questions.
2. Describe the advantages and disadvantages of practical examinations.

3. Describe the advantages of multiple-choice questions.
4. Explain observational checklists.
5. Describe the criteria for the selection of evaluation techniques and devices.
6. Describe OSCE with examples.
7. Describe the types of reliability used for an assessment tool.
8. Describe the disadvantages of multiple-choice questions.
9. Explain Likert attitude scale.
10. List the purposes of educational evaluations and explain the qualities of an evaluation tool.
11. Describe the scope of evaluation.
12. Describe the validity of assessment tools.
13. Mention the criteria for the selection of evaluation methods.
14. Discuss the multiple-choice questions/items.

Short Answer Questions

1. Define evaluation.
2. Mention the parts of a multiple-choice question with an example.
3. Give one example for any type of rating scale.
4. Write any two characteristics of MCQ.
5. List down the characteristics of a Likert scale.
6. Define the Objective Structured Clinical Examination (OSCE).
7. Define summative and formative evaluation.
8. Mention the advantages of essay type questions.
9. Discuss the purposes of short answer questions.
10. Discuss the characterstics of checklist.

Multiple-Choice Questions (MCQs)

1. What do you mean by term *evaluation*?
   (a) Process of finding out the level of achievement based on predecided criteria
   (b) Measurement of quantity of pupil's attainment in a subject
   (c) By the use of some test check the performance of students
   (d) Testing the quality and quantity of students
2. Evaluation of students' performance is based on which law?
   (a) Law of effect
   (b) Law of motivation
   (c) Leadership law
   (d) Both (a) and (b)
3. Evaluation is a
   (a) Static process
   (b) Continuation process
   (c) Motivational process
   (d) Helpful only for students
4. Evaluation process involves
   (a) Teacher
   (b) Learner
   (c) Question
   (d) Teacher and learner

5. Evaluation process involves the maximum use of
   (a) Motivation
   (b) Learning
   (c) Knowledge
   (d) Insight
6. What do you mean by term *measurement*?
   (a) Quantifying and describing of pupil's achievement
   (b) It is a tool for measuring evaluation
   (c) It shows a measurement as 50 out of 100
   (d) All of these
7. Is measurement a part of evaluation?
   (a) Evaluation includes measurement and a wider process of judgement
   (b) Measurement includes evaluation and a wider process of judgement
   (c) Measurement includes evaluation and a narrow process of judgement
   (d) Evaluation includes measurement and a narrow process of judgement
8. Validity of an instrument varies with
   (a) Influence of extraneous variables
   (b) Difficult levels of items
   (c) Both (a) and (b)
   (d) Expert opinion
9. Validity of a measurement tool means
   (a) The accuracy with which a test measures whatever it is intended to measure
   (b) The inaccuracy is tested in this method to remove error
   (c) It is a degree of consistency of result when measured by particular instrument
   (d) It is a test–retest method
10. Reliability of a measurement tool means
    (a) A test measures whatever it is intended to measure
    (b) Consistency with which test measures a given variable
    (c) Both (a) and (b)
    (d) None of these
11. Which one of the following is the type of validity of a measurement tool?
    (a) Reality, concurrent, parallel, content, predictive validity
    (b) Content, reliability, face, predictive, content validity
    (c) Predictive, face, concurrent, content, construct validity
    (d) Face, construct, concurrent, reliability, content validity
12. What should be the quality of a good measurement tool?
    (a) Validity
    (b) Reliability
    (c) Practicability
    (d) All of these
13. Student evaluation is for what?
    (a) Motivation
    (b) Feedback
    (c) Certification of competence
    (d) All of these

14. Validity is measurement in
   (a) Degree: high, moderate, low
   (b) Levels: level 1, level 2, level 3
   (c) Present or absent
   (d) Consistent or nonconsistent
15. Approaches/methods used for establishing reliability of a measurement tool include
   (a) Mean, median and mode
   (b) Test–retest method and split half method
   (c) Mean, median, mode and range
   (d) Geometrical mean and test–retest method

Answers of the Multiple-Choice Questions

1. (a), 2. (d), 3. (b), 4. (d), 5. (a), 6. (a), 7. (a), 8. (c), 9. (a), 10. (b), 11. (c), 12. (d), 13. (d), 14. (c), 15. (b)

FURTHER READING

Adams, R. J., Doig, B. A., & Rosier, M. J. (1991). *Science learning in Victorian schools: 1990, ACER Monograph No. 41*. Hawthorn, Vic.: Australian Council for Educational Research.

Black, P., & Wiliam, D. (1998). Assessment and classroom learning. *Assessment in Education*, 5, 7–74.

Bloom, B. S., Hastings,T., & Madaus, G. (1971). *Handbook on formative and summative evaluation of student learning*. New York: McGraw-Hill.

Bowling, A. (2002). *Research Methods in Health: Investigating health and health services*. Buckingham, UK: Open University Press.

Bridge, P. D., Musial, J., Frank, R., Roe, T., & Sawilowsky, S. (2003). Measurement practices: Methods for developing content-valid student examinations. *Med Teach*, 25, 414–421.

Brown, G., & Pendlebury, M. (1992). *Assessing active learning part 1: Core materials*. Sheffield, UK: CVCP Universities' Staff Development and Training Unit.

Brown, G., & Pendlebury, M. (1992). *Assessing active learning part 2: Illustrative examples of the core materials*. Sheffield, UK: CVCP Universities' Staff Development and Training Unit.

Brown, S., Rust, C., & Gibbs, G. (1994). *Strategies for diversifying assessment in higher education*. Oxford, UK: Oxford Centre for Staff Development.

Burns, R. (2000). *Introduction to research methods*. London, UK: Sage.

Case, S. M., & Swanson, D. B. (2001). *Constructing written test questions for the basic and clinical sciences* (3rd ed.). Philadelphia, PA: National Board of Examiners.

Crooks, T. J. (1988). The impact of classroom evaluation practices on students. *Review of Educational Research*, 58, 438–481.

Crossley, J., Humphries, G., & Jolly, B. (2002). Assessing health professionals. *Med Educ*, 36, 800–804.

Crow, L. D. (1951). *Introduction to education: Fundamental principles and practices*. New York: American Book Company.

Doig, B. A., Piper, K., Mellor, S., & Masters, G. (1994). *Conceptual understanding in social education, ACER Research Monograph No. 45*. Melbourne, Vic.: Australian Council for Educational Research.

Gronlund, N. E. (1968). *Constructing achievement tests*. Englewood Cliffs, NJ: Prentice Hall Inc.

Haladyna, T. M. (1999). *Developing and validating multiple-choice test items* (2nd ed.). Mahwah, NJ: Lawrence Erlbaum Associates.

Harden, R., & Gleeson, F. (1979). Assessment of clinical competence using an objective structured clinical examination (OSCE). *Med Educ*, 13, 41–54.

Harlen, W., & James, M. (1996). *Creating a positive impact of assessment on learning*. New York: Paper presented at the annual meeting of the American Educational Research Association.

Heidgerkan, L. E. (1966). *Teaching and learning in schools of nursing* (3rd ed.). Philadelphia: J B Lippincott Co.

Henrysson, S. (1971). Gathering, analyzing, and using data on test items. In R. L. Thorndike, (Ed.) *Educational measurement* (2nd ed., pp. 130–159). Washington, D.C.: American Council on Education.

Hopkins, C. D., & Antes, R. L. (1990). *Classroom measurement and evaluation*. Itasca, IL: Peacock.

Izard, J. (1991). *Assessment of learning in the classroom*. Geelong, Vic.: Deakin University.

Izard, J. (1997). *Trial testing and item analysis in test construction*. Paris: International Institute for Educational Planning.

Linn, R. L., & Gronlund, N. E. (2000). *Measurement and assessment in teaching* (8th ed.). Upper Saddle River, NJ: Prentice-Hall.

Masters, G. N., Lokan, J., Doig, B., Khoo, S. T., Lindsey, J., Robinson, L., et al. (1990). *Profiles of learning: The basic skills testing program in New South Wales, 1989*. Hawthorn, Vic.: Australian Council for Educational Research.

Mehrens, W. A., & Lehmann, I. J. (1984). *Measurement and evaluation in education and psychology* (3rd ed.). New York: Holt, Rinehart and Winston.

Oosterhoff, A. (2003). *Developing and using classroom assessments* (3rd ed.). Upper Saddle River, NJ: Pearson Education.

Osterlind, S. J. (1998). *Constructing test items: Multiple-choice, constructed-response, performance, and other formats* (2nd ed.). Norwell, MA: Kluwer Academic Publishers.

Ross, K. N. (1992). *Sample design procedures for a national survey of primary schools in Zimbabwe. Issues and methodologies in educational development #8*. UNESCO: IIEP.

Royal College of Nursing (2008). *Advanced nurse practitioners: An RCN guide to the advanced nurse practitioner role, competencies and programme accreditation*. London: Royal College of Nursing.

Rushforth, H. (2007). Objective structured clinical examination (OSCE): Review of literature and implications for nursing education. *Nurse Educ Today*, 27, 481–490.

Rust, W. B. (1973). *Objective testing in education and training*. London, UK: Pitman Education Library.

Tinkelman, S. N. (1971). Planning the objective test. In R. L., Thorndike. *Educational measurement* (2nd ed., pp. 46–80). Washington, D.C.: American Council on Education.

Waldner, M., & Olson, J. (2007). Taking the patient to the classroom: Applying theoretical frameworks to simulation in nursing education. *International Journal of Nursing Education Scholarship*, 4(1), 1–14.

Ward, H., & Barratt, J. (2005). Assessment of nurse practitioner advanced clinical practice skills: Using the objective structured clinical examination (OSCE). *Primary Health Care*, 15(10), 37–41.

Wass, V., Van der Vleuten, C., Shatzer, J., & Jones, R. (2001). Assessment of clinical competence. *Lancet*, 357, 945–9.

Withers, G. (1997). *Item writing for tests and examinations*. Paris: International Institute for Educational Planning.

10

Information, education and communication for health

Educate and inform the whole mass of the people. They are our only sure reliance for the preservation of our liberty.
—**Thomas Jefferson**

LEARNING OBJECTIVES

This chapter is designed to enable the reader to

- Understand the concept of health behaviour and health education
- Discuss the objectives, principles, scope and importance of health education
- Describe the purposes, principles and steps in planning health education
- Explore meaning, methods, advantages and disadvantages of individual, group health education
- Appraise the factors contributing in the success of communicating the messages and methods and media used for it
- Define and classify the mass media
- Identify the importance and methods of mass media communication

KEY TERMS

INTRODUCTION

Information, education and communication (IEC) are interrelated. Information is the knowledge derived from study, experience or instruction. It can also be defined as a collection of facts or data. Education is both the acquisition of knowledge and experience and the development of skills, habits and attitudes that help a person lead a full and meaningful life. Communication is the interaction between two or more persons that involves the exchange of information between the sender and the receiver. Therefore, information, education and communication are closely related to health and play a vital role in creating awareness about health, mobilizing people and making them knowledgeable about health-related factors through efficient mass communication methods. IEC has two principal functions, i.e. informative and persuasive, which are essential for bringing about prerequisite social mobilization and facilitating participatory development towards the health of an individual, family and community.

HEALTH BEHAVIOUR

Health behaviour is an action taken by a person to maintain, attain or regain good health and to prevent illness. Health behaviour reflects a person's health beliefs. Some common health behaviours are exercising regularly, eating a balanced diet and obtaining necessary inoculations.

In other words, health behaviour is any activity undertaken by an individual, regardless of the actual or perceived health status for the purpose of promoting, protecting or maintaining health, whether or not such behaviour is objectively effective towards that end.

Individual behaviours such as staying physically active and eating a balance diet can contribute to good health. Other behaviours such as smoking, heavy drinking and illicit drug use can have detrimental health effects. Ultimately, health behaviours are individual choices that people make. However, these behaviours are influenced by the social and economic environments where individuals work, live, learn and earn.

Various strategies made to influence the behaviour of individuals and groups will vary greatly and depend on some specific concerned health problems and its distribution in the population as well as on the characteristics and acceptability of the available methods that help in preventing and controlling that health problem. It is clear that education is necessary, but education alone is insufficient to achieve the desired health behaviour and ultimately optimum health. In addition to acquiring knowledge through education, other factors such as biological, psychological, social, cultural factors, socioeconomic status and health beliefs of the people may influence the health behaviour of an individual (Box 10.1).

While people may aspire towards a healthier lifestyle, the initiation and maintenance of health behaviours result from an interaction of social, psychological, biological and environmental factors. In recent years, the emerging discipline of health psychology has tried to explain why people engage in unhealthy behaviours and inform the development of health behaviour interventions. Research suggests that intentions to change a behaviour, while often a prerequisite of change, can be insufficient to produce sustained change. Starting and maintaining behavioural change can be aided by psychological characteristics and processes. These include the belief that one has the psychological resources to undertake the desired behaviour (self-efficacy) and the individual's ability to use self-regulatory strategies (Box 10.2). Box 10.3 shows how these can be translated into practice for quitting smoking and healthier eating.

I. HEALTH BELIEF MODEL

Health belief model is helpful in predicting the health behaviour of individuals. It is a psychological model that attempts to explain and predict health behaviours. It focuses on attitude and beliefs of

---

BOX 10.1 FACTORS INFLUENCING HEALTH BEHAVIOUR

- Knowledge
- Biological factors
- Psychological factors
- Social factors

- Socioeconomic status
- Cultural factors
- Health belief of the people

BOX 10.2 PSYCHOLOGICAL FACTORS CONTRIBUTING TO SUCCESSFUL HEALTH BEHAVIOUR CHANGE

Self-efficacy

Self-efficacy is the belief that one has the capability to undertake the actions to bring about particular outcomes. Self-efficacy can be enhanced by:

- Experience of succeeding at the behaviour. To promote safer sex practices, teenagers might be encouraged to role-play asking a partner to use a condom.
- Modelling or observing others by successfully undertaking the target behaviour. To promote self-efficacy in children to eat healthily, they might be encouraged to observe other children eating fruits and vegetables.

Self-regulation

Self-regulation includes a number of processes that aid the implementation of behaviour.

- Setting and reviewing realistic goals to implement behaviour. The goal of walking to work to increase physical activity may be more achievable than going to the gym which requires effort and financial outlay.

- Formation of implementation intentions specifying the context in which the person is going to engage in the behaviour. If swimming is the target behaviour then the person might identify the day of the week, the time and the place he or she will swim.
- Identifying barriers and ways to overcome them. Someone trying to quit smoking might identify that they always smoke with a social drink. The smoking cessation charity QUIT advises smokers to overcome this by having a different drink from their usual, and holding it in the hand in which they usually hold their cigarette, along with other practical suggestions.
- Monitoring performance. Tools such as diaries to record attempts at the behaviour can be helpful in identifying both successes and failures to reach the goal which can then be used to develop further strategies.
- Feedback on performance from others can contribute to strategies to implement behaviour.

BOX 10.3 HEALTH PROMOTION STRATEGIES

Smoking

Population level interventions

- Media information campaigns about the harms of smoking can motivate and support behaviour change. The *get unhooked* campaign tries to raise smokers' self-efficacy by communicating that they can stop as well as provide information about support to give an immediate way to turn motivation into behaviour.
- Incentives: smokers are encouraged to quit by imposing taxes on cigarettes, while general practitioners are offered incentives to promote smoking cessation in their patients.

Individual level interventions

- Medical treatments include nicotine replacement therapy to reduce withdrawal symptoms and medicines such as bupropion to reduce cravings.
- Psychological support such as the telephone counselling services provided by QUIT. This aims to help smokers understand their smoking behaviour and increase consciousness of their smoking; minimize their reasons to continue smoking and maximize reasons to stop; and plan their quitting attempt using psychological support from friends and family and medical treatments.

Healthy eating

Population level interventions

- *Food labelling:* The Food Standards Agency (FSA) labelling scheme gives fat, saturates, sugars and salt

a traffic-light-colour-coded label indicating its level in the product. Red labels indicate high levels, amber levels indicate medium levels and green labels indicate low levels. Some retailers also colour code calories. Since Sainsbury's introduced the traffic light labels, they have identified sales increase of mainly green-labelled products and decrease of mainly red-labelled products across ranges including sandwiches, ready meals and dairy desserts.

- *Advertising bans:* Regulatory agencies have announced a ban on adverts for foods high in fat, salt and sugars around children's programmes. Such advertising affects children's food preferences and consumption.
- *Signalling:* Health researchers and pressure groups suggest public institutions should signal what a healthy diet is by providing it for their patients. Fast food outlets in hospitals and machines vending sweets, crisps and fizzy drinks in schools have the opposite effect.

Individual level interventions

- *The Food Dudes* intervention is based on the model of, and rewards for, healthy eating. Children between 5–7 years of age see healthy eating modelled in a video in which a group of slightly older children are shown eating and enjoying vegetables while encouraging the viewers to do the same. Rewards include Food Dudes lunch boxes and stickers.

individuals. It was developed in the 1950s by a group of social psychologists, Hochbaum, Rosenstock and Kegels, working for US Public Health Service with a view to improve the public use of preventive services. This model was developed in response to the failure of the free Tuberculosis Health Screening Programme. The principal components of the health belief model are as follows (Fig. 10.1):

- *Individual perception:* Individual perception includes the following aspects:
  - *Perceived susceptibility:* Belief that disease state is present or likely to occur. Family history may make the individual feel at high risk.
  - *Perceived seriousness:* Perception that the state or condition of disease is harmful and has serious consequence. For example, HIV/AIDS.
  - *Perceived threat:* Perceived susceptibility and perceived seriousness combined to determine perceived threat.
- *Modifying factors:* Modifying factors in the health belief model includes the following variables:
  - *Demographic variables:* Include age, sex, race and ethnicity, for example, an infant does not perceive the importance of diet; an adolescent may perceive peer approval as more important than family approval.
  - *Sociopsychological variables:* Social pressure or influence from peers or other reference groups may encourage preventive health behaviours even when individual motivation is low.
  - *Structural variables:* Knowledge about the target disease and prior contact with it are presumed to influence the preventive behaviour.
  - *Cues to action:* Cues can be external or internal. Internal cues include feelings of fatigue, uncomfortable symptoms or thoughts.
- *Likelihood of action:* The health belief model includes the following likelihood of action:
  - *Perceived benefit:* Belief that health action is of some value. For example, refraining from smoking to prevent lung cancer and eating nutritious foods and avoiding snacks to maintain weight.
  - *Perceived barrier:* Belief that health action would be associated with hindrance. It includes cost, inconvenience, unpleasantness and lifestyle changes.

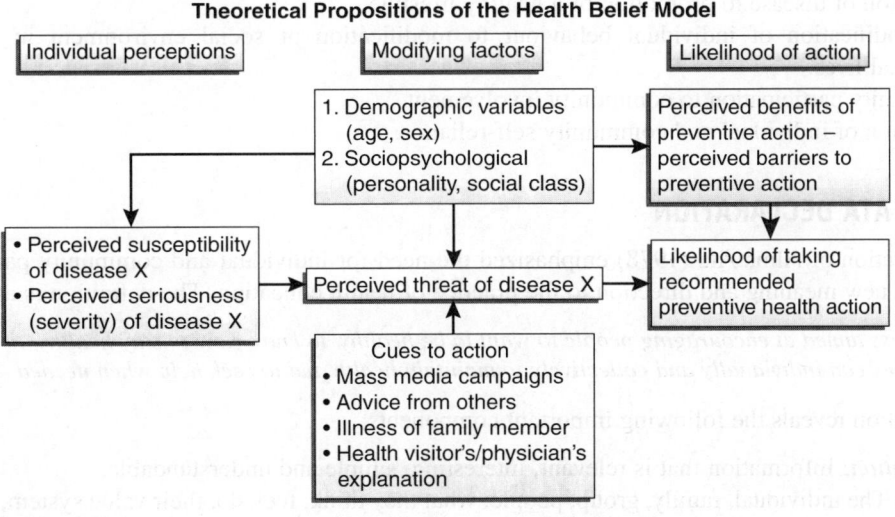

FIGURE 10.1

Health belief model.

HEALTH EDUCATION

According to the World Health Organization, the health is the state of complete physical, psychological, social and spiritual well-being and not merely an absence of disease or infirmity. Education is a process, the chief goal of which is to bring about changes in human behaviour. Every individual has access to a type of education that permits maximum development of his potential and capabilities.

Health education is a term frequently used by health care professionals. It aims at achieving individual and community health. Health education is the translation of what is known about health into desirable individual and community behaviour patterns by means of an educational process.

Health education is not simply giving information or instructions on health matters to patients or people at large. It is much more than that. Like general education, it is a process of communication of information on health and disease to individuals, family groups and communities to learn and adopt a lifestyle that promotes help.

According to World Health Organization, health education is like a general education which is concerned with changes in knowledge of people in its most usual forms, it concentrates on developing such practices as are believed to bring the best possible state of well-being.

A similar but more clear and comprehensive definition that is adopted by the National Conference on Preventive Medicine in USA is health education is a process that informs, motivates and helps people to adopt and maintain healthy practices and lifestyles, advocates environment changes as needed to facilitate this goal and conducts professional training and research to the same end.

John M. Last defines health education as the process by which individuals and groups of people learn to behave in a manner conducive to promotion, maintenance or restoration of health. Further, it is any combination of learning opportunities and teaching activities designed to facilitate voluntary adaptations of behaviour that are conducive to health.

Health education is the part of health care that is concerned with promoting healthy behaviour. Historically, health education has been committed to disseminating information and change human behaviour. In the Alma Ata declaration adopted in 1978, the emphasis has shifted from:

- Prevention of disease to promotion of a healthy lifestyle.
- The modification of individual behaviour to modification of social environment in which an individual lives.
- Community participation to community involvement.
- Promotion of individual and community self-reliance.

I. ALMA ATA DECLARATION

The declaration of Alma Ata (1978) emphasized the need for individual and community participation and gave a new meaning and direction to the practice of health education. The definition is as follows:

A process aimed at encouraging people to want to be healthy, to know how to stay healthy, to do what they can individually and collectively to maintain health and to seek help when needed.

This definition reveals the following important components:

- *Information:* Information that is relevant, interesting, simple and understandable.
- *Patient:* The individual, family, group, people; what they think, feel, do, their value system, readiness to learn and bring in desired changes in their lifestyle and environment.

- *Social environment:* Sociocultural and economic supports, barriers which may promote or inhibit behaviour changes for health promotion.
- *Health education content:* The content about health and disease, favourable and nonfavourable lifestyle, environment, proper use of resources and health care facilities, etc.
- *Communication methods:* Means for dissemination of and receiving information that can help in understanding, motivating and bringing in desired changes for healthy living.

II. AIMS OF HEALTH EDUCATION

The definition adopted by WHO in 1969 and the Alma Ata declaration adopted in 1978 provide a useful basis for formulating the aims and objectives of health education. These are as follows:

- To help the people understand that health is the most valuable community asset, and to help them achieve optimum health by their own activities and efforts.
- To develop a sense of responsibility for improving their health as individual members of families and communities.
- To develop scientific knowledge, attitude, skills on health matters to enable people to develop correct habits.
- To educate people for proper use of health services in whatever forms it is made available to them by the government.
- To alter behaviour that may have directly or indirectly influenced the occurrence or spread of diseases in a given setting, a culturally relevant health education programme can be planned only after understanding the behaviour in all its manifestations.
- To promote the greater possible fulfilment of inherited powers of the body and the mind and happy adjustment of an individual in the society.
- To provide a person with appropriate knowledge to enjoy decent health and also knowledge about the occurrence and spread of disease thus enabling him to adopt relevant preventive measures.
- To create in him an interest in his own health and well-being.
- To create in him an interest for the health of other members of his family as well those living in his surroundings.
- To create in him a desire to support health education programmes in his area.

In a nutshell, the focus of health education is on people and action. Its goal is to make realistic improvements in the basic quality of life.

III. OBJECTIVES OF HEALTH EDUCATION

The main objectives of health education are as follows:

- To inform people or disseminate scientific knowledge about prevention of disease and promotion of health.
- To motivate people to change their habits and lifestyle that are harmful to their health and also motivate people to adopt habits and ways of living conducive to healthy living.
- To guide the people who need help to adopt and maintain healthy practices and lifestyle by showing proper community resources.

IV. PRINCIPLES OF HEALTH EDUCATION

Health education encompasses two activities: teaching and learning. Teaching is ineffective without learning. Both the health educator and the patient are responsible for bringing about a change in health knowledge, health attitude and behaviour. Some essential principles of health education are discussed below (Fig. 10.2).

- *Credibility of message:* It is the degree to which the message to be communicated is perceived as trustworthy by the receiver.
- *Creating interest among participants:* It is a psychological principle that people are unlikely to listen to things that are not of their interest. If a health programme is based on the felt needs, people will participate in the programme willingly.
- *Motivating the participants:* Motivation is like a petrol engine that drives the mental engine. It is the fundamental desire in every person to learn. Motivation is contagious; one motivated person may spread motivation throughout the group.
- *Enhance comprehension of content:* It means health education should be based on the level of understanding, education and literacy of people at whom the teaching is directed. Teaching should be within the mental capacity of the audience.
- *Ensure reinforcement:* Repetition at intervals is necessary to promote learning. Without reinforcement and feedback, students can go back to the preawareness stage.
- *Encourage active participation:* Participation is a key word in health education. It is based on the psychological principle of learning. Health education should aim at encouraging people to work actively with health workers and others in identifying their own health problems and also in developing solutions. The Alma Ata declaration states, 'the people have a right and duty to participate individually and collectively in the planning and implementation of their health care'.
- *Learning by doing:* Teaching is effective when individuals actively participate in health education. Learning becomes active and quicker if the individuals are made active physically as well as psychologically.

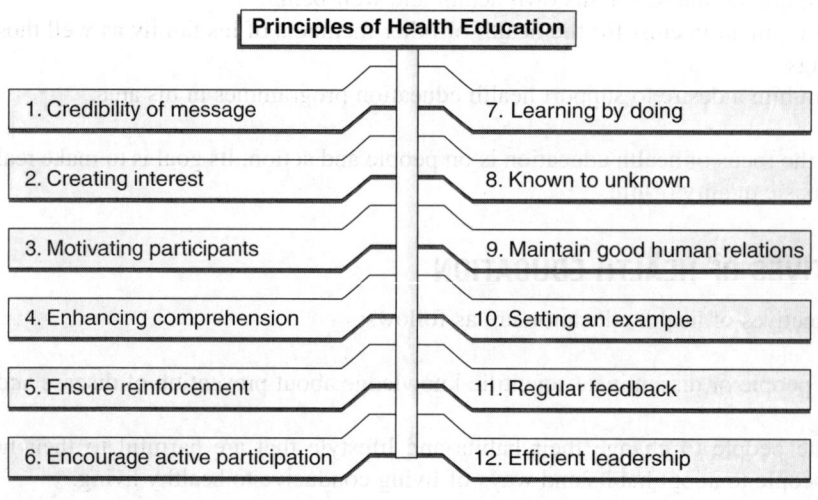

FIGURE 10.2

Principles of health education.

- *Known to unknown:* It is based on the *appreciative mass theory of learning.* The people in a community know something and the health educator enlarges this knowledge. If the health educator links new knowledge with the old knowledge, it can enhance learning.
- *Maintaining good human relations:* Sharing of information, ideas and feelings happens most easily between people who have a good relationship.
- *Setting an example:* The health educators should set a good example in the topic they are dealing with as it fosters better understanding.
- *Regular feedback:* Feedback is one of the key concepts of the system approach. The health educator can modify the elements of the system in light of the feedback from his audience. For effective communication, feedback is of paramount importance.
- *Efficient leadership:* Leaders are agents of change and they can be made use of in health education work. Psychologists have shown and established that we learn best from people we respect and regard. The essential attributes of a leader are as follows:
  - Understands the needs of the community.
  - Provides proper guidance.
  - Takes initiative.
  - Is receptive to the views and suggestions of people.
  - Identifies himself with the community.
  - Is selfless, honest, impartial, considerate and sincere.
  - Is easily accessible to people.

Local leaders in a village community are the village leader or *numberdar* and the school teacher.

V. SCOPE OF HEALTH EDUCATION

The scope of health education extends beyond the conventional health sector. It covers every aspect of individual, family and community health. Health education has limited impact when directed from general education; most of the needed information must be integrated into the educational system (by way of books, classroom material, etc.) and must have the young population as the principal target. The basic scope of health education is as discussed below (Fig. 10.3).

- *Human biology:* Understanding health demands an understanding of human biology, i.e. the structure and functions of the body; how to keep physically fit; the need for exercise, rest and sleep; the effect of alcohol, smoking and drugs on the body, etc. Reproductive biology is also an important part of current interests. The best place to teach human biology is school. It is only in school, through its sequential health curriculum, that we can provide a continuous in-depth learning experience for millions of students.
- *Nutrition:* The aim of nutrition education is to guide people to choose optimum and balanced diets, remove prejudices and promote good dietary habits. Nutritional problems such as ignorance about breast feeding, weaning and traditional food allocation pattern within families can be best solved by nutrition education. In recent years, the link between dietary habits and diabetes, cancer and heart diseases has been established. Thus, nutrition education is a major intervention for the prevention of malnutrition, promotion of health and improving the quality of life.
- *Hygiene:* This has two aspects: personal and environmental. The aim of personal hygiene is to promote standards of personal cleanliness within the setting of conditions where people live. Environmental hygiene has two aspects: domestic and community. All environmental sanitation programmes should include health education.

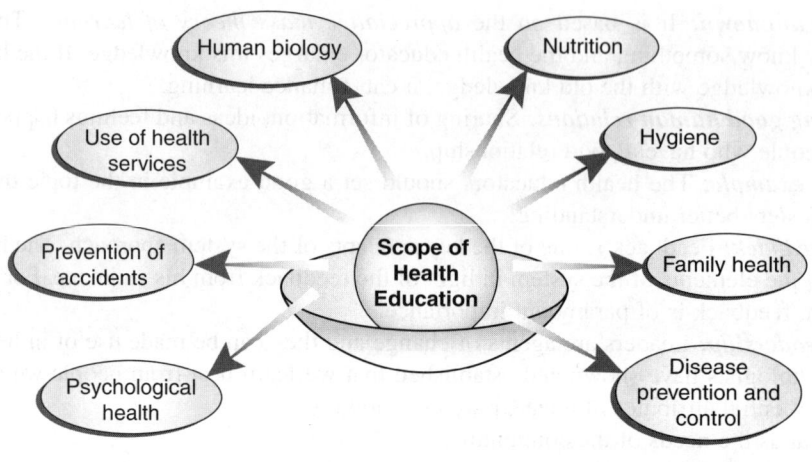

FIGURE 10.3

Scope of health education.

- *Family health:* The family is the first defence as well as the chief reliance for the well-being of its members. Health largely depends on the family's social and physical environment and lifestyle and behaviour of the members. The role of the family in health promotion and in the prevention of disease, early diagnosis and care of sick is of crucial importance. One of the main tasks of health education is to promote family self-reliance, especially regarding the family's responsibilities in child bearing, child rearing, self-care and in influencing their children to adopt a healthy lifestyle.
- *Disease prevention and control:* Drugs alone will not solve health problems. Without health education, a person may fall sick again and again from the same disease. Educating the people about the prevention and control of locally endemic diseases is the first of the eight essential activities in primary health care.
- *Psychological health:* Psychological health problem can occur everywhere. There is a tendency to an increase in the prevalence of psychological diseases when there is a change in society from agriculture to an industrial economy and when people move from the warm intimacy of a village community to the isolation found in big cities. The aim of health education is to help the people to keep psychologically healthy and to prevent a psychological breakdown.
- *Prevention of accidents:* Accidents are a feature of the complexity of modern life. Accidents can occur in home, road and place of work. The predominant factor in accidents is carelessness that can be tackled by health education.
- *Use of health services:* Many people, particularly in rural areas, do not know what health services are available and many more do not know what signs indicate a visit to a doctor is necessary. Studies indicate that public attitude towards health services is still apprehensive. There is a communication gap between the public and state health administration in the form of feedback for further improvement of health services. One of the declared aims of health education is to inform people about the health services available in their community, how they can utilize them and the use of the health care resources.

VI. IMPORTANCE OF HEALTH EDUCATION

Health education is considered an important part of community health services. Community health nurses are in a strategic situation to provide need-based health education to patients in various settings. They come in direct contact with their patients and have the opportunity to make direct observation of their health and learning needs and plan and implement health education as a part of their nursing care plans.

The importance of teaching families about personal hygiene, environmental sanitation and care of the sick was realized by leaders in nursing during the middle and late 19th century. Health education efforts were also felt necessary because of the realization that health could not be protected or promoted through regulatory approaches. Currently, health education, as mentioned earlier, is considered as an important and powerful tool, all the more because of varied factors discussed below.

- The ultimate aim of health care is to promote, protect and maintain health and not only treat the disease. This requires people to have sufficient knowledge and bring in a change in the health behaviour. This is possible through continuous and sustained health education.
- Shortened hospital stays with early ambulation require the preparation of patients and their family members for their convalescence and care they may have to undergo at home. This is done through health education as part of the total nursing care from the time of admission till the time of discharge.
- There has been increase in long-term and chronic illnesses and disabilities and both the patients and families require a thorough understanding of the disease, related problems and treatment through well-planned and organized health education programmes.
- The consumer protection and human rights movements imply the need and importance of health education to become informed and act according to existing situations.
- The goal of health for all lays emphasis on self-care, self-help and sufficiency, which determines the need for health education to bring in a change in health knowledge, attitude and behaviour.
- For effective utilization of services that are planned and provided to the people through infrastructure in rural and urban areas, consumer participation is very important. This is made possible through education of people at large and specific groups in particular.

PLANNING FOR HEALTH EDUCATION

Health education cannot be planned in a vacuum. It is planned in connection with a specific health programme or health service. Therefore the specifics of health education strategy in a group have to be formulated in accordance with its sociocultural, psychosocial, physical, economic and situational characteristics. The planner should be fully conversant with the health education needs of the particular programme for which health education is to be planned.

It is essential to plan the health education activities before they are implemented so that desired objectives of the health education may be achieved more appropriately and efficiently. Planning is the process of making thoughtful and systematic decisions about what needs to be done, how it has to be done, and by whom and with what resources. Planning is central to health education and health promotion activities (Box 10.4). If planning is not done, it will not be clear how, when and where the health education tasks have to be carried out.

> **BOX 10.4 KEY QUESTIONS TO ASK WHEN PLANNING**
>
> - What will be done?
> - When will it be done?
> - Where will it be done?
>
> - Who will do it?
> - What resources are required?

I. PURPOSE OF PLANNING IN HEALTH EDUCATION

The main purposes of planning in health education are as follows:

- Planning enables matching resources to the problem intended to solve through health education.
- Planning helps in using resources more efficiently so that the best use of scarce resources may be ensured.
- Planning helps in avoiding duplication of activities. For example, you would not offer health education on the same topic to households at every visit.
- Planning helps in prioritizing needs and activities. This is useful because the community may have a lot of problems but not the resources or the capacity to solve all these problems at the same time.
- Planning enables thinking about how to develop the best methods to solve a problem.

II. PRINCIPLES OF PLANNING IN HEALTH EDUCATION

Planning is not a haphazard activity but follows certain specific principles or rules that must be considered while planning health education so that the desired objectives may be achieved. The basic principles of planning in health education are as follows:

- *Focus on actual current needs and context of community:* It is important that plans are made with the needs and context of the community in mind. Health education should try to understand what is currently happening in the community one works in.
- *Plan for basic needs and interest of the community:* Consider the basic needs and interests of the community. If the local needs and interests are not kept under consideration, the plans may not be effective.
- *Planning with actual beneficiaries of health education:* Plan with the people involved in the implementation of an activity. If people are included in planning, they will be more likely to participate and the plan will be more likely to succeed.
- *Identify and use all relevant community resources:* It is essential that the health educator identify all the relevant resources that are locally available which could be used for benefit of people receiving the health education.
- *Follow principle of flexibility:* Planning should be flexible, not rigid. One should be able to modify the plans when necessary. For example, you would have to change your priorities if a new problem needing an urgent response arose.
- *A realistic plan not hypothetical:* The planned activity should be achievable and take into consideration the financial, personal resources available and time constraints. Planning must be realistic; do not plan unachievable activities.

III. STEPS IN PLANNING HEALTH EDUCATION

Planning is a continuous process. It does not just happen at the start of a project. Health education must be well planned to actually improve and promote individual, family and community health. Planning can be thought of as a cycle that has six steps as explained below (Fig. 10.4).

- *Needs assessment:* Conducting needs assessment is the first and probably the most important step in any successful planning process. Sufficient time should be given for each needs assessment and the time required depends on the nature and urgency of the problem being assessed. Needs assessment is the process of identifying and understanding the health problems of the community and their possible causes. The problems are then analyzed so that priorities can be set for any necessary interventions. The information collected during needs assessment serves as a baseline for monitoring and evaluation at a later stage.
- *Identify priorities:* After identifying the needs and resources of the community, the next step is to identify their priorities because each community may have several problems but the most urgent have to be given top priority in health education. For example, a selected community has a higher incidence of goitre than other health problems. Here planning health education for goitre becomes the top priority than other nonserious potential health problems.
- *Set the goals and objectives:* In planning the process of health education, setting goals and objectives is the third and most essential step because these goals and objectives serve as consciously thought baseline parameters to be achieved during health education. These goals and objectives must be realistic and can be achieved in the stipulated period and available resources.
- *Develop strategies:* Prior to the implementation of the health education intervention one must plan, develop and evaluate the several alternative strategies to achieve the set goals and objectives of health education because each problem and target community is quite unique. Therefore, before implementation of health education intervention one must develop robust strategies to efficiently benefit the target community.

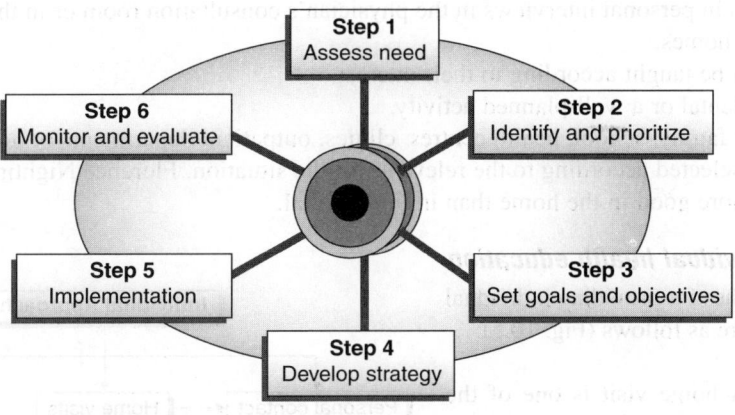

FIGURE 10.4

Steps in planning health education activities.

- *Implementation:* This is the core phase of the health education process which includes carrying out the planned strategies so that the set goals and objectives of health education may be achieved.
- *Monitor and evaluation:* This the final step of the planning process of health education where continuous monitoring as well as end evaluation is carried out to ensure the degree to which stated goals and objectives have been achieved.

HEALTH EDUCATION WITH INDIVIDUAL, GROUP AND COMMUNITIES

Health education can be carried out at various levels:

- Individual level
- Group level
- Community level
- Mass level

I. HEALTH EDUCATION WITH INDIVIDUAL

Individual health education is an important part of the health education process which includes the exchange of opinions, feelings, ideas or information with another person. Nurses are routinely engaged in providing individual health education to their patients, patient's family in hospitals as well as the community. It can be more powerful than other methods of communication in bringing about health-related behavioural change. Individual health education approach provides the opportunity to create mutual understanding between the two people: the one providing the health education and the receiver. In addition, they more closely interact and give and receive feedback immediately. It also creates the opportunity to discuss problems that are sensitive and need special handling, for example discussions on sexuality. Individual level health education may have the following characteristics:

- It helps the individuals to learn and assimilate health information to modify change their behaviour.
- It may be given in personal interviews in the physician's consultation room or in the health centre or in the people's homes.
- Individuals can be taught according to their interest.
- It may be incidental or a well-planned activity.
- It can be in the family, school, health centres, clinics, outpatient departments or hospital wards.
- Topics can be selected according to the relevance of the situation. Florence Nightingale said that the nurse can do more good in the home than in the hospital.

Methods of individual health education

The basic approaches for providing individual health education are as follows (Fig. 10.5):

- *Home visits:* A home visit is one of the best approaches for individual health education because it can become one of the best opportunities for health education

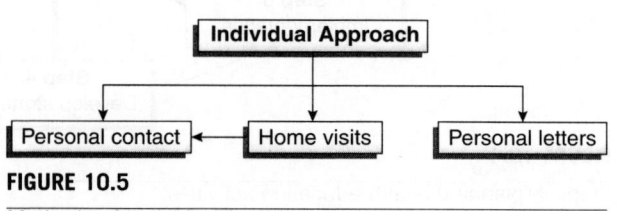

FIGURE 10.5

Methods of individual health education.

with individuals and their families. Health workers will be able to visit all homes in their communities regularly, especially if there are significant problems that have been identified. Home visits are important to understand the real background of families, their living conditions and the environment in which they live. The basic purposes of the home visit in individual health education are given in Box 10.5.

- *Personal contacts/counselling:* Personal contacts or counselling (one-to-one communication) is a helping process where one person explicitly and purposefully gives his or her time to assist people explore their situations and act on a solution. The process includes several steps through which the counsellor first understands the problem and then helps people to understand their problems. After this the counsellor needs to work together with the person to find solutions that are appropriate to their situation. Counselling involves helping people to make decisions and gives them the confidence to put their decisions into practice.
- *Personal letters:* Personal letters may also be used for individual health education, where health educators may get an opportunity to dispatch letters or printed education material to the people in a target community. This method is quite cost effective and people at a distance may be approached through this method of individual health education.

Advantages of individual health education

- The health educator can discuss, argue and persuade the individual to change his or her behaviour.
- It provides an opportunity to ask questions in terms of specific interests.
- Individuals get an opportunity to clarify their doubts more promptly and easily.

Limitations of individual health education

- We can reach only a small number of people who come in contact with us.
- It is time-consuming and an expensive method of health education.
- It needs more efforts by the health educator.

II. GROUP HEALTH EDUCATION

Group health education may be a useful way to deliver health education messages in an efficient manner. The group can provide support and encouragement to its members so they are able to maintain healthy behaviour. A well-organized group permits sharing of experiences and skills so that people are able to

---

BOX 10.5 PURPOSE OF HOME VISITS FOR INDIVIDUAL HEALTH EDUCATION

- *Establish rapport:* Make and keep a good relationship with families in the community
- Detect and try to improve troublesome situations at an early stage
- *Follow-up opportunities:* Check the progression of sick people
- Educate the family on how to help a sick person
- Observe the environment and behaviours that affect the health of the family
- Identify barriers to possible behavioural change
- Provide health education whenever possible
- Inform people about important community events in which their participation is needed
- Appreciate the fact that people may feel free to talk more openly with health providers when they are in their own homes

learn from each other. This makes it possible to pool the resources of all members. Examples of positive group activity to resolve problems include the following:

- One person in a group may not have enough money to afford the visit to a doctor for the care of an old woman in the end stage of illness. However, a group of people could contribute enough money to meet that need.
- Members of a group can give money, labour or materials to one of their members in times of personal or family crisis. They can also support the promotion of community health through projects such as developing a safe water supply or building a latrine.

Group health education may be successful because of helpful behaviour of the group or may be a failure because of coexisting nonhelpful behaviour of group members as presented in Box 10.6.

A. Methods of group health education

The choice of the right method of health education is very important in health teaching and the subject must be according to the group's interests. We have to select a suitable method of health education; some of the successful methods for group health education are given below (Fig. 10.6).

There are a variety of methods that can be used for health education of people especially in the group and community. It is very important to select the most effective method. Some of the guidelines helpful in selecting an effective method are as follows:

- One must consider the objectives and content of health education, i.e. what is the domain and its level which is a predominant part of the content and the intended behavioural change.
- One must consider the merits and demerits of the methods while selecting the method for the purpose at that time.
- Methods selected must meet health educational objectives, create participant interest, encourage their active participation and motivate them to know more and bring in a modification/change in health behaviour.

The methods of health education teaching are discussed below:

- **Lecture method:** It is a very old method of teaching. The word lecture is derived from the Latin word *lectare* meaning 'to read aloud.' A lecture may be defined as an educational presentation usually

---

BOX 10.6 TYPES OF GROUP BEHAVIOUR CONTRIBUTING IN HEALTH EDUCATION

Helpful behaviour
Making suggestions, encouraging each other to talk, responding politely to the suggestions of others, helping make points clear, giving information, showing concern for each other, volunteering to help with work, attending meetings regularly and on time and thanking each other for suggestions given.

Nonhelpful/nonfunctional behaviour
- *Blocking:* Interfering with group process, diverting attention by citing personal experiences unrelated to the problem, disagreeing and opposing a point without reason. Arguing too much on a point the rest of the group has resolved, rejecting ideas and preventing a decision.
- *Aggression:* Blaming others, showing hostility.
- *Seeking recognition:* Calling attention to oneself by excessive talking and boasting.
- *Withdrawing:* Becoming indifferent or passive and whispering to others.
- *Dominating:* Excessive manipulation or authority and interrupting or undermining the contribution of others.

delivered by an instructor to a group of individuals with the use of instructional aids and training devices.

- *Group discussion:* A group is an aggregation of people interacting in a face-to-face situation. It is a very effective method of health communication.
- *Demonstrations:* It is a carefully prepared presentation to show how to perform a skill or procedure. For example, explaining how to perform lumbar puncture. The demonstrator ascertains that the audience understands how to perform it. The demonstrator involves the audience in the discussion. Clinical teaching in hospitals is based on demonstrations. This method has a high motivational value.
- *Panel discussions:* They can be extremely effective methods of education provided they are properly planned and guided.
- *Symposium:* It is a series of speeches on a selected subject. Each person presents an aspect of the subject briefly. There is no discussion during the presentation of the topic. The audience may raise questions at the end. The chairperson makes a comprehensive summary at the end of the session.
- *Workshops:* Workshops are a noble experiment in education. They consist of a series of meetings (usually four or more) with an emphasis on individual work within the group with the help of a consultant. Workshops are divided into two groups and each group chooses a chairman and a recorder. Workshops provide each participant with an opportunity to improve his effectiveness as a professional worker.
- *Conferences and seminars:* It contains a large component of commercialized continuing education, where a group of people collect to share their ideas. Conferences and seminars may be successfully used for a group education.

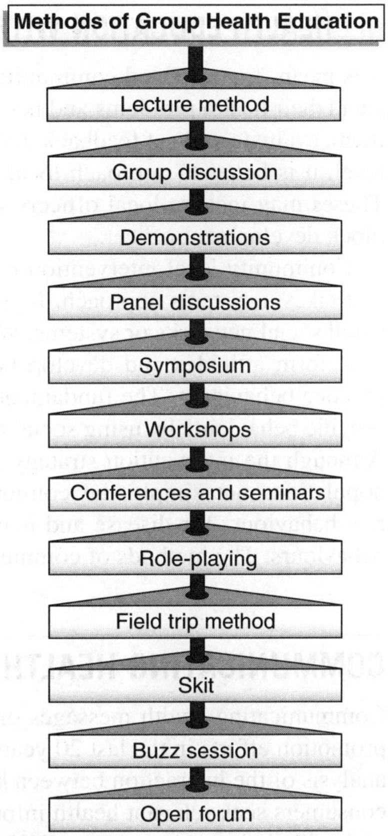

FIGURE 10.6

Methods of group health education.

- *Role-playing:* Role-playing or sociodrama is based on the assumption that many values in a situation cannot be expressed in words, and communication can be more effective if the situation is dramatized by the group.
- *Field trip method:* In this method, an educational tour is organized for a group to have first-hand information through direct observation of a place, object, etc. It has an additional benefit of group interaction and entertainment during travelling time.
- *Skit:* It refers to a brief, rehearsed, dramatic presentation. It may evoke emotional involvement and stimulate discussion and the thinking process. The limitations of this method are that it requires preparation and rehearsal time.
- *Buzz session:* In this method, a large group is divided into several small groups to meet simultaneously to discuss either the same issue or problem or different aspects of the same issue or problem. These small groups, after their discussion is over, meet in large groups and pool their findings and recommendations. The final report is presented in front of the whole group.
- *Open forum:* It refers to the public meetings which are held for various purposes in the community, for example, *gram sabha.* In this method, participants are asked to air their problems, views, etc. Thus, it helps in identifying people's health concerns.

III. HEALTH EDUCATION WITH COMMUNITY

It is meant for a defined community and is not only to create awareness but also to help people understand their health problems and needs, find alternative solutions to their problems and needs, implement them, evaluate and get feedback and accordingly do the needful. For health education at the community level, it is better to approach local leaders who are influential and who have the people's confidence. Theses may include local officers such as *patwari, numberdar, panchayat sarpanch*, police officer or block development officer.

Community level intervention combines the community organization and social marketing strategy that takes a systems approach. Its foundation is an assumption that individuals make up the large and small social networks or systems. Within these social networks or systems, individuals acquire information, form attitudes and develop beliefs. Also, within these networks, individuals acquire skills and practice behaviours. The fundamental programme goal of community level intervention is to influence specific behaviours by using social networks to consistently deliver disease risk reduction interventions. Although the intervention strategy is community based, community level interventions target specific populations not simply the community in general. The patient populations have identified shared risk behaviours for disease and may also be defined by race, ethnicity, gender or other health-related behaviours. The methods of community health education are the same as the group education methods.

COMMUNICATING HEALTH MESSAGES

Communicating health messages or health communication has become increasingly centred to health promotion efforts in the last 20 years. Health communication is a very broad field of study that includes analysis of the interaction between health care providers and consumers in the delivery of care, the way consumers seek relevant health information, the provision of social support, the preserving and sharing of health information using different media and information terminologies, the sharing of health information for informed health care decisions making use of communication to coordinate interdependent activities between the health care providers, the administration of personnel and resources within complex health care systems and the development of health communication campaign interventions for health education and health promotion.

Strategic health communication efforts are effective at influencing behaviour. They draw on social, psychology, health education, mass communication and marketing to develop and deliver influential health promotion and prevention messages that appeal to unique audience capabilities and orientations.

Health communication has been broadly defined by Everett Rogers, a pioneer in the communication field as any type of human communication concerned with health. Communicating a health message encompasses the study and use of communication strategies to inform and influence individual and community decisions that enhance health. McGuire mentioned that a successful accomplishment of communicating health messages depends on the following factors:

- Characteristics of the message source (e.g. attractiveness, credibility)
- Design of the message (e.g. organization, style)

- Channel characteristics (e.g. directness)
- Characteristics of the person who receives the message (e.g. mood, education).

I. FACTORS CONTRIBUTING TO THE SUCCESSFUL COMMUNICATION OF HEALTH MESSAGES

The process of communicating the health message must have the following specific attributes for successful communication:

- *Clarity of message:* The message should be clear to the audience. In other words, it should be easy for them to point out the actions expected to be taken, the incentives or reasons for taking those actions as well as evidence for the incentives and any background information or definitions. Elements that can help or hinder clarity include the following:
  - Language (vocabulary, lingo) and reading level
  - Pace/speed
  - Amount of content (avoid trying to cram in too much)
  - Background (text, graphics, music, etc.) and repetition
- *Accuracy of message:* The message delivered for health education must be accurate and fateful without the presence of any error because the accuracy of a message sent during health education has immense value in the successful achievement of objectives of health education.
- *Availability of appropriate resources to deliver the health message:* It must be ensured that there is availability of appropriate resources for communicating the health message because the target people must be able to have access and availability of these resources to receive the health message.
- *Consistency in delivering the health message:* There must be a provision that the health message is delivered consistently to the target people so that their motivation can help them achieve the desired goals or objectives of health education.
- *Health message must be cultural, competent and appropriate:* Each society or group of people has set cultural values; therefore, it must be ensured that the health message delivered is culturally appropriate to avoid undue problems and hindrances of health message delivery.
- *Validity and reliability of the health message:* The health message to be delivered must be valid and reliable for the content and methods of message delivery so that the desired purpose of health education may be achieved.
- *Constant repetition and re-enforcement:* There must be constant repetition and re-enforcement for communication of the health message whenever required because that helps in bringing a permanent change in the health behaviour of individuals who are reluctant to accept the expected change in their health behaviour.
- *Understandability of the health message to be communicated:* The language and the content of the health message to be delivered must be understandable to the recipients so that the desired purpose may be achieved. For example, supplying a health educational pamphlet in a local language to the target people may serve the purpose and people can appropriately understand the health message conveyed to them.
- *Feasibility of the health message:* It must to be ensured that the health message to be delivered is feasible in terms of time, money and resources available.

- *A realistic message:* Messages must be realistic. This means they should not make extreme claims or use extreme examples, avoid highly dramatic episodes and provide accurate (not misleading) information.

The messengers' factors contributing to the successful communication of the health message. The following essential messengers' factors may contribute to the successful communication of a health message. These factors may further enhance the credibility of the messenger:

- *Power:* The strength and positive enforcement the messenger (health educator) is communicating the message to recipients with. This helps in seeking the attraction and faith of the recipients.
- *Perceived expertise:* Expertise is the key success in the communication of the message to the target audience because it provides the messenger with an ability to handle all types of complexity in the communication of a message as well in the question–answer session with the message recipients.
- *Perceived honesty:* Honesty in the messengers provides them with the sincerity to accomplish the task of communication of the health message.
- *Attractiveness of messenger:* Attractiveness of the messenger does have some significant value in communication of the health message because it is a universal truth that everyone likes to see and interact with a person who is attractive and good looking.
- *Being similar to the target audience:* Starting the communication of a health message with similar target audience helps the messenger to easily accommodate with the similar new audience and situations.

II. METHODS AND MEDIA FOR COMMUNICATING THE HEALTH MESSAGE

Truly persuasive health communication messages are difficult to create, regardless of the change one is trying to elicit in the target population. Appropriate methods and media are essential to be used for the communication of a health message. The main methods and media used for communicating the health messages are described below (Box 10.7).

A. Individual methods

Individual interaction may be accomplished using the following methods for communicating the health message:

- *Interview:* It refers to a presentation in which one or more individual answers questions posed by one or more interviewers in front of the audience.

BOX 10.7 METHODS AND MEDIA FOR COMMUNICATING THE HEALTH MESSAGE

Individual/group methods and media	Mass methods and media
Individual interactions: Interview, dialogue, personal letters and home visits.	*Performing arts:* Music songs, dramas, skits, puppet show, poetry, speech, gossip, jokes, etc.
Lecturer method: Media used is chalk and talk, flip charts, flannel charts, exhibition charts, posters, etc.	*Visual arts:* Paintings, certain printed literature handicrafts and costuming.
Group discussion, demonstrations, panel discussion, symposium, workshops, conference, seminars, role playing, field trip method, skits buzz session and open forum.	The common media used are television, radio, internet, printed material, direct material, posters and health museum and exhibitions.

- *Dialogue:* In this method, two expert members have a dialogue about a particular health issue, topic or problem between them in front of the audience for their benefit.
- *Personal letters:* They may also be used for individual health education where the health educator may get an opportunity to dispatch letters or printed education material to the people in a target communality. This method is quite cost effective and people at a distance may be approached through this method of individual health education.
- *Home visit:* It is one of the best approaches for individual health education because it can become one of the best opportunities for health education with individuals and their families. Health workers will be able to visit all homes in their communities regularly, especially if there are significant problems that have been identified.

B. Group methods

It is convenient to use the group approach in communicating the health message to a group of people. The basic essential methods that may be used for communicating health messages to a group of people are as follows:

- *Lecture method:* The lecture method is a very old method of teaching. The word *lecture* is derived from the Latin word *lectare* meaning 'to read aloud'. A lecture may be defined as an educational presentation usually delivered by an instructor to a group of individuals with the use of instructional aids and training devices. The lecture method has certain limitations when used for group health education purposes such as participants are involved to a minimum extent, learning is passive, it does not stimulate thinking or problem-solving capacity and the health behaviour of listeners is not necessarily affected. The following guidelines must be followed while using the lecture method:
  - The health educator requires speaking ability and expertise in subject matter.
  - The content needs to be organized well and the topic should be based on a subject of current interest or health needs of the group.
  - The preferable size of the group should be 30–45 persons for a single lecture.
  - The time limit should not be more than 45–50 minutes for a long lecture or 15–20 minutes for a short lecture.
  - Questioning must be encouraged among participants while imparting information to clarify concepts.
  - Ensure attention of the audience by using appropriate audiovisual aids.
- *Group discussion:* A group is an aggregation of people interacting in a face-to-face situation. It is a very effective method of health communication. In a group discussion, the members should observe the selected rules such as express ideas clearly and concisely, listen to what others say, not interrupt when others are speaking, make only relevant remarks, accept criticism gracefully and help reach the conclusion. Group discussion is successful if the members know each other beforehand when they can discuss freely. However, there are certain limitations of group discussions such as those who are shy may not take part in the discussion while some others may dominate the discussion. Thus, there may be unequal participation of members in a group discussion and unless properly guided some members may deviate from the subject and make the discussion irrelevant.
- *Demonstrations:* It is a carefully prepared presentation to show how to perform a skill or procedure, for example, lumbar puncture. The demonstrator ascertaining that the audience understands how to perform it. The demonstrator involves the audience in a discussion. This method has a high motivational value. Demonstration has the following advantages:
  - Dramatizes by arousing interest of the participants.
  - Persuades the onlookers to adopt recommended practices.

- Upholds the principal of *seeing is believing* and *learning by doing.*
- Can bring desirable changes in the behaviour pertaining to the use of new practices.
- Clinical teaching in hospitals is based on demonstrations.
- This method has a high motivational value.

- *Panel discussions:* Panel discussions can be extremely effective methods of education, provided they are properly planned and guided. The main guidelines to be followed for using panel discussions in communicating the health message are as follows:
  - It consists of a chairperson or a moderator and 4–8 speakers.
  - The chairperson opens the meeting, welcomes the group and introduces the panel speakers.
  - He introduces the topic briefly and invites the panel speakers to present their point of view.
  - It needs only qualified speakers who have an in-depth knowledge a about particular targeted topic.
  - Planning consumes a lot of time and energy.

- *Symposium:* It is a series of speeches on a selected subject; each person presents an aspect of the subject briefly. There is no discussion. The audience may raise questions in the end. The chairperson makes a comprehensive summary at the end of the session. The following guidelines must be followed to use the symposium in communicating the health message to a group of people:
  - Each person or expert presents an aspect of the subject, briefly.
  - There is no discussion among the symposium members unlike in panel discussion.
  - At the end of presentation the audience can ask question, clarify their quarries, and give their views and comments.
  - The chairperson makes comprehensive summary at the end of the entire session.

- *Workshops:* Workshops are noble experiments in education. They consist of a series of meetings (usually four or more) with an emphasis on individual work, within the group, with the help of the consultant and divided into two groups. Each group chooses a chairperson and a recorder. The workshops provide each participant with an opportunity to improve their effectiveness as a professional worker.

- *Conferences and seminars:* It contains a large component of commercialized continuing education. The following guidelines must be followed in using conferences and seminars to communicate health messages:
  - It contains a large component of material for a day or two on a given topic or a selected group of topic or on a selected group of topics.
  - The report prepared is also circulated later as a material of reference and awareness.
  - There is a moderator for discussion on each person's presentation.
  - It is a very effective but costly method.
  - It needs proper planning to arrange a seminar.
  - Usually held on a regional, state or national level.
  - It covers a single topic in depth or can be broadly comprehensive.
  - They use a variety of formats to aid the learning process from self-instruction to multimedia.

- *Role-playing:* Role-playing or sociodrama is based on the assumption that many values in a situation cannot be expressed in words and the communication can be more effective if the situation is dramatized by the group. The limitations of role-playing are that group members may be too shy to participate and the intended content may or may not surface. The following guidelines must be followed for using role-play to communicate the health message to a group of people:
  - Used to practice real life situations.
  - The size of the group is thought to be best at about 25 participants.

- It is used to provide a discussion of the problem of human relationship.
- It is a particularly useful educational device for school children.
- It is followed by a discussion of the problem.

- *Case study method:* In this method, a particular event, health situation or condition is presented in detail to a group of participants. It is followed by discussion or written activity. The group is then helped to discuss its various aspects, identify related problems and factors, suggest alternative solution to deal with the event/health situation/condition.
- *Field trip method:* In this method, an educational tour is organized for a group to get first-hand information through direct observation of a place, object, etc. It has the additional benefit of group interaction and entertainment during travelling time.
- *Skit:* It refers to a brief, rehearsed, dramatic presentation. It may evoke emotional involvement and stimulate discussion and the thinking process. The limitations of this method are that it requires preparation and rehearsal time.
- *Buzz session:* In this method, a large group is divided into several small groups to meet simultaneously to discuss either the same issue or problem or different aspects of the same issue or problem. These small groups, after their discussion is over, meet in large groups and pool their findings and recommendations. The final report is presented in front of the whole group.
- *Open forum:* It refers to the public meetings held for various purposes in the community, for example: *gram sabha.* The participants are asked to air their problems, views, etc. Thus, it helps in identifying people's health concerns.

C. Mass methods and media

Mass media refers collectively to all media technologies that are intended to reach a large audience via mass communication. Broadcast media transmit their information electronically and comprise television, film and radio, movies, internet, CDs, DVDs and other devices like cameras and video consoles. Alternatively, print media use a physical object as a means of sending their information, such as newspapers, magazines, brochures, newsletters, books, leaflets and pamphlets. Outdoor media is a form of mass media which comprises billboards, signs, placards placed inside and outside commercial buildings and objects like shops and buses, flying billboards (signs in tow of airplanes), blimps and skywriting. Public speaking and event organizing can also be considered as forms of mass media.

USING MASS MEDIA

A message can be communicated to a mass audience by many means. No health worker or health team member can mount an effective health education programme for the whole community except through mass media of communication. The evolution of the media has been rapid. Up until the early 1920s mass communication largely depended on what was printed, posters, pamphlets, books periodicals and newspapers. Then came the radio and with it a new dimension of experience. Later, the radio and TV came close to the warmth and motivational effect of a person-to-person communication. They have become a part of the public of modern civilization. Recently, more advanced electronic mass media such as video consoles, CDs, DVDs, movies and internet have grown rapidly and become popular means of mass education. Today, these advanced electronic mass media have superseded all other mass media. However, other printed and folk mass media have their own importance and significance in mass health education.

I. DEFINITIONS OF MASS MEDIA

It is defined as a one-way communication that is useful in transmitting messages to the people even in the remotest places.

Mass media is those means of communication that reach and influence large numbers of people, especially newspapers, popular magazines, radio and television.

Mass media are those media that are created to be consumed by large number of people worldwide and also a direct contemporary instrument of mass communication.

II. CLASSIFICATION OF MASS MEDIA

Mass media may be classified as follows:

- *Electronic media:* Electronic media may include television, film and radio, movies, internet, CDs, DVDs and other devices like cameras and video consoles.
- *Performing media:* This includes music, songs, dramas, skits, puppet shows, poetry, speech, gossip and jokes.
- *Visual media:* Paintings, handicrafts, costumes, certain printed literature such as books, pamphlets, leaflets, brochures, newsletters, journals, magazines and newspaper make up the visual media.

III. IMPORTANT AGENCIES OF COMMUNICATION

- The press associations collect and distribute news and pictures to newspapers, TV and radio stations and news magazines.
- Syndicates offer background news and pictures, commentary and entertainment features to the newspapers, TV, radio and magazines.
- The advertising agencies serve their business patients on the one hand and mass media on the other. The advertising department of companies and institutions serve in merchandizing roles and the public relations departments serve in information roles.
- The public relations counselling firms and publicity organizing offer information on behalf of their patients.
- Research individuals and groups help and guide mass communicators to more effective paths.

IV. IMPORTANCE OF MASS MEDIA

- The importance of mass media today is immense. Never before in mankind's history have the media had such a significant impact on our lives and behaviour. This is due to rapid development in modern science and technology.
- From early childhood, children sit in front of the TV for hours, the succession of pictures is watched by the eyes that serves as an opening into the world and it becomes imprinted on minds that are still impressionable. A few years later, when going to school, newspaper headlines and magazines covers arrest the eyes. Out of this plethora of images, what will remain in the minds of the child are pictures of war, violence, women's body whether clothed or not, sporting exploits, the photos of film stars or political stars, etc.
- In the last few decades, the society has experienced a radical change due to mass media appearance. Some of the used systems of communication are the radio, TV and internet. At the moment, thanks to these means we enjoy good communication with people in other countries.

- They also provide a great facility to obtain data on several subjects.
- Political factions use the media to influence possible members into joining their groups.
- Media connect the world to the individuals and reproduce the self-image of the society.
- They have a strong social and cultural impact on the society.
- It is important to say that these innovations also have bad effects as with new technology the old customs are lost.

V. METHODS OF MASS MEDIA COMMUNICATION

The common methods used for mass media communication are television, film and radio, movies, internet, CDs, DVDs and other devices like cameras and video consoles. Alternatively, print media use a physical object such as newspapers, magazines, brochures, newsletters, books, leaflets and pamphlets as a means of sending their information.

A. Television

TV has become the most popular of all media. It is effective in not only creating awareness, but also to an extent influencing public opinion and introducing new ways of life. The importance of the television is given below:

- It is a good source of entertainment.
- It keeps our knowledge up to date.
- Advertisements inform general public about various health programmes and new ideas.
- It provides us with latest information.
- It contributes positively to the education of the society and provides awareness to the people.

B. Radio

It is found nearly in every home. In many developing countries, the radio has a broader audience than television as it can also be seen in the remotest of villages. The radio transmission serves as a vital agency of mass education if used effectively as it is also approachable by poor people. Example, the Government is promoting Kangaroo Mother Care for preterm and low birth weight babies through radio these days. Most common advantages of the radio are as follows:

- It can be valuable aid in *putting across* useful information in the form of straight talks, plays questions and answers and quiz programmes.
- It is cheaper and portable.
- It is good for mass education.
- Radio programmes with dramatic effects can arouse positive emotions and reinforce positive attitude.
- It keeps our knowledge up to date.
- It is also a good source of entertainment, news, sports and traffic events.
- People can listen to the radio even by closing their eyes as it is only audible.

C. Newspapers

The newspaper today plays a vital role in human affairs. Its importance has not been diminished by the appearance of radio or TV. Men no longer have to travel to get information. Though the radio and TV convey important news and messages quicker than the newspaper, it not only gives more detail about a particular incident but also contains more new items and is easy to carry. The importance of newspapers is as follows:

- They play an important part both in the national and international areas. They give us news and views. The way a man wants food for his belly, he also needs news for his mind to keep pace with the world.
- They refresh our knowledge and ideas.
- They broaden our outlook and change views.
- They educate the common people.
- They shape the opinions of the common people of a country by influencing public opinion.
- They are critics of administration, justice and laws.
- They remove the barriers separating man from man.
- They are advocates of liberty, equality and fraternity.
- They enforce the right and redress the wrong.

D. Internet

Technically, the internet is all the computers in the world that are connected including the technologies (routers, servers etc.) as well as wires and antennas that keeps all the computers talking to each other. This is a fast growing communication media and has a large potential to become a major health education tool. The importance of the internet for mass communication of health message is as follows:

- The internet is the gigantic library, as well as a worldwide message board, telephone network and publishing medium. It is open 24 hours a day and you can find anything you want there.
- In-depth and up-to-date information, current events and blogs about any subject are available.
- The foremost target of internet has always been communication and internet has excelled beyond expectations.
- Information is probably the biggest advantage the internet is offering.
- Entertainment is another popular reason and many people prefer to use internet for downloading games, chatting, etc. Chat rooms are popular because users can meet new and interesting people. Internet has been successfully used by people to find life partners. When people surf the web, there are numerous things, e.g. music, hobbies, news, that can be found and shared on the internet.
- Many services are provided on the internet such as online banking, job seeking, purchasing tickets for your favourite movie, hotel reservations, etc.
- E-commerce is the concept used for any type of commercial manoeuvring or business deal that involves the transfer of information across the globe through the internet. This is the phenomenon associated with any kind of shopping on the internet.
- The disadvantages of the internet are as follows:
  - *Theft of personal information:* Your personal information such as name, address, credit card details may be available to others on the internet.
  - *Spamming:* It refers to sending unwanted e-mails in bulk, which provides no purpose and needlessly obstructs the entire system.
  - *Virus threat:* A virus is a programme that disrupts the normal functioning of your computer system.
  - *Pornography:* It is the biggest threat related to your children's healthy mental life.

E. Printed material

Magazines, pamphlets, booklets and handouts have long been in use for health communication. They are aimed at those who can read. Their usefulness lies in the fact that they can convey detailed information. They can be produced in bulk for very little cost and can be shared by others in the family and community.

F. Direct mailing

It is a new innovation in health communication in India. The intention is to reach remote areas of the country with the printed word (e.g. folders and newsletters, booklets on family planning, immunization and nutrition). These are directly sent to the village leaders, literate people, *panchayats* and local bodies and those who are considered as opinion leaders. Direct mailing has been successful mass media in creating public awareness. It is possibly the most impersonal means of mass communication.

G. Posters, billboards and signs

These media are intended to catch the eye and create awareness. Therefore, the message to be communicated must be simple and artistic. Posters are not expensive when one considers that they are seen by a large number of people. Motives such as humour and fear are introduced in the posters to hold the public's attention. In places where the exposer time is short (streets), the message on the posters should be short, direct and simple so it could be easily understood (e.g. at bus stops, railway stations, hospitals and health centres). Posters can represent more information. The right amount of matter should be put up in the right place and at the right time. The life of a poster is usually short; they should be changed frequently otherwise they will lose their effect.

H. Health museums and exhibitions

Properly organized health museums and exhibitions can attract a large number of people by presenting a large variety of ideas and increase knowledge and awareness. Photographic panels attract more persons than graphic panels. This is because photos give a humanized touch to the communication. Three-dimensional models with lighted visuals are even more effective than photos. In exhibitions, there is a big element of personal communication through workers who explain each item on the exhibit. Printed literature explaining the exhibits is often freely distributed. Health exhibitions and museums thus offer a package of both personal and impersonal methods of communication.

I. Folk media

Culture is preserved and promoted by tradition to a considerable extent. Tradition is the handing down of beliefs, experiences and customs from one generation to the next especially in the oral form or by a process of traditional performances and communication. All over the world, the vehicle that has passed on tradition and customs and which has been contributing to national culture for generations is folklore. Folklore is comprised of oral folklore such as folk songs and ballads, customary folklore such as folk dances and material folklore such as crafts, arts and costumes.

Folk media in terms of mass communication ought to refer to the totality of communication which takes within its compass not only the electronic media, but also folk (indigenous) media such as *keertan*, *katha*, folk songs, dance, dramas and puppet shows having roots in our culture. Muslims have their own traditional folk forms like *ghazal* and *qawwali*.

Importance of folk media. Folk media in India has contributed a great deal in developing this vast subcontinent into a single culture entity inspite of cultural diversities created by linguistic and regional subnationalism. Though a large number of cultures blossomed in different regions of this multilingual and multiracial country, they all contributed to a pan-Indian culture representing what is often characterized as unity in diversity.

- Traditional media, whatever the form and region, has been imparting information, education and invoking respect for social and ethical values through the stories drawn from them. Thus, traditional media is a means of changing values, attitudes and norms to provide a proper information generally from the same source, like *Vedas, Puranas* and the epics *Ramayana* and *Mahabharata*.
- It is a method of promoting certain behaviour acts, patterns, techniques and facilities that people may use to solve problems.
- Being close to the people at the local level, these channels are potentially useful in the service of social concerns. Folk media is the personal form of entertainment and communication. This is important because behavioural changes are most easily brought about by personal interaction.
- Another advantage of folk media is they attract the people who might not attend educational meetings. Skills and new knowledge may be added to the old forms that are already familiar and dear to the people.
- It deals with values such as status of the family, education and standards of living that are related to family life.
- It is a means of changing values, attitudes and norms to provide a proper climate for social and economic progress.

Limitations of folk media, on the other hand, include the dangers in overloading certain traditional channels with too many messages of an instrumental nature. Channels could only be loaded according to their capacity and with respect, in particular, to cultural, religious or other sensitively integral elements. Sociologists and anthropologists could help planners define these sensitive factors affecting such limitations.

Selection and criteria for using folk media. The following points may be considered in the selection of folk media:

- Concern for plasticity of the medium or capacity of a particular form to be loaded with specific innovative messages. Examination of religious or social functions attributed to the medium should be made so as to not distort its special role. In some cases, examination may reveal such use to be unacceptable. However, it has been found that religious themes can be interpreted in the modern context providing impetus for social change.
- It should be determined whether the medium has an age or individuality (in which case the positive identification of audience with the actor can be the agent of change), or whether it is entirely nonindividual. It has sometimes been found that certain messages can be best expressed without the personalities of actors in evidence during a performance as in puppet shows, mask presentations and giant figures.
- It should be noted whether a particular medium or any aspect of its traditions and features could be used by or extended to a mass media presentation. If so, is this desirable in relation to both a medium and the message?
- Are the required resources, talent, materials and texts available for extensive utilization of the medium?
- Does the selected medium have entertainment value and/or artistic appeal?
- Is it unique enough to prove a valuable communication channel?
- Is the form of the proposed medium flexible enough to incorporate a sufficiently broad range of content materials such as family planning and other developmental messages?
- Is the medium sufficiently versatile to reach varied audiences? To properly assess this criterion, the country must be in a position to assess the range of traditional media and their suitability for audiences according to local and provincial make-up.
- Is the selected medium relevant to the intended audience?

REVIEW QUESTIONS

Long-Answer Questions

1. Explain the methods of selection of media for the public education programme in a rural area.
2. Write a short note on health education.
3. Describe the methods of health education.
4. Plan and conduct a health education session for a group of people in the community on the topic immunization.
5. Explain the planning of health education.
6. Describe the principles of health education.
7. Explain the uses of mass media.
8. Describe the methods of communicating the health message.
9. List the different mass media used for health education.
10. Describe the importance of health education.
11. Discuss the importance of information, education and communication in the Indian context.
12. Explain the aims of health education.
13. Define health education and list the principles of health education.
14. Elaborate the following: (a) Principles of health education. (b) Steps in planning of health education programme. (c) Role of nurse in health education.
15. Elaborate the following: (a) Define mass media. (b) What are the advantages and disadvantages of mass media? (c) Mention the different methods and media which can be used in delivery of health education.

Short-Answer Questions

1. Define mass media.
2. List down four types of mass media.
3. List factors influencing health behaviour.
4. Discuss in brief the principles of health education.
5. Discuss scope of health education.
6. Write down the steps in planning health education.
7. Discuss briefly the methods of group health education.

Multiple-Choice Questions (MCQs)

1. IEC stands for
   (a) Information, entertainment, communication
   (b) Information, exhibition, communication
   (c) Information, education, communication
   (d) Informal, education, communication
2. Communication is derived from the word
   (a) Community
   (b) Communist
   (c) Common
   (d) Connect

3. Purpose of communication is
   (a) To understand and exchange ideas
   (b) To interpret and explain to the people
   (c) To improve interpersonal relationship
   (d) All of these

4. Medium of giving information is known as
   (a) Sender
   (b) Message
   (c) Channel
   (d) Feedback

5. Another name of intrapersonal communication is
   (a) No talk
   (b) Self-talk
   (c) Group talk
   (d) Two-way talk

6. Body language used by a communicator during imparting information is an example of
   (a) Verbal communication
   (b) Nonverbal communication
   (c) Formal communication
   (d) Informal communication

7. Lecture as a method of teaching is an example of
   (a) One-way communication
   (b) Two-way communication
   (c) Formal communication
   (d) Informal communication

8. Formal communication is also known as
   (a) Horizontal
   (b) Vertical
   (c) Cylindrical
   (d) Straight

9. Which of the following communication is an example of telecommunication?
   (a) Television
   (b) Radio
   (c) Internet
   (d) All of these

10. Which of the following are principles of effective communication?
    (a) Have clarity of idea
    (b) Use two-way communications
    (c) Have adequacy of the message
    (d) All of these

11. Which of the following is not the principle of effective communication?
    (a) Have credibility in communication
    (b) Be sensitive to receiver's needs, feelings and perceptions
    (c) Use any language you like
    (d) Be a good listener

12. Which one of the following is barrier of communication?
    (a) Mutual understanding
    (b) Concise message
    (c) Wrong channel
    (d) All of these
13. Barriers in communication can be overcome by
    (a) Mutual trust and confidence
    (b) Clarifying the ideas
    (c) Using appropriate channel
    (d) All of these
14. IEC department in Punjab state level is situated at
    (a) Patiala
    (b) Faridkot
    (c) Chandigarh
    (d) Ludhiana
15. Who is responsible for IEC (information, education and communication) activities at block level?
    (a) Child development project officer
    (b) Block extension educator
    (c) Medical officer
    (d) Sarpanch

Answers of the Multiple-Choice Questions

1. (c), 2. (b), 3. (d), 4. (c), 5. (b), 6. (b), 7. (a), 8. (b), 9. (d), 10. (d), 11. (c), 12. (c), 13. (d), 14. (c), 15. (b)

FURTHER READING

Bundy, D., Guya, H. L. (1996). Schools for health, education and the school-age child. *Parasitology Today*, 12(8), 1–16.

Canadian Population Health Initiative. (2004). *Improving the health of canadians*. Ottawa: Canadian Institute for Health Information.

Centers for Disease Control & Prevention. (2007). *National health education standards*. Retrieved May 1, 2009 from http://www.cdc.gov/HealthyYouth/SHER/standards/index.htm.

Christian, M. (1984). Morbidity and mortality of car occupants: Comparative survey over 24 months. *British Medical Journal*, 289, 1525–1526.

Coalition of National Health Education Organizations. (1999). *Introduction. Health education code of ethics*. Chicago, IL. Retrieved May 1, 2009 from http://www.cnheo.org/code1.pdf.

Cottrell, R. R., Girvan, J. T., & McKenzie, J. F. (2009). *Principles and foundations of health promotion and education*. New York: Benjamin Cummings.

Dahlgreen, G. & Whitehead, M. (2006). *European strategies for tackling social inequities in health: Levelling up part 2*. Geneva: World Health Organization.

Donatelle, R. (2009). *Promoting healthy behavior change. Health: The basics* (8th ed., p. 4). San Francisco, CA: Pearson Education, Inc.

Fee, E., & Brown, T. M. (2005). The Public Health Act of 1848. *Bulletin of the World Health Organization*, 83(11), 866–867.

Hill, G., Millar, W., & Connelly, J. (2003). "The great debate": Smoking, lung cancer, and cancer epidemiology. *Canadian Bulleting of Medical History*, 20(2), 367–386.

Hrudey, S., & Hrudey, E. J. (2004). *Safe drinking water, lessons from recent outbreaks in affluent nations*. London, UK: IWA Publishing.

Joint Committee on Terminology. (2001). Report of the 2000 Joint Committee on Health Education and Promotion Terminology. *American Journal of Health Education*, 32(2), 89–103.

Kann, L., Brener, N. D., & Allensworth, D. D. (2001). Health education: Results from the School Health Policies and Programs Study 2000. *Journal of School Health*, 71(7), 266–278.

Last, J. (2001). *A dictionary of epidemiology* (4th ed.). Oxford University Press.

Luo, W., Morrison, H., de Groh, M., Waters, C., DesMeules, M., Jones-Mclean, E. et al. (2007). The burden of adult obesity in Canada. *Chronic Disease in Canada*, 27(4), 135–144.

Luo, Z. C., Kierans, W. J., Wilkins, R., Liston, R. M., Uh, S. H., & Kramer, M. S. (2004). Infant mortality among First Nations versus non-First Nations in British Columbia: Temporal trends in rural vs. urban areas, 1981–2000. *International Journal of Epidemiology*, 33, 1252–1259.

Macintyre, S. (2007). *Inequalities in health in Scotland: What are they and what can we do about them?* Glasgow: Medical Research Council Social & Public Health Sciences Unit.

Mass media. (2010). *Oxford English Dictionary*. online version.

McKenzie, J., Neiger, B., & Thackeray, R. (2009). *Health education and health promotion. Planning, implementing, & evaluating health promotion programs* (5th ed., pp. 3–4). San Francisco, CA: Pearson Education, Inc.

Mowat, D. & Butler-Jones, D. (2007). Public health in Canada: A difficult history. *Healthcare papers*, 7(3), 31–76.

National Advisory Committee on SARS and Public Health. (2003). *Learning from SARS: Renewal of public health in Canada*. Ottawa.

Pan American Health Organization. (2001). *Promoting health in the Americas: Annual report of the Director 2001*. Washington, D.C.

Park, K. (2009). *Text book of preventive and social medicine* (18th ed., pp. 760–764). Jabalpur: Banarsidas Bhanot.

Patterson, S. M., & Vitello, E. M. (2006). Key influences shaping health education: Progress toward accreditaion. *The Health Education Monograph Series*, 23(1), 14–19.

Potter, P. (2009). *Fundamentals of nursing*. Vol. 1, 5th ed. pp. 445–446.

Prabarkar, G. N. (2004). *Text book of community health nursing* (pp. 528–533). New Delhi: Peepee Publications.

Reidpath, D. D. & Allotey, P. (2003). Infant mortality rate as an indicator of population health. *Journal of Epidemiology and Community Health*, 57(5), 344–346.

Rutledge, R., Lalor, A., Oller, D., Hansen, A., Thomason, M., Meredith, W., et al. (1993). The cost of not wearing seat belts. A comparison of outcome in 3396 patients. *Annals of Surgery*, 217(2), 122–127.

Sharma, D. K. (2008). *Communication and education technology* (1st ed., pp. 357–376). Jalandhar: Lotus Publishers.

Waldram, J., Herrign, D. A., & Young, T. K. (1995). *Aboriginal health in Canada: Historical, cultural and epidemiological perspective*. Toronto: University of Toronto.

Witschi, H. (2001). Profile in Toxicology: A short history of lung cancer. *Toxicological Sciences*, 64, 4–6.

World Health Organization. (1946). *Constitution of the World Health Organization*. Retrieved on January 3, 2008, from http://www.who.int/library/collections/historical/en/index3.html.

World Health Organization. (1998). List of Basic Terms. *Health Promotion Glossary* (pp. 4). Retrieved May 1, 2009 from http://www.who.int/hpr/NPH/docs/hp_glossary_en.pdf.

World Health Organization. (2007). Achieving health equity: From root causes to fair outcomes. Interim Statement. *Commission on Social Determinants of Health*.

Yan, D. (2004). Public Health in Canada: Considerations on the history of neglect. *McMaster University Medical Journal*, 2(1), 34–37.

Lesson plan on course equivalency, transcript and credit system

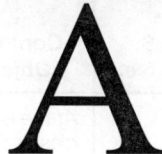

LESSON PLAN

Subject	:	Nursing Education
Topic	:	Course equivalency, transcript and credit system
Group of students	:	M.Sc. (N) First year
No. of students	:	25
Name of student teacher	:	Ms Kumud Kumari
Method of teaching	:	Lecture cum discussion method
Date of teaching	:	12/12/12
Time of teaching	:	10.00 am
Language	:	English
Duration	:	25 minutes
AV Aids	:	PowerPoint presentation (PPT), flannel board and flash cards
Venue	:	M.Sc. (N) First year classroom
Supervisor	:	Dr Suresh K. Sharma

Previous knowledge of the group: Students have basic knowledge regarding course equivalency, transcript and credit system in B.Sc. Nursing.

General objective: At the end of teaching, students will be able to develop knowledge about course equivalency and transcript and credit system.

Specific objective: At the end of the teaching, students will be able to

- Define course equivalency, transcript and credit system.
- Explain the steps of course equivalency.
- Elaborate the implications for implementation and assurance of standards.
- Describe the items of transcript.
- Explain the credit system.
- Explain the continuing nursing education credit system.

S. No.	Contributory Objectives	Time	Content	Teaching and Learning Activities	
				AV Aids	**Evaluation**
	At the end of the class students will be able to . . .				
1.		1/2 min	Good afternoon to all of you. My name is Ms Kumud Kumari. The topic of my presentation is course equivalency, transcript and credit system.	Verbally	
2.	Define course equivalency	2 min	**Course equivalency** • *Course equivalency* is the term used in higher education, describing how a course offered by one college or university relates to a course offered by another. • If a course is viewed as equal or better than the course offered by the receiving college or university, the course can be noted as an equivalent course.	LCD	What is course equivalency?
3.	Explain the steps of course equivalency	2 min	**Process** • The university/board from where the student has acquired the qualification shall duly fill up the transcript performa. • The duly filled transcript performa will be placed before the equivalency committee meeting; the recommendation with regard to equivalency status will be informed thereafter to the concerned candidates. • The equivalency process can take 2–3 months to complete.	Flannel board	What is the process of course equivalency?
4.	Explain the principles of course equivalency	1 min	**Principles of course equivalency** • Courses are regarded as equivalent if they have the same intended learning outcomes and consequently the same graduate profile. • Equivalent courses should therefore have the same overall educational aims and assess their achievement at the same standard.	LCD	What are the principles of course equivalency?

S. No.	Contributory Objectives	Time	Content	Teaching and Learning Activities	
				AV Aids	Evaluation
5.	Elaborate the implications for the implementation and assurance of standards	5 min	**Implications for implementation and assurance of standards** • Assurance of standards. • Course structures and subject material. • Academic programmes office • Admission standards. • Teaching standard and support. • Learning environment and support. • Transfer between equivalent courses. • Monitoring and evaluation.	LCD	List down the steps of implementation and assurance of standards.
6.	Define the transcript	2 min	**Transcript** • A nursing school/college transcript contains academic career record from the nursing school and college or university. • Transcripts are needed to confirm the equivalency of the course. • It itemizes all sorts of academic information.	LCD	What do you mean by a transcript?
7.	Describe the items of a transcript	5 min	**What is contained in a transcript?** • Name of student. • Previous school names, addresses and phone numbers. • List of courses you took—usually by year. • Dual enrollment and/or any honors—as applicable. • Your class grades (either letter or numeric). • Total GPA (grade point average). • Number of credits taken/achieved per semester and year. • Grade scale used by that school. • State proficiency exams (if any). • Graduation date and degrees achieved. • Classes you had learning experiences.	LCD	What are the items of a transcript?

Continued

S. No.	Contributory Objectives	Time	Content	Teaching and Learning Activities	
				AV Aids	**Evaluation**
8.	Explain the credit system	5 min	**Credit system** • A course credit (often credit hour, or just credit or 'unit') is a unit that gives weightage to the value, level or time requirements of an academic course taken at school or other educational institution. • Students in a school or university earn credits for the successful completion of each course for each academic term. • The state or the institution generally sets a minimum number of credits required to graduate. • Various systems of credits exist: one per course, one per hour/week in class, one per hour/week devoted to the course (including homework), etc. • The credit system is basically a division of hours of the whole syllabus unitwise. The credit system (total hours) are different for different courses. Also the requirement is also different in different courses.	LCD	What is the credit system?
9.	Explain the continuing nursing education credit system	2 min	**Continuing Nursing Education (CNE) credit system** • The percentage of staff fulfilling the CNE requirement, which is 15 credit points per year, has risen from 70 to 85%. • Nursing staff have also shown appreciation of an annual record of their CNE achievement as it provides a kind of recognition of their professional activities. • In general, one CNE point is allocated for an hour's learning activity, which may consist of a talk, workshop, seminar and conference, related to patient care issues and/or nursing professional development.	LCD	What is CNE credit system?
10.	Summarize the topic	1/2 min	Today in the class I have discussed the definitions, steps, principles of course equivalency, transcript and credit system. **References** **Assignment** Develop course equivalency, transcript and credit system for B.Sc. Nursing programme.	Verbally Flash cards	

Comprehensive review (multiple-choice) questions

1. Nurse is communicating with the patient; she asks the patient: 'What's your name? Are you having keen interest in watching cricket? Where's your home? Who are all in your family?' This communication may be termed as
   (a) Incongruence
   (b) Underloading
   (c) Invalidation
   (d) Overloading

2. Communication which involves gestures for sending and receiving messages is known as
   (a) Symbolic communication
   (b) Verbal communication
   (c) Nonverbal communication
   (d) Therapeutic communication

3. A patient complaints that nurse is giving him less attention. The lack of attention may be categorized under which of the following type of communication barrier?
   (a) Environmental barrier
   (b) Physiological barrier
   (c) Psychological barrier
   (d) Social barrier

4. Which one of the following could be an appropriate intervention to overcome the environmental barrier in a communication?
   (a) Maintaining the distance between sender and receiver
   (b) Maintaining the low room temperature
   (c) Keep background noise at lowest possible level
   (d) Keeping dim light

5. A nurse is providing discharge teaching to a patient; this communication may be categorized under which type of communication?
   (a) One-to-one communication
   (b) One-way communication
   (c) One-to-many communication
   (d) Mass communication

6. Hidden area of Johari window depicts area which is
   (a) Known to self and others
   (b) Known to self only
   (c) Known to others only
   (d) Not known to self and others

7. As per Johari window, by seeking feedback from others, one strives to
   (a) Increase both the open area and the blind area
   (b) Increase the open area and decrease the blind area
   (c) Decrease both the open area and the blind area
   (d) Decrease the open area and increase the blind area

8. As per Johari window, during whole of our life, one should work towards increasing the
   (a) Open area
   (b) Blind area
   (c) Hidden area
   (d) Unknown area

9. As per Johari window, on facing the challenges of life, one strives towards decreasing the
   (a) Open area
   (b) Blind area

433

(c) Hidden area
(d) Unknown area

10. A nurse manager promotes sharing of knowledge and ideas with the others, considering assumptions of Johari's window; she is trying to expand the
    (a) Blind area
    (b) Open area
    (c) Hidden area
    (d) Unknown area

11. To build an effective team, Nursing Superintendent should
    (a) Hold formal and informal meetings
    (b) Fill desirable performance appraisal
    (c) Take periodic rounds
    (d) Appoint supervisors

12. Following are the examples of group except
    (a) Nurses' union
    (b) Audience watching movie
    (c) People attending health Mela
    (d) Mob

13. Interaction among the group members is always
    (a) Physical
    (b) Firm and rigid
    (c) Reciprocal and mutual
    (d) Informal and social

14. Our social behaviour is usually influenced by
    (a) Our blood group
    (b) Social norms
    (c) Socio-economic status
    (d) Occupational status

15. All are true about self-concept except
    (a) Present since birth
    (b) Dynamic
    (c) Evolves with time
    (d) Affected by one's body image

16. Self-analysis of the client is best exhibited in which type of counselling?
    (a) Impersonal
    (b) Directive
    (c) Nondirective
    (d) Eclectic

17. Most cost-effective and practical approach to counselling is
    (a) Directive
    (b) Nondirective
    (c) Impersonal
    (d) Eclectic

18. In Indian nursing institutes, the immediate assistance available to the nursing student facing any problem is usually
    (a) A teacher
    (b) A Counsellor
    (c) Parents
    (d) Friends

19. A counsellor should possess following attributes except
    (a) Sound health
    (b) Professional degree
    (c) Integrated personality
    (d) Religious faith

20. Crisis situation is often considered as
    (a) Anticipated
    (b) Sudden
    (c) Manageable
    (d) Insignificant

21. Retirement of a physically active elderly person is an example of which of the following type of crisis?
    (a) Situational crisis
    (b) Maturational crisis
    (c) Significant crisis
    (d) Insignificant crisis

22. Which of the following educational philosophy focuses on development of academic standards and improves the mind and work ability of a child?
(a) Essentialism
(b) Existentialism
(c) Reconstructionism
(d) Progressivism

23. Which of the following is the basic concept of idealism?
(a) Human spirit is the most important element in life
(b) It does not believe in standard, permanent and eternal values
(c) It propagates for the truth and reality in daily life
(d) Nature itself is a total system that contains and explains all existence

24. The principle of Learning by Doing is followed by
(a) Idealism
(b) Realism
(c) Naturalism
(d) Pragmatism

25. 'Man is nothing else but what he makes of himself' is the first principle of
(a) Existentialism
(b) Essentialism
(c) Perennialism
(d) Idealism

26. The concept of 'curriculum must be based on abilities, interest and capabilities of students' is believed in which of the following educational philosophy?
(a) Naturalism
(b) Realism
(c) Pragmatism
(d) Essentialism

27. Which of the following is/are the component(s) of educational objectives?
(a) Condition
(b) Criteria
(c) Order
(d) All of above

28. Which of the following are the recommended steps of lesson planning?
(a) Preparation . . . Presentation . . . Generalization . . . Comparison . . . Application . . . Recaptulization . . .
(b) Preparation . . . Presentation . . . Comparison . . . Generalization . . . Application . . . Recaptulization . . .
(c) Preparation . . . Comparison . . . Presentation . . . Generalization . . . Application . . . Recaptulization . . .
(d) Application . . . Preparation . . . Comparison . . . Presentation . . . Generalization . . . Recaptulization . . .

29. Co-operating in group activities is an example of which domain of learning?
(a) Cognitive
(b) Psychomotor
(c) Affective
(d) None of the above

30. Which of the following is/are the characteristic(s) of educational objectives?
(a) Specific
(b) Attainable
(c) Measurable
(d) All of the above

31. Memory and reasoning are emphasized in which domain of learning?
(a) Cognitive
(b) Psychomotor
(c) Affective
(d) All of the above

32. The abbreviation 'PBL' stands for
(a) Problem-based language
(b) Problem-based learning
(c) Programme-based language
(d) Programme-based laboratory

33. The blueprint of nursing care rendered by a nursing student to a selected patient, for a particular period by following nursing process approach, with an intention to develop comprehensive nursing care abilities is better called as
(a) Nursing assignment
(b) Nursing conference
(c) Nursing rounds
(d) Nursing care study

34. Recording and reporting should consider the following principles except:
(a) Written promptly
(b) Concise and complete
(c) Preferably oral
(d) Significant

35. When a group of multidisciplinary professional persons come together for problem solving and interchange of ideas, that method is called as
(a) Nursing care study
(b) Health team conference
(c) Individual conference
(d) Nursing rounds

36. Process recording essentially involves
(a) Teaching–learning of the patient
(b) Verbatim of conversation of patient and nurse
(c) History taking by nursing student
(d) Evaluation of nursing care

37. Which one of following is not a type of projected visual aid?
(a) Opaque projector
(b) Slide projector
(c) Film strip
(d) Flip chart

38. Angle of plane mirror to the vertical plane in microprojector is
(a) 35°
(b) 45°
(c) 55°
(d) 65°

39. To show small image directly from book you can use
(a) Microprojector
(b) Transparencies
(c) Epidiascope
(d) Stereograph

40. How many photographs can be used in a stereograph?
(a) Single
(b) Double
(c) Triple
(d) Quadruple

41. Sand material, soil and mud can be used in preparation of the following AV aid:
(a) Sketching
(b) Puppets
(c) Both (a) and (b)
(d) None of them

42. To get first-hand information you will use which of the following teaching aid/method?
(a) Field trips
(b) Puppets
(c) Cartoons
(d) None of them

43. Which one of the following is not a projected visual aid?
(a) Stereograph
(b) Models
(c) Microfilm
(d) Epidiascope

44. How many strips are present in a filmstrip?
(a) 12–14
(b) 15–20

(c) 20–25

(d) 30–35

45. What is the other name of pie diagram?

(a) Circle diagram

(b) Triangle diagram

(c) Oval diagram

(d) Rectangle diagram

46. What is the purpose of making narrative chart?

(a) To show relationship between two systems

(b) To show development of a significant issue

(c) To present transitions or cycle

(d) All of above

47. Line of authority is shown by which of the following mean?

(a) The chain chart

(b) The flow chart

(c) The tree chart

(d) None of them.

48. Which one of the following is not a characteristic of audio devices?

(a) Authenticity

(b) Two-way communication

(c) Audition

(d) Emotional impact

49. Which one of the following is not a limitation of audio devices?

(a) Adjustment

(b) Emotional impact

(c) Administrative problems

(d) Inability attract continuous attention

50. Phonograph recording falls under which type of educational aids?

(a) Audio aids

(b) Audio visual aid

(c) Projected aid

(d) Nonprojected aid

51. The objective of using an AV aid in teaching is to

(a) Clarify content

(b) Add interest

(c) Increase audience attention

(d) All of the above

52. AV aids should be used only when they

(a) Require a definite purpose

(b) Require little or no explanation

(c) Catch audience's attention

(d) All of the above

53. Which of the following is not a guideline for effective use of AV aids?

(a) Overuse of AV aids

(b) Aids that require no explanation

(c) Aids that are appropriate to topic

(d) Aids that serves a definite purpose

54. AV aids should be used depending upon which of the following?

(a) Objectives of training programme

(b) Nature of subject matter being taught

(c) Nature of audience

(d) All of the above

55. Which one of the following is not an audio aid?

(a) Radio

(b) Television

(c) Microphone

(d) Filmstrips

56. Which of the following falls under nonprojected AV aids?

(a) Charts

(b) Blackboard

(c) Models

(d) All of the above

57. Mock-ups and specimens are the examples of which type of following AV aid?

(a) Activity aids

(b) Projected aids

    (c) 3-D nonprojected aids
    (d) Audio aids

58. What is/are the use(s) of AV aids in teaching?
    (a) Improve and make teaching effective
    (b) Make learning interesting
    (c) Stimulate curiosity
    (d) All of the above

59. Which of the following is/are the characteristic(s) of a good AV aids?
    (a) Meaningful
    (b) Purposeful
    (c) Up to date
    (d) All of the above

60. Which of the following is not true about planning for use of AV aids?
    (a) Plan well in advance
    (b) Plan for the use of variety of AV aids
    (c) The size of the audience is not to be anticipated
    (d) Anticipate the problem and avoid them

61. Which of the following is the most commonly available aid in the classroom situation?
    (a) Bulletin board
    (b) Blackboard
    (c) Flannel board
    (d) Notice board

62. Exact visual real life situations may be presented using which of the following AV aids?
    (a) Illustrations
    (b) Paintings
    (c) Drawings
    (d) Photographs

63. Which of the following type of board that provides a suitable place for display of students' creative works?
    (a) Lobby stand board
    (b) Notice board
    (c) Bulletin board
    (d) Exhibition board

64. Which of the following is the main limitation of blackboard?
    (a) Poor eye contact
    (b) Cannot be preserved
    (c) Visually attractive
    (d) All of the above

65. Which one of the following AV aids is preferred when we want to compare two types of data?
    (a) Simple bar graph
    (b) Double bar graph
    (c) Pie graph
    (d) Histogram

66. A two-dimensional frequency density diagram is known as
    (a) Line graph
    (b) Pie graph
    (c) Histogram
    (d) Pictorial graph

67. Metaphorical presentation of reality can be done by using which of the following?
    A V aid:
    (a) Pictogram
    (b) Sketches
    (c) Cartoon
    (d) Illustrations

68. Direct contact with real life situation can be achieved by using which of the following teaching strategy?
    (a) Puppet show
    (b) Field trips
    (c) Drama
    (d) Simulation

69. Organization of knowledge can be represented by using which type of visual aid?
    (a) Concept mapping
    (b) Pictogram
    (c) Line graph
    (d) Cartoon

70. Nursing theories are usually represented by using which of the following?
    (a) Allograms
    (b) Concept mapping
    (c) Linear diagrams
    (d) Publications

71. Information represented within a format of interlocking geometric shapes is known as
    (a) Spider concept map
    (b) System concept map
    (c) Mandala concept map
    (d) Problem solution map

72. Concept of Concept Mapping was first used by
    (a) Joseph D Novak & team
    (b) Taylor & Wros
    (c) All & Haycke
    (d) Edgar Dale

73. The board with one side marker pen writing and the other side with interchangeable letters is called
    (a) Paging board
    (b) Lobby stand board
    (c) Reception board
    (d) Tariff board

74. The board which helps in three-dimensional demonstrations with objects on a vertical surface is
    (a) Cork board
    (b) Magnetic board
    (c) Paging board
    (d) Exhibition board

75. Which one the following is the advantage of blackboard?
    (a) Does not require electricity
    (b) User friendly
    (c) Can used with lights on
    (d) All of the above

76. Which of the following is not the guideline for using transparency?
    (a) Use all capital letters
    (b) Use no more than four to six words per line

    (c) Use no more than four to six lines per transparency
    (d) All of above

77. Which type of the following presentational aid is three dimensional?
    (a) Model
    (b) Graph
    (c) Picture
    (d) Board

78. To show the relative proportion of a data you will prefer to use which of the following?
    (a) Pie graph
    (b) Diagram
    (c) Bar graph
    (d) Line graph

79. Which of the following is not a type of graphic aid?
    (a) Object
    (b) Picture
    (c) Diagram
    (d) Graph

80. The problem is constructed; the solution and the supporting reasons can be indicated by the student quickly and easily with minimum amount of writing is
    (a) Matching type
    (b) Practical examination
    (c) Problem situation test
    (d) Oral examination

81. Which of the following presentational aid is most difficult to execute effectively?
    (a) Handouts
    (b) Projections
    (c) Film and video
    (d) Graphics

82. The best graphic used for showing quantitative comparison among variables is
    (a) A bar graph
    (b) Line graph

(c) Circle graph
(d) Diagram

83. Which type of map is best to use as teaching aid?
(a) Brightly coloured
(b) Detailed
(c) Simple
(d) Commercially prepared

84. Which one of the following is a major drawback of using visual aid during a lecture?
(a) Over simplify complex information
(b) Can distract audience from message
(c) Distract the speaker who handle them
(d) Are hard to carry to class

85. Pre-requisites for validity and reliability are
(a) Objectivity, specificity
(b) Relevance
(c) Both (a) and (b)
(d) Incomprehensiveness

86. Which one of the following is indirect method of observation of practical skills?
(a) Real practical test
(b) Simulated practical test
(c) Project method
(d) None of the above

87. Practical examination is used to evaluate, which of the following learner's skills?
(a) Communication skills
(b) Psychomotor skills
(c) Cognitive skills
(d) All of the above

88. The scaling techniques are used to measure, which of the following attribute?
(a) Attitude
(b) Behaviour
(c) Both (a) and (b)
(d) None

89. Scale can be validated on the grounds of
(a) Logic
(b) Opinion of jury
(c) Both (a) and (b)
(d) None of the above

90. The characteristic of cardinal scale is
(a) It interprets the order of scale scores
(b) It has equal units of measurement
(c) It interprets the distance between scores
(d) All of the above

91. If the scale measures what it is intended to measure, it is said to be
(a) Reliable
(b) Accurate
(c) Valid
(d) Genuine

92. In test–retest method
(a) The same population is subjected to two or more types of scales
(b) The same scale is applied twice to the same population
(c) The scale may be divided into two equal parts
(d) The same scale is given to different populations

93. Graphic scale is a type of
(a) Ratio scale
(b) Rating scale
(c) Interval scale
(d) None

94. Scale designed in the manner of {Excellent ——Very good——Good——Average—— Poor} is a type of
(a) Nominal scale
(b) Rating scale
(c) Ordinal scale
(d) Interval scale

95. Which of the following is/are the type of Numerical Rating scale(s)?
   (a) Itemized rating scale
   (b) Specific rating scale
   (c) Specific category rating scale
   (d) All of the above

96. Rating scale can be
   (a) Observational
   (b) Descriptive
   (c) Systematic
   (d) None

97. Which of the following is not an attitude scale?
   (a) Point scale
   (b) Differential scale
   (c) Likert scale
   (d) Check list

98. Which of the following scales permit degrees of agreement or disagreement?
   (a) Thurstone scale
   (b) Likert scale
   (c) Both of the above
   (d) None of the above

99. In which of the following scale, only the strictly related items are included?
   (a) Likert scale
   (b) Thurston scale
   (c) Point scale
   (d) None of the above

100. Which thing should be kept in mind by the teacher while preparing a checklist?
   (a) The kinds of behaviour are important to record
   (b) The kinds of objectives are to be evaluated
   (c) Both (a) and (b)
   (d) None of the above

101. Which method of evaluation should be used when we are interested in ascertaining the presence or absence of a particular trait?
   (a) Q-sort scaling technique
   (b) Checklist
   (c) Point scale
   (d) Semantic differential scale

102. A complete checklist should be given to each student for
   (a) Discussing the strength and weakness of the performance
   (b) Formulating a plan to improve the performance
   (c) Both (a) and (b)
   (d) None of the above

103. Peer Appraisal Method is used in
   (a) Evaluation
   (b) Assessment
   (c) Both (a) and (b)
   (d) None of above

104. In Peer Appraisal Method evaluation is done by
   (a) Fellow students
   (b) Teacher
   (c) Student himself
   (d) Both (a) and (c)

105. Anecdotal Record includes brief description of
   (a) Observed behaviour
   (b) Teaching
   (c) Evaluation
   (d) Assessment

106. Anecdotal Record is used by
   (a) Teacher
   (b) Student
   (c) Peer group
   (d) Both (a) and (b)

107. Anecdotal Record should contain record of
(a) Each incident
(b) Single incident
(c) More than one incident
(d) Both (a) and (b)

108. Anecdotal Record should contain
(a) Negative aspect
(b) Positive aspect
(c) Both (a) and (b)
(d) None of above

109. Anecdotal Record include
(a) Observed event
(b) Comments of teacher
(c) Signature of teacher and student
(d) All of above

110. Anecdotal Record can be used by student for
(a) Self-appraisal
(b) Peer assessment
(c) Both (a) and (b)
(d) None of above

111. Sociometry is used to study
(a) Interaction of children
(b) Behaviour of children
(c) Observed incident
(d) Both (a) and (b)

112. Sociometry and sociogram is special method of obtaining the information through:
(a) Oral question
(b) Written response
(c) Analyzing the records
(d) All of above

113. Cumulative Record is account of:
(a) Learning process
(b) Child's history
(c) Teaching process
(d) Teacher–student interaction

114. Cumulative Record should contain
(a) Cord sheet in envelop
(b) Printed folder
(c) Booklet
(d) All of above

115. Critical Incident Record include:
(a) Total period of observation
(b) Number of incident
(c) Effective and ineffective behaviour
(d) All of above

116. Question Bank contains questions which are pretested for
(a) Reliability
(b) Validity
(c) Practicability
(d) All of above

117. Purpose of question bank is
(a) To improve the teaching learning process
(b) To improve evaluation process
(c) To provide question to student
(d) Both (a) and (b)

118. Subject matter in the lesson plan should be
(a) Well selected
(b) Sequentially organized
(c) Both (a) and (b)
(d) Incoherent

119. Assignment prescribed should be
(a) Comprehensive
(b) Clear and creative
(c) Appropriate
(d) All of above

120. Evaluation includes which of the following aspects?
(a) Quantitative and qualitative assessment
(b) Value judgment
(c) Both (a) and (b)
(d) None of the above

121. Which is not the component of internal assessment?
     (a) Subject-wise assessment
     (b) Favouritism towards student
     (c) Assessment of cocurricular activities
     (d) Assessment of personality traits

122. Which of the following is not an appropriate nonverbal communication?
     (a) Humour
     (b) Gestures
     (c) Tics
     (d) Expressions

123. Which of the following personality traits is not assessed in internal assessment?
     (a) Cooperation
     (b) Initiativeness
     (c) Leadership
     (d) Supervision

124. Kalyani magazine is one of the IEC activity related to
     (a) Leprosy
     (b) AIDS
     (c) Cancer
     (d) Malaria

125. Advertisement of ORS on television is to create awareness regarding management of
     (a) Dengue
     (b) Diarrhoea
     (c) Fever
     (d) Polio

126. 'Do Boond Zindagi Ki' is related to campaign against
     (a) Malaria
     (b) Polio
     (c) Tetanus
     (d) Whooping cough

127. The slogan 'Poora Course Pakka Ilaj' is against
     (a) Yaws
     (b) Kala azar
     (c) Tuberculosis
     (d) Leprosy

128. Tuberculosis day is observed on:
     (a) 2nd October
     (b) 24th September
     (c) 24th March
     (d) 7th April

129. Complete the slogan 'Chune Se Na Gandhon Se _____ Avaidh Sambhandon Se'.
     (a) Malaria
     (b) AIDS
     (c) Hepatitis
     (d) TB

130. 'Hum Do Hamare Do' is a slogan to promote
     (a) Education
     (b) Employment
     (c) Small family norms
     (d) Water supply

131. Promotion of iodized salt is to prevent
     (a) Polio
     (b) Goiter
     (c) Anemia
     (d) Blindness

132. 'Bulandi' is a character to create awareness regarding
     (a) Goiter
     (b) Anemia
     (c) AIDS
     (d) Leprosy

133. ARSH clinic is to create awareness regarding
    (a) Child health
    (b) Care of antenatal mother
    (c) Adolescent health
    (d) Elderly health

134. *'Nanhi Chhan'* is an effort to
    (a) Save trees
    (b) Save girl child
    (c) Save male child
    (d) Save mother

135. Which movie showed example of telecommunication?
    (a) Kahani
    (b) 3-Idiots
    (c) Agent Vinod
    (d) Ra-one

136. *'Balika vadhu'* serial is based on
    (a) Female foeticide
    (b) Dowry
    (c) Child marriage
    (d) Domestic violence

137. National Cancer awareness day is observed on
    (a) 5th August
    (b) 1st October
    (c) 7th November
    (d) 19th February

138. *'MDT Khao Kusht Bhagao'* is slogan regarding treatment of
    (a) Malaria
    (b) Leprosy
    (c) Dengue
    (d) Tetanus

139. Advertisement given on Doordarshan by ASHA is to create awareness regarding
    (a) Institutional deliveries
    (b) Tetanus injection
    (c) Iron and folic acid tablets
    (d) All of above

140. Advertisement regarding blood examination for fever is to detect
    (a) Dengue
    (b) Malaria
    (c) Typhoid
    (d) All of above

141. Main aim of IEC is to
    (a) Educate people
    (b) Change behaviour of people
    (c) Communicate health message
    (d) All of above

142. *'Afsar Bitia'* is a TV show to
    (a) Promote health of girl child
    (b) Promote education of girl child
    (c) Stop female feticide
    (d) Stop dowry system

143. Abbreviation 'MMU' stands for
    (a) Mandatory Medical-aid Unit
    (b) Mobile Medical Unit
    (c) Medical Means Used
    (d) None of these

144. New schemes related to health can be communicated by
    (a) Publishing in newspaper
    (b) Broadcasting on radio
    (c) IEC by health personnel
    (d) All of above

145. People can be motivated to donate blood by
    (a) Giving them money
    (b) Threatening them
    (c) Requesting them
    (d) Behaviour change

146. Most effective mean to intimate regarding any epidemic is
    (a) Booklet
    (b) Role-play
    (c) Health magazine
    (d) Radio and TV

147. Advertisement regarding breastfeeding helps to
(a) Provide immunity to child
(b) To realize mother its need and importance
(c) Prevent malnutrition of child
(d) All of above

148. Physical barriers to communication are
(a) Unpleasant climate
(b) Unwanted sound
(c) No proper channel
(d) All of above

149. What are the new strategies adopted by the government as a part of IEC activities in RCH programme?
(a) Use of top-down approach
(b) Camp-oriented approach
(c) Cash incentives for sterilization cases
(d) Enhancing the budget for RCH programme

150. What are the main components of the IEC campaigns under RCH programme?
(a) Contraceptive methods
(b) Eye donation fortnight
(c) Gender and sexuality issues
(d) Community participation

151. National fund for IEC material in RCH programme was assisted by which health agencies?
(a) UNICEF
(b) WHO
(c) World Bank
(d) World Bank and European Commission

152. What are the newer schemes undertaken by RCH2 Programme?
(a) Janani Suraksha Yojana
(b) Janani Shishu Suraksha Karyakaram
(c) Mata kaushalya Scheme
(d) All of the above

153. Under RCH programme, IEC sessions related to child health include
(a) Session on EMR obstetric care
(b) Session on ARI and diarrhoeal diseases
(c) Session on infection control
(d) Session on FRUs

154. Under RCH programme, Community Participation will be elicited through which group of people?
(a) NGO's
(b) Panchayats
(c) Mahila Mandals
(d) Both (b) and (c)

155. Awareness regarding eye donation among the community people is guided by which festival under NPBC?
(a) Fortnight celebration
(b) Mass awareness
(c) Eye donation camp fest
(d) Nakshtarya festival

156. Who are the target population for IEC activities under National AIDS Control Program (NACP)?
(a) Adolescent and young adults
(b) Pregnant women
(c) HIV positive people
(d) All of the above

157. Which of the following is the communication dimension under IEC strategies for NACP?
(a) Behaviour change communication
(b) One-way communication
(c) Meta communication
(d) Symbolic communication

158. How many dimensions are there for communication framework under NACP?
(a) Four
(b) Two
(c) Three
(d) Six

159. What is communication?
    (a) Information technique
    (b) Talk
    (c) Health education
    (d) Meeting

160. Modern method of communication is
    (a) E-mail
    (b) Telephone
    (c) Mobile
    (d) Radio

161. Which of the following factor(s) affects the communication?
    (a) Knowledge
    (b) Experience
    (c) Interest
    (d) All of above

162. Which of the following is the main advantage of communication?
    (a) In-time help
    (b) Motivation
    (c) Participation
    (d) Learning

163. Abbreviation 'BCC' stands for
    (a) Behaviour chance communication
    (b) Behaviour change counselling
    (c) Behaviour change communication
    (d) None of above

164. Strategies of BCC are
    (a) Increase knowledge
    (b) Reduce stigma and discrimination
    (c) Promote services for prevention care and support
    (d) All of above

165. MIS stands for
    (a) Management information system
    (b) Multiple information system
    (c) Management informed system
    (d) None of above

166. Which of the following is/are the phase(s) of MIS?
    (a) Input
    (b) Process
    (c) Output
    (d) None of above

167. At which of the following level(s) BCC is strategy implemented?
    (a) Intrapersonal level
    (b) Interpersonal level
    (c) Community level
    (d) All of above

168. BCC is based on
    (a) Scientific based
    (b) Client centric
    (c) Service linked
    (d) All of above

169. What are the principles of education?
    (a) Credibility, participation
    (b) Interest, motivation
    (c) Feedback
    (d) All of above

170. Which of the following is the basic need to Abraham's Maslow hierarchy of needs?
    (a) Love
    (b) Security
    (c) Hunger
    (d) Self-esteem

171. Which of the following is the correct Chinese proverb?
    (a) If I hear, I remember
    (b) If I hear, I know
    (c) If I do, I remember
    (d) If I hear, I forget, if I see, I remember, if I do, I know

172. Which is the individual approach for education?
    (a) Personal contact
    (b) Home visits

(c) Personal letters
(d) All of above

173. Which of the following is folk media?
(a) Wall painting
(b) Newspaper
(c) Puppet show
(d) Television

174. Visual aids improve learning about up to
(a) 50%
(b) 30%
(c) 80%
(d) 10%

175. What is the correct measurement for flash cards?
(a) 25 × 30 cm
(b) 20 × 10 cm
(c) 10 × 15 cm
(d) 15 ×15 cm

176. Which of the following is the group approach of teaching?
(a) Lecture
(b) Discussion
(c) Panel discussion
(d) All of above

177. What is the ideal size of a poster?
(a) 20 × 30 inches
(b) 20 × 15 inches
(c) 10 × 15 inches
(d) 28 × 22 inches

178. How many flash cards can be used for single time?
(a) 2–5
(b) 5–10
(c) 10–12
(d) 20–30

179. Which of the following is the mass approach of dissemination of health education?
(a) TV
(b) Newspaper
(c) Both (a) and (b)
(d) None

180. Which of the following is a three-dimensional AV aids?
(a) Blackboard
(b) Slides
(c) Models
(d) Radio

181. What is full form of KAP?
(a) Knowledge, aptitude, practice
(b) Know, aptitude, patience
(c) Knowledge, attitude, practice
(d) Know, attitude, practice

182. Who have given this definition 'education is self-realization and service to people?'
(a) Mahatma Gandhi
(b) Vivekananda
(c) Guru Nanak Dev
(d) Plato

183. Which of the following is/are the domain(s) of educational objectives?
(a) Cognitive domain
(b) Affective domain
(c) Psychometric domain
(d) All of above

184. Which of the following is elements specific educational objective?
(a) Act
(b) Content
(c) Criteria
(d) All of above

185. Which is the correct sequence of stages of group dynamics?
    (a) Forming, storming, norming, performing
    (b) Forming, norming, storming, performing
    (c) Forming, storming, performing, norming
    (d) Forming, performing, storming, norming

186. Which are the components of triangular process of education?
    (a) Pupil
    (b) Teacher
    (c) Social environment
    (d) All of above

187. Which one of the following is not an example of type of education?
    (a) Informal
    (b) Formal
    (c) Nonformal
    (d) Western

188. Panel discussion is which type of educational approach?
    (a) Group approach
    (b) Mass approach
    (c) Individual approach
    (d) None

189. What is the full form of CBE?
    (a) Communication based education
    (b) Community based education
    (c) Competency based education
    (d) Criteria based education

190. Who have given this definition 'by "education", I mean an all-round drawing out of the best in child and man–body–mind and spirit?'
    (a) Shri guru Nanak dev ji
    (b) Chanakya
    (c) M. K. Gandhi
    (d) R. N. Tagore

191. Automatism is the component of which domain of learning?
    (a) Domain of communication skill
    (b) Domain of intellectual skill
    (c) Domain of practical skill
    (d) Domain of intelligent skill

192. Which of the following is/are the division(s) of health education?
    (a) Nutrition
    (b) Family health
    (c) Mental health
    (d) All of above

193. What is the full form of OBE?
    (a) Odd based education
    (b) Oval based education
    (c) Outcome based education
    (d) Outreach based education

194. Item analysis helps in judging
    (a) Quality of test
    (b) Worth of test
    (c) Both (a) and (b)
    (d) None of the above

195. Major advantage of objective type test is
    (a) Provide objectivity, reliability and validity
    (b) Cost is high when administer to large group
    (c) Guessing is possible when distracters not plausible
    (d) Construction of items require greater skills

196. Which of following test is able to assess the intellectual domain of the students?
    (a) Multiple-choice questions
    (b) Problem situation test

(c) Essay-type test
(d) All of the above

197. What type of tests should be given to students for individual comparison?
(a) Oral test
(b) Project assignment
(c) Consistent tests
(d) Standardized impersonal tests

198. The procedure used to judge the quality of an item is
(a) Formative analysis
(b) Systemic analysis
(c) Item analysis
(d) Standard analysis

199. Degree to which a given item discriminates among students who differ sharply in their functions is measured by
(a) Item analysis
(b) Difficulty index
(c) Standard deviation
(d) Discrimination index

200. Objective type questions are used to assess which domain?
(a) Knowledge
(b) Attitude
(c) Skill
(d) Practice

Answers

1. d, 2. c, 3. c, 4. c, 5. a, 6. b, 7. b, 8. a, 9. c, 10. b, 11. a, 12. d, 13. c, 14. b, 15. a, 16. c, 17. d, 18. a, 19. d, 20. b, 21. b, 22. a, 23. a, 24. c, 25. a, 26. b, 27. d, 28. b, 29. c, 30. d, 31. a, 32. b, 33. d, 34. c, 35. b, 36. b, 37. d, 38. b, 39. c, 40. b, 41. a, 42. a, 43. b, 44. a, 45. a, 46. b, 47. b, 48. b, 49. a, 50. a, 51. d, 52. d, 53. a, 54. d, 55. d, 56. d, 57. c, 58. d, 59. d, 60. c, 61. b, 62. d, 63. d, 64. b, 65. b, 66. c, 67. b, 68. b, 69. b, 70. c, 71. a, 72. a, 73. b, 74. d, 75. d, 76. a, 77. a, 78. a, 79. a, 80. c, 81. c, 82. b, 83. a, 84. b, 85. c, 86. c, 87. b, 88. c, 89. b, 90. c, 91. c, 92. b, 93. b, 94. b, 95. d, 96. b, 97. d, 98. b, 99. a, 100. c, 101. b, 102. c, 103. c, 104. a, 105. a, 106. a, 107. b, 108. c, 109. d, 110. c, 111. d, 112. d, 113. b, 114. d, 115. d, 116. d, 117. d, 118. c, 119. d, 120. c, 121. b, 122. c, 123. d, 124. c, 125. b, 126. b, 127. c, 128. c, 129. b, 130. c, 131. b, 132. c, 133. c, 134. b, 135. b, 136. c, 137. c, 138. b, 139. d, 140. d, 141. d, 142. b, 143. b, 144. d, 145. d, 146. d, 147. d, 148. d, 149. d, 150. c, 151. d, 152. d, 153. b, 154. d, 155. a, 156. d, 157. a, 158. c, 159. a, 160. a, 161. d, 162. a, 163. c, 164. d, 165. a, 166. d, 167. d, 168. d, 169. d, 170. c, 171. d, 172. d, 173. c, 174. c, 175. a, 176. d, 177. d, 178. c, 179. c, 180. c, 181. c, 182. c, 183. d, 184. c, 185. b, 186. d, 187. d, 188. a, 189. c, 190. c, 191. c, 192. d, 193. c, 194. c, 195. a, 196. b, 197. d, 198. c, 199. d, 200. a

Index